Nursing:
a knowledge base
for practice

GW00372140

Nursing: a knowledge base for practice

Edited by

Abigayl Perry
BSc (Hons) Soc, MSc(Econ), FETC, SRN

and

Moya Jolley
MA(Ed), BSc(Econ), Dip Ed, RNT, SRN, Dip in Nursing (Lond)

Edward Arnold
A division of Hodder & Stoughton
LONDON MELBOURNE AUCKLAND

© 1991 Abigayl Perry and Moya Jolley

First published in Great Britain 1991
Reprinted 1992
British Library Cataloguing in Publication Data
Perry, Abigayl
  Nursing.
  1. Medicine. Nursing. Theories
  I. Title II. Jolley, Moya
  610.7301

  ISBN 0-340-51492-2

Whilst the advice and information in this book is believed to be
true and accurate at the date of going to press, neither the author
nor the publisher can accept any legal responsibility or liability for
any errors or omissions that may be made.

Typeset in Great Britain by TecSet Ltd, Wallington, Surrey
Printed and bound in Great Britain for Edward Arnold, a division
of Hodder and Stoughton Limited, Mill Road, Dunton Green,
Sevenoaks, Kent TN13 2YA by Biddles Ltd, Guildford.

Foreword

As nursing becomes more academic and places a greater emphasis on research-based clinical care, it becomes increasingly important to provide texts that encourage students to read writings from the wide range of sciences that underpin nursing both as a discipline and as a practical skill. The editors and writers of this textbook have tried to do just this. They have used a scholarly approach to both nursing and the related sciences, but they have at no time lost sight of the fact that nursing is practice-based. The book commences and concludes with a chapter on nursing. The opening chapter discusses knowledge for nursing and the concluding chapter centres on nursing knowledge – the ultimate objective. The intervening chapters assist readers in reaching that objective.

I commend this book for pre- and post-registration students of all branches of nursing. I have no doubt that this text will benefit existing nursing students and those entering 'Project 2000 schemes'. I am also convinced that it will be a valuable text for those nurses following post-registration courses. Above all, I hope that those reading it will develop not only their knowledge but their skill in patient and client care.

Margaret D Green
Deputy General Secretary/Director of Education
Royal College of Nursing

Contents

List of contributors

Paul Barber MSc, BA, RGN, RMN, RNMS, RNT
Lecturer, Interpersonal Skills and Group Dynamics, Institute of Advanced Nursing Education, Royal College of Nursing, London

Anne Betts MSc, BSc(Hons), RGN, RNT
Lecturer, Physiology, Institute of Advanced Nursing Education, Royal College of Nursing, London

Jane Chapman BSc(Hons), RGN
Senior Nurse, Research and Quality Assurance, Harrow Health Authority

Kim Manley MN, RGN, Dip in Nursing (Lond), RCNT
Lecturer, Nursing, Institute of Advanced Nursing Education, Royal College of Nursing, London

Suzanne McBean BSC(Hons), RGN, RHV, NDN Cert, Dip N Ed
Director of Health Promotion, Highland Health Board, Scotland. Formerly Lecturer, Health and Community Studies, Institute of Advanced Nursing Education, Royal College of Nursing, London

Alan Myles MA(Ed), RGN, Dip Ed, RNT
Principal Lecturer, Education Studies, Institute of Advanced Nursing Education, Royal College of Nursing, London

Abigayl Perry BSc(Hons) Soc, MSc(Econ), FETC, SRN
Independent Writer and Researcher

Jane Robinson PhD, MA, MIPM, RGN, ONC, RHV, HVT, Cert Ed
Professor and Head of Department, Nursing Studies Department, University of Nottingham

Mary Watkins RMN, RGN, Dip in Nursing (Lond), Dip N Ed, MN
Senior Nurse, Education and Management, Education Centre, Derriford Hospital, Plymouth

Mary Watts MA, BSc, SRN, RMN, Dip in Nursing (Lond), PGCEA, RNT, Dip Counselling

Lecturer in Behavioural Sciences, Department of Social Sciences, City University, London

The Editors

Abigayl Perry   BSc(Hons) Soc, MSc(Econ), FETC, SRN
Independent Writer and Researcher

Moya Jolley   MA(Ed), BSc(Econ), SRN, Dip Ed, RNT, Dip in Nursing (Lond)
Lecturer, Institute of Advanced Nursing Education, Royal College of Nursing, London

Introduction

Our intention in the production of this book is to provide a text for a wide range of students which addresses the main concerns of nursing as an applied science. It seeks to examine psychological, social, physical and political aspects of nursing practices and health care. As the curriculum at basic nurse education level broadens and deepens, and as modular, post basic and degree programmes become ever more popular, the need for nursing texts which embrace and reflect integrated and holistic approaches becomes increasingly apparent. This collection explores a broad range of nursing knowledge and issues, adopting a multi-dimensional approach throughout.

Though there is no national advanced curriculum, we are confident that the subjects selected for this book represent a defensible core for an explicit nursing knowledge base. Each chapter is capable of standing alone, while also contributing to the structure of the book as a whole. The writers have organised their chapters around key elements in their subjects. Many of these disciplinary concerns are shared; particularly the control/dependency debate in the health education and social science chapters. These discussions confront the mind/body polarity in clinical diagnosis, treatment and patient care (Chapters 3, 7 and 8) and argue against rigid and 'context-bound' interpretations of nurses and their practices (Chapters 6 and 9). The introductory and concluding chapters have deliberate connections: Chapter 10 develops the philosophical and humanistic issues generated in Chapter 1, applying the theory to differing research processes, client groups and areas of nursing practice. Both theorists move with considerable facility between the dimensions of theoretical knowledge and practice settings: the difference is one of emphasis, that is from theory to practice (Chapter 1) and the practice-theory-practice spiral, as in Chapter 10.

These shared concerns will enable readers to view particular relationships such as the learned helplessness of patients (and nurses), from the differing realities of physical being, feeling states, social roles and the resources or power available to individuals and groups. Other multi-disciplinary themes, albeit in different measure, include professional responsibility, personal identity and autonomy, power, politics, health beliefs and caring strategies.

All the contributors refer to the theory/practice divide in nursing and the problematic links between nursing actions and the clinical and health outcomes of patients or clients. Chapters 2 and 5, on

research and physiology respectively, make clever use of the
questioning approach to guide the reader through different
dimensions of the 'application problem'. It is to the credit of these
authors that sophisticated data on body systems, diagnostic tests and
comparative research methods will have a direct appeal to those new
to these areas as well as those wishing to develop further expertise.
The education topic (Chapter 4) makes excellent use of experiential
learning exercises throughout. Brainstorming activities or 'spring
board' questions are used to explore key concepts such as health,
nursing, prevention and modes of communication, enabling
educators and students to clarify the educational intentions of present
and future courses.

Stylistically the chapters diverge, producing a degree of textual
variation and avoiding the problem of dull uniformity, sometimes
seen in nursing texts in the past. For example, Paul Barber's
discussion on caring (Chapter 8) flows from a symbolic interactionist
perspective. This is an intimate account of his experiences as a
hospital patient, paralleled by professional insights into the
nurse-patient relationship. Mary Watts's material on psychology
(Chapter 7), based upon her research on shared learning in nursing,
draws together data derived from social survey methods. Chapters 7
and 8 provide accounts of applied research which highlight important
aspects of the 'scientific method' discussed in Jane Chapman's
chapter on research-mindedness (Chapter 2) and the 'flexibility' in
research thinking and planning advocated by Kim Manley and Mary
Watkins in the opening and concluding essays.

Suzanne McBean (Chapter 3), Abigayl Perry (Chapter 6) and Jane
Robinson (Chapter 9) conduct the reader through various theoretical
models and critiques in the search for explanations of nursing and
health, ideologies and structures. An alternative framework can be
seen in the education topic (Chapter 4) which uses an empirical,
functional or descriptive approach. Here, Alan Myles's discussion
focuses on descriptions of the theoretical and administrative
mechanisms of curriculum design in response to the most significant
policy change seen so far in late twentieth century nursing. Using a
similar framework (Chapter 5) Anne Betts describes homeostasis and
many health disorders in relation to an individual's health
opportunities, including environmental as well as personal factors.

The fundamental purpose of this volume is to provide a resource
book for students which will have relevance at pre-registration,
diploma and degree levels of nurse education: to provide a text which
will stimulate student thinking, generate debate, and encourage
further exploration of the content material presented: and, most
importantly of all, cause its readers to re-examine their own
professional beliefs and values. We hope that, if these purposes are

achieved, this text will fulfil the ultimate aim of all nursing texts, that of assisting nurses in raising standards of care.

Abigayl Perry and Moya Jolley
1990

Acknowledgements

The editors would like to extend their grateful thanks to all the contributors to this book. Their expertise, generosity in time and energy, as well as enthusiasm and commitment has made this book possible.

Thanks go also to Miss Margaret Green for writing the Foreword; to Mr Josef Keith for preparing the Index; and to Miss Hazel Wigmore in assisting in manuscript preparation.

Appreciation and thanks are also extended to Miss Helen Thomas, Assistant Librarian in the Library of Nursing at the RCN, for her meticulous work in checking and preparing references; and to Mrs Jean Smith for her tireless efforts, great patience and support in the preparation of the final typescript.

1 Knowledge for nursing practice

Introduction

'The definition of a knowledge base for a discipline begins with the separation of that knowledge which is important to the discipline and that which is not' (Visintainer, 1986). But what is meant by knowledge; who should judge the relevance of that knowledge, and what knowledge base is important to nursing? This book provides some insight into aspects of knowledge considered relevant to nursing by its various authors. However, it is the aim of this chapter that the nature of knowledge itself be examined, and that certain themes pertinent to the practice of nursing be considered in relation to knowledge; namely theory, philosophy, power, professionalism and, finally, accountability.

Knowledge/Knowing

According to Walker and Avant (1988) 'knowledge is the product of knowing'. It is both, 'experiential and summative'. However 'knowing' something does not necessarily mean that what is known is understood. For example, one can know that it is necessary to monitor for sugar in the urine of patients who are taking steroids, but this is quite different from knowing why increased urine sugar can occur in such patients.

Knowledge itself can be defined in several ways:

- familiarity gained by experience of person, thing, fact (Concise Oxford Dictionary, 1976)
- theoretical or practical understanding of a subject (Concise Oxford Dictionary, 1976)
- philosophically-certain understanding as opposed to opinion (Concise Oxford Dictionary, 1976), or a 'justified true belief' (Runkle, 1985)
- the sum or range of that which can be perceived or learned (Walker and Avant, 1988)

From these definitions, it can be seen that even in lay terms knowledge does not just comprise 'facts' and 'information' but also 'experience' and 'understanding'. Therefore the knowledge base of

1

anything, be it a discipline, profession, or any activity, encompasses experiences and understanding in addition to facts.

Know-how and know-that

Johnson (1968) states that 'knowledge differs in *kind* not amount. It is the difference between *knowing that* and *knowing how*, and *knowing why*, and *knowing what*'.

Within nursing several other authors have differentiated between types of knowledge dividing it into two types, '*know-how*' and *know-that*' (Meleis, 1985; Benner, 1984). These divisions in turn stem from descriptions of knowledge from other disciplines, particularly philosophy (Ryle, 1949; Polanyi, 1958; Kuhn, 1970). 'Know-how' consists of practical expertise and skills, for example knowing when a surgical patient is deteriorating, or knowing how to give an injection, how to identify a patient's strengths and weaknesses, how to mutually agree goals with patients, or how to build up a therapeutic relationship with clients. All these examples demonstrate practical knowledge, that knowledge which is used every day in practice settings.

In contrast, 'know-that' knowledge encompasses theoretical knowledge, that found in textbooks, and 'includes formal statements about interactional and causal relationships between events' (Benner, 1984); examples in nursing would include knowledge that social isolation is a contributing factor to sensory deprivation in acutely ill patients (Goldberger, 1966), that significant life crisis can predispose individuals to pathological change (Parkes *et al.*, 1969; Creed, 1981), or that individuals experience various stages following bereavement or in anticipation of it (Kübler-Ross, 1970; Parkes, 1986).

Often 'know-how' knowledge is acquired through practice and experience, and often cannot be theoretically accounted for by 'know-that' knowledge.

Practical knowledge

Benner (1984) considers that practical knowledge is gained over time and describes six areas of practical knowledge that can be observed in experts.

* *Graded qualitative distinctions* These are distinctions that are made on the basis of perceptual recognition; they cannot be reduced to minute variables and are not context-free. Examples given by Benner include judgements of muscle tone in the

premature infant, or the degree of cyanosis or respiratory distress.

- *Common meanings* are developed by nurses working with common issues. The meanings are developed over time.

- *Assumptions, expectations and sets* relate to practical situations where nurses have 'learnt to expect a certain course of events'.

- *Paradigm cases and personal knowledge* are particular situations that stand out in the practitioner's mind and which alters the practitioner's subsequent understanding and perception of future clinical situations.

- *Maxims* are 'cryptic' instructions which only make sense if there is already a deep understanding of the situation.

- *Unplanned practices* These are practices that nurses may have been delegated and have taken on because they are constantly at the bedside, and have, as a result, become highly skilled. Benner calls this unplanned delegation as 'delegation by default'. She provides an example in the intensive care nurse who has become highly skilled in the titration and weaning of vasodilator and anti-arrhythmic drugs.

Benner asserts that the expert nurse perceives the situation as a whole and that expertise is based on experience, and 'many hours of direct patient observation and care'. Also, that the 'knowledge embedded in this clinical expertise is central to the advancement and the development of nursing science'. This practical knowledge, she considers, has much to offer to the development of nursing theory if it were to be described and studied. (See Chapter 10.)

Theoretical knowledge

This type of knowledge is probably what most of us have come to accept as being the lay meaning of the word 'knowledge' and can be defined more precisely as that which is systematically organised into general laws and theories (Carper, 1978). This is considered in more depth under the heading of 'knowledge and theory' (see p. 5).

Carper's 'patterns of knowing'

Carper (1978) was one of the first nurses to consider the nature of knowing in nursing. She considers that there are four types:

- Empirics
- Aesthetics
- Personal knowledge
- Ethical knowledge

Scientific knowledge, or as Carper describes it 'empirics', concerns the 'science of nursing', and its purpose is to describe, explain and predict phenomena. Empiricism is a characteristic of science and can be defined as 'the process wherein evidence rooted in objective reality and gathered through the human senses is used as the basis for generating knowledge' (Polit and Hungler, 1987). It is this type of knowledge which is often considered as being synonymous with knowledge itself. Examples of this type of knowledge in nursing can be derived from descriptive, explanatory and predictive studies, and some examples are illustrated in Fig. 1.1.

Assessment tools developed in nursing frequently demonstrate all three types of theory. Such tools are derived from describing the factors commonly associated with a particular phenomenon, for example pain, incontinence or decubitus ulcers; these factors may then be weighted due to more positive correlations between some factors than others as found, for example, in the Glasgow coma scale, or various pressure sore tools. Such tools may also be predictive in the way they identify particular high-risk groups such as the possible victims of child abuse, depression or alcoholism. Problem-solving approaches to decision making are also very good examples of the application of a scientific and rational approach to the prescription of nursing actions.

Aesthetics involves knowledge which relates to the 'art of nursing' and examples demonstrating this type of knowledge include Benner's (1984) work on 'the intuitive expert practitioner' and the six types of practical knowledge described earlier (pp. 2-3).

Descriptive
Factors which affect intensive care nurses' job satisfaction (Manley, 1989)
An ethnographic study of new model Griffiths Management (Strong and Robinson, 1988)

Explanatory
Cannula related infection is influenced by covering or exposing the cannula site (Petrosino *et al.*, 1988)

Predictive
Pre-operative information will reduce post-operative analgesia requirements. (Hayward, 1975)

Fig. 1.1 Examples of descriptive, explanatory and predictive studies from which empirical knowledge can be derived.

Personal knowledge relates to the 'way that nurses view themselves and the client' and is concerned with the 'therapeutic use of self' (Carper, 1978). This type of knowledge is the most difficult to master and teach. Examples demonstrating the need to develop this type of knowledge can be seen in the work of Barber (1986) and Burnard (1988).

Finally, ethical knowledge encompasses 'the understanding of different philosophical positions about what is good, right and wrong'. This type of knowledge develops from considering areas of ethical enquiry and analysing moral decision-making, for example from the perspectives of Jeremy Bentham's (1748–1832) utilitarianism or Immanual Kant's (1724–1804) idealism.

Figure 1.2 summarises and defines Carper's four types of knowing and their definition. Associated theories, and possible ways of generating and testing theories which relate to each knowledge type are also suggested. Chapter 2 considers more closely the role of research in relation to theory generation and testing.

Carper considers each pattern of knowing to be fundamentally separate although interrelated and interdependent. The view that each type of knowledge is interrelated and complementary is also shared by Heron (1981), and supported by Burnard (1987). Heron, however, proposes four types of knowledge:

- Propositional belief (relates to values, beliefs and similar to Carper's ethical knowledge)
- Practical knowledge (synonymous with 'know-how' knowledge)
- Experiential knowledge (similar to Carper's 'personal knowledge')
- Propositional knowledge (synonymous with 'knowing that'/ textbook knowledge)

However these types of knowing are seen by Heron to be phases that are passed through in the stated order above. These phases relate to each other in a cyclical process similar to the nursing process, and each may need to be revisited several times before knowledge becomes meaningful.

Knowledge and theory

Theory provides one method for generating knowledge. The word 'theory' is often used loosely by the layman to mean 'the content covered in the classroom, as opposed to the actual practice of performing nursing activities' (Polit and Hungler, 1987); or even the opposite of the practical or useful (Chinn and Jacobs, 1987). If this is how theory is viewed by practicing nurses, it is no wonder that so

Carper's types of knowing	Definition	Related theories	Suggested studies for theory generation and testing	Methods
EMPIRICS (The science of nursing)	objective factual generalisable publically verifiable	**Predictive** – predicts precise relationships between dimensions/ characteristics of a phenomenon/ differences between groups	**Experimental** – manipulation of some variable to determine its effect on another variable	e.g. experimental/ control groups, pre/post testing
		Explanatory – specifies relationships between dimensions/characteristics of individuals, groups, situations or events	**Correlational** – measurement of dimensions or characteristics of phenomena in their natural states	e.g. interviews, surveys
		Descriptive – describes/classifies specific dimensions/characteristics of individuals, groups, situations or events	**Descriptive/Exploratory** – observation of a phenomenon in its natural setting	qualitative e.g. grounded theory/ethnography quantitative methods
AESTHETIC (The art of nursing)	empathy understanding perceiving	Theories concerned with **technical** skills needed for practice Theories concerned with **perception** of what is significant in an individual's behaviour	Standard 'scientific' methods indicated above **Phenomenology** – where the emphasis is on **understanding** the individual's definition of the situation. **Constructivist** methodology	
PERSONAL KNOWLEDGE	subjective concrete existential promotion of wholeness and integrity	The therapeutic use of self The nature of the interpersonal process	Standard 'scientific' methods Inquiry reflecting humanistic existential perspectives	
ETHICAL KNOWLEDGE	moral knowledge	Theories concerning values Theories of methods used to solve ethical dilemmas and formulate moral judgements		ethical enquiry

Fig. 1.2 Carper's knowledge types, their definition and possible research methodologies for theory testing and generation. (Adapted from Carper, 1978.)

much concern and confusion exists about the nature and purpose of nursing theory. Theories are often misconstrued for the reason that they are considered to be the product of academic theorising which takes place in academic institutions far removed from practice settings. In fact theories 'represents a scientist's best effort to describe and explain phenomena' (Polit and Hungler, 1987). Theories therefore *do* serve some purpose, as they help us make sense of what we observe and perceive by suggesting relationships between concepts. Such statements of relationships between variables are termed propositions. All these characteristics are nicely brought together in Riehl and Roy's (1980) definition of a theory:

'a logically interconnected set of propositions used to *describe*, *explain*, and *predict* a part of the empirical world'

In taking this argument further, a theory about sensory deprivation in acute hospital settings may *describe* the scenarios associated with the development of sensory deprivation in patients; *explain* the relationships between factors, for example that social isolation hastens the effects of sensory deprivation; and finally in their most sophisticated form, allow us to prescribe nursing actions which we can confidently *predict* will reduce the occurrence of sensory deprivation, for example we may predict that turning the lights off at night and muting the telephone bell will maintain normal sensory patterns.

Theories developed in other disciplines may be used in nursing to describe and explain some phenomena observed in practice, for example Engel (1962) developed a middle-range theory in psychology which relates psychosocial stressors to the physiological state of 'fight and flight', i.e. sympathetic nervous system arousal. This theory can be used in nursing to prescribe nursing care in, for example, the person who has recently suffered a myocardial infarction. Such a person may be particularly vulnerable to cardiac arrhythmias as a result of increased circulating adrenaline, secondary to sympathetic arousal. This arousal could, according to Engel's theory, result from exposure to psychosocial stressors. If the person is of a highly independent nature then it may be more stressful psychologically if dependence is enforced in activities of living, rather than allowing the person to continue with his or her own self-care.

Similarly theories from sociology, for example symbolic interactionism (grand theory), have been used by nurse theorists such as Riehl-Sisca (1989) and Wiedenbach (1964) to suggest how interaction between client and nurse can be understood. Theories developed in nursing are less well developed because theory building has been a much more recent development than in the fields of psychology and sociology. Chapters 6 and 7 consider sociological and psychological theories as a source of nursing knowledge in more depth.

Theory generation and refinement

Dickoff and James (1968) reiterate the importance of the *purpose* of theory in that nursing must generate theory that will serve to achieve its purposes and goals. Consequently this determines how Dickoff and James propose that theory is generated. They suggest four levels of theory generation, the fourth level entitled 'situation-producing' theory being the most sophisticated. This level of theory is practice orientated because it involves the prescription of nursing actions to achieve desired outcomes. For this reason, Walker and Avant (1988) go on to suggest that fourth level theory is really therefore 'practice' theory. Each of the lower levels of theory act as a basis for the next, so contributing to the development of theory with 'prescriptive' status. Walker and Avant (1988) considered that these four levels 'roughly paralleled the acts of description, explanation, prediction and control'. However before 'practice' theory can be developed Dickoff and James state that the three other levels of theory have to be passed through. Figure 1.3 links the four levels of theory to Avant and Walker's terms with an example from the well known area of information giving in pre-operative patients (Haywood, 1975; Boore, 1978). These examples are used to illustrate the sort of theory generated at each level and demonstrates how the four levels of Dickoff and James may be applied.

First level theory (factor-isolating) is therefore concerned with the identification of factors and variables, and their subsequent definition. Dickoff, James and Wiedenbach (1968) consider that the generation of first level theory, i.e. that of isolating and naming factors, is one that is so basic that it is often overlooked. Johnson

Level 1 Factor-isolating DESCRIPTION	Patients appear anxious prior to operation. Patients have little knowledge of what to expect following their operation. Anxiety is defined.
Level 2 Factor-relating EXPLANATION	Anxiety may be related to knowledge of what to expect following operation.
Level 3 Situation-relating PREDICTION	Giving information pre-operatively may reduce anxiety.
Level 4 Situation-producing CONTROL	Information will be given preoperatively for the specific purpose of reducing anxiety.

Fig. 1.3   Dickoff and James's (1968) four levels of theory, their corresponding description by Walker and Avant (1988) and examples using the work of Hayward (1975) and Boore (1978).

(1978; cited Adam, 1985) also supports the view that nurses may be neglecting the first levels of theory development. Fawcett (1978) too considers that basic descriptive studies could provide 'the baseline data crucial for theory building' but have been neglected in preference to experimental studies which predominantly have been favoured as a research approach for theory testing even though a firm theoretical foundation is often lacking. The directory and classification of nursing diagnosis (Gordon, 1982) may be a useful tool for starting to define concepts important to nursing at this level.

Second level theory tries to explain the situation by identifying possible relationships between factors; and several other propositions could be made in relation to the example in Fig. 1.3.

Third level theory predicts what may occur if factors are varied or manipulated.

With fourth level theory, control of the situation can be achieved where 'nursing intervention has a high probability of accomplishing desired goals' (Leddy and Pepper, 1989). In Fig. 1.3 the example given for fourth level theory demonstrates a specific nursing intervention which could be prescribed to meet a specifically stated goal. It is Dickoff and James's (1968) major contention that 'all theory exists finally for the sake of practice (since in a sense every lower level of theory exists for the next higher level and the highest level exists for practice . . .)'. If Dickoff and James's view of theory is to be accepted then nursing knowledge will commence with the generation of theory at first level where various phenomena need to be described and defined. Such phenomena important to the focus of nursing could be said to have begun to be described by various nursing theorists. To understand how nursing models can help identify nursing knowledge it is important to understand not only Dickoff and James's view of theory generation but also Walker and Avant's (1988) perspective. The latter authors classify theory development literature into four levels:

- Meta-theory
- Grand theory (sometimes called Macro- or Molar theory)
- Middle-range theory
- Practice theory

Such a classification was earlier proposed by Merton (1967).

Meta-theory is concerned with philosophical and methodological aspects of theory building in nursing: for example philosophical issues about the relationships between nursing theory, the philosophy of science and nursing knowledge; or methodological examples, for example the work of Dickoff and James described earlier (Walker and Avant, 1988; Suppe and Jacox, 1985).

Grand theories are those theories we know as nursing models. They define nursing broadly and abstractly from a global perspective, describing 'the whole of nursing's concern' (Chinn and Jacobs, 1987). Fawcett (1984) defines such theories as 'conceptual frameworks'. According to Walker and Avant (1988) grand theories 'have made an important contribution in conceptually sorting out nursing from the practice of medicine by demonstrating the presence of distinct nursing perspectives'. However, because of the vague terminology used and the lack of clear interrelationships between concepts at this stage in their development, most are untestable (Suppe and Jacox, 1985; Walker and Avant, 1988).

Middle range theories, although still abstract, contain elements of grand theories but have less scope and less variables, therefore making them more appropriate for testing (Walker and Avant, 1988).

The last level identified by Walker and Avant is practice theory as described under the situation-relating theory of Dickoff and James (1968).

Nursing models, theory and classification

Most nursing theories or models (both the words theory and model are used because it depends on the definitions and criteria used) can be classified as grand theory because they are very abstract, and 'give some broad perspective to the goals and structure of nursing practice' (Walker and Avant, 1988). Another name synonomous with grand theory is global theory; and Fawcett (1984) uses the term 'conceptual model' in the same context.

Nursing theory, according to Chinn and Jacobs (1987), 'ought to guide practice, generate new ideas, and differentiate the focus of nursing from other professions'. Walker and Avant (1988) agree with this view.

All nursing models or theories state something about the following four concepts (Fawcett, 1984; Levine, 1988):

- **Man** or the **individual**
- **Society** or the **environment** of care
- **Health**
- **Nursing**, its nature and role

In fact these four concepts, or 'constructs' to be more correct (constructs being more abstract and including a number of concepts), are fundamental to nursing knowledge, and therefore form the building blocks of the Project 2000 curriculum (see Chapter 4). What one's values and beliefs are about these four constructs (i.e. one's philosophy) will determine the knowledge required for practice. In fact many teams of nurses have used such a framework to develop their ward/unit/team philosophies, before considering which model of nursing is congruent with their own views. Such an approach links knowledge to philosophy and this is the reason that we return to this subject later.

If the values and beliefs associated with the four constructs fundamental to all nursing models determine what specific knowledge is central to nursing, although in each nursing setting there are likely to be differences in how roles are perceived, then for that reason it is worthwhile trying to make sense of the large number of nursing models that currently exist. Are there any common themes for example that would allow nursing models to be classified according to the underlying theories that contribute to them?

All nursing theories have been derived inductively and/or deductively, that is to say that other theories developed outside nursing have been applied to nursing (deduction) and introduced into individual theorist's models to be combined with the theorist's own experiences and observations in nursing (induction). Orlando (1961) is a rare exception in that her theory is almost exclusively inductive, i.e. based only on her observations and experiences as a nurse.

Several classifications of nursing theory exist. Johnson (1974) and Riehl and Roy (1980) classify nursing models according to the origin of their underpinning theories:

- **Developmental** those based on developmental theories
- **System** those based on systems theory
- **Interaction** those based on interaction theories

Leddy and Pepper (1989) introduce another dimension. They do not classify nursing models but instead classify the theories that form the basis of nursing models, according to how changes are explained in the inter-relationships between humans, health, environment and nursing. The following four groups result:

- **Stress and adaptation theories**
- **Growth and development theories**
- **Systems theory**
- **Rhythm theories**

There is some commonality between the two classifications, but what is interesting is that if all these theories have contributed to nursing models then does this therefore suggest the knowledge which is important to nursing? Figure 1.4 defines the characteristics of each of Leddy and Pepper's four groups, examples of theories that fall into these groups and corresponding nursing models that use these underlying theories.

Classification group	Focus	Examples of nursing models using these theories	Examples of theories within group
STRESS AND ADAPTATION	Cause and effect	Roy's Adaptation Model (1984)	Seyle's Stress Theory (1976) Engle's Stress Theory (1962) Helson's Adaptation Theory (1964)
GROWTH AND DEVELOPMENT	Positive linear growth towards maximum potential	Peplau's Interpersonal Model (1952)	Sullivan's Interpersonal Development Theory (1963) Maslow's Psychosocial Theory (1968) Kohlberg's Moral Reasoning Developmental Theory (1981)
SYSTEMS THEORY	Interrelationship between parts. Change in one part effects the whole	Rogers' Theory of Unitary Human Beings (1989) Johnson's Behavioral Systems Model (1980)	General Systems Theory, von Bertalanffy (1981)
RHYTHM	Predictable cyclical patterns e.g. circadian rhythm	Rogers' Science of Unitary Human Beings (1989)	Theories about biological rhythm and sleep-wake patterns

Fig. 1.4 Leddy and Pepper's classification of theories which contribute to nursing models with examples. (Adapted from Leddy and Pepper, 1989.)

Leddy and Pepper go on to consider how each of these groups would define man, health, nursing and the environment in different ways. From such a viewpoint it is the implications for nursing that are important to address, because they will dictate the knowledge basis for nursing. For example, if models based on systems theory are used, then within the nurse-patient relationship both patient and nurse would be mutually affected by any change, therefore changes in one partner of that relationship will have an effect on the other and vice versa. This supports the value of aesthetic knowledge and knowledge of self as proposed by Carper (1978). Nursing models based on stress and adaptation theories suggest that nurses need knowledge of how to help clients reduce stressful external stimuli, and how to enhance their coping strategies. Models based on growth and development would mean that nurses, using them depending on the setting, would need to assess and recognise where clients were placed in their psychological, social, psychosexual, moral, cognitive and interpersonal development, before they could help the client move forward. It is often assumed that both clients, relatives and students can grasp complex moral issues without considering at what stage they are in their moral reasoning, using either Kohlberg's (1981) or Gilligan's (1982) moral reasoning and developmental stages.

Although all theories can be criticised, it is important to remember the previous point made about the nature of theory, that is, that theory is the theorists' best efforts to try and describe and explain the phenomena observed.

Some implications that rhythm theories have for nursing concern the maintenance and enhancement of biological cycles, for example the maintenance of differences between day and night, i.e. 'diurnal rhythm'. Knowledge of such biological rhythms (Chapter 5) is particularly relevant to acute nursing settings, where continuous nasogastric feeding may be common practice through the night, and any fall in hourly urinary outputs are automatically responded to by pleas to the doctors for diuretics. Orlando (1961) considers that automatic responses in themselves are potentially harmful to clients because they have not been made deliberately and/or are not based on sound decision making.

Two classifications of nursing models have been focused on here for the purpose of elucidating what could be considered as nursing knowledge for practice. However there are others, and before leaving this topic the classification proposed by Meleis will be considered. Meleis (1985) has classified nursing models into 'schools of thought' which relate to some extent to their chronology, the backgrounds of the theorists, and the broader social times during which they were developed. Each of the schools of thought have been associated with a particular question which determines the main focus of the models. If considered carefully, these questions can also throw some light on what knowledge is important to nursing. The three schools of thought are;

- **Needs theorists**
- **Interaction theorists**
- **Outcome theorists**

According to Meleis, needs theorists asked the question *What do nurses do*?; interaction theorists asked the question *How do nurses do whatever it is they do*?; and outcome theorists asked the question *Why*?

Needs theorists based their models on theories by Maslow and the developmental theorist Erikson. Examples of needs theorists are Henderson (1966) and Orem (1985). The focus of this school of thought is on problems, deficits and needs, with nursing fulfilling the role of meeting needs. Although breaks from the medical model can be seen the focus is still very much on illness, with perceptions of the client or influences of the environment absent.

The interactionist school of thought represented by theorists such as Peplau (1952), and King (1981) developed from the needs school and was influenced by the many social and cultural changes of the 1950s and 1960s. These are described more fully by Meleis. The characteristics of the interactionists are that nursing is seen to be an interaction process which is deliberate and involves helping and caring. Caring is considered to be humanistic rather than mechanistic. The nurse-patient relationship is considered to be therapeutic, which means that the nurse would use him or herself in a therapeutic way. To achieve this the nurse needs to consider, clarify and evaluate his or her own values (knowledge of self). Illness is considered to be an 'inevitable human experience' (Meleis, 1985), one from which the individual can grow and learn. The theories underpinning this school relate to humanism, interactionism and phenomenological (where experiences of the world are central) and existential (where individuals are considered unique beings able to make choices) philosophies.

The outcome school theorists are concerned with the outcome of care. Examples include Rogers (1970) and Roy (1984). Building on the 'what' and 'how' they focus on the recipient of care and his or her harmony with the environment; the goal of nursing care being to bring back 'some balance, stability, and preservation of energy, or enhancing the individual and the environment' (Meleis, 1985).

Knowledge and philosophy

'Philosophy provides a point of view: it is a belief construct, a speculation about the nature and value of things'

(Bevis, 1982)

Philosophy is the 'seeking after wisdom or knowledge, especially that which deals with ultimate reality, or with the most general causes and principles of things and ideas and human perception and knowledge of them, physical phenomena and ethics' (Concise Oxford Dictionary, 1976).

A major concern of philosophy is the study of the nature of knowledge – this is called epistemology. Examples of epistemological questions could be, How one comes to know? or What is knowledge? In most other disciplines and in nursing to date the most valued approaches to developing knowledge have been the 'Scientific-Empirical' approach (Chinn and Jacobs, 1987). Chalmers (1982) however considers that this 'ideology of science' as it functions in society contains 'the dubious concept of science and the equally dubious concept of truth'. He further supports this belief with examples from behavioural psychology 'which encourages the treatment of people as machines' and 'the extensive use of the results of I.Q. studies in our educational system'. Chalmers states that 'bodies of knowledge such as these are defended by claiming or implying that they have been acquired by means of the "scientific method" and therefore must have merit'.

Philosophers do not have criteria which differentiate between knowledge that is scientific and that which is not. Each area of knowledge should be analysed for what it is, and for its purpose by considering the following questions:

* What is the aim of knowledge? (Chalmers states that this is different from what the aim is commonly thought to be or presented as)
* What methods are used to accomplish the aims?
* To what degree have the aims been successfully accomplished?

(Chalmers, 1982)

This line of thought therefore focuses on knowledge itself, not whether knowledge can be claimed to be scientific or not. There have been many criticisms initially from outside nursing (Chalmers, 1982) and latterly from inside nursing (Suppe and Jacox, 1985) about the traditional approach to science and views about the nature of scientific knowledge (i.e. philosophy of science). Before these changes can be examined in more detail it is important to differenti~~e between philosophy and science. Figure 1.5 indicates more clearly how philosophy differs from empirical science.

Bergendal (1983) considers 'Such words as 'knowledge' and 'science' as not well defined' and goes on to state that 'one prevailing opinion is that knowledge and science are basically much the same'. Bergendal also states that another common opinion is that science is 'true' knowledge, the supreme form of knowledge. Science can be thought of in two ways: firstly as a body of knowledge, i.e. empirical knowledge which is the 'outcome' of methods used to generate knowledge; and secondly as a 'process' which relates to the logical and systematic methods used to generate knowledge. According to Suppe and Jacox (1985) the problem central to the philosophy of science is understanding the nature of scientific knowledge. The following brief overview will illustrate how this has changed over time.

Historical aspects of the philosophy of science

Aristotle, the Greek philosopher and a pupil of Plato, lived during the period 384–322 B.C. He studied the whole field of knowledge and considered that knowledge was derived from deductive logic. He considered that 'the scientist was primarily a passive observer of what was' (Fitzpatrick, 1989). This view about knowledge continued until

PHILOSOPHY	EMPIRICAL SCIENCE
After Bevis (1982)	
Explores values	Describes facts
Looks at wholes and relationships with other wholes	Reduces phenomena to component parts to study, describe and explain how they operate
Answers questions why and queries the worth of experience	Answers how, when and where
Provides a value system for ordering priorities and selecting from various data	
After Sarter (1988)	
Unlimited totality 'the entire universe'	Domain delineated and definite

Fig. 1.5 Differing characteristics of philosophy and empirical science.

the sixteenth century when Francis Bacon, the famous English philosopher and a founder of modern science, rejected Aristotle's view of knowledge generation in favour of the inductive method. Bacon considered that the purpose of science was to improve 'man's lot on earth' and 'if we wanted to understand nature then we must consult nature and not the writings of Aristotle' (Chalmers, 1982). This could only be achieved by inductive methods. Such methods involve producing universal statements by generalising from repeating organised and careful observations of specific situations or phenomena (i.e. induction is defined as an approach which produces generalisations from specific situations, and deduction the reverse; the application of general principles to specific situations through the use of logical argument). To clarify induction and deduction Fig. 1.6 provides an example of both.

Empiricism is an approach that considers all knowledge to be derived from experience via pure observation and collection of facts through the senses. This approach was strongly supported by the English philosopher John Locke in the seventeenth century. Rationalism is an opposing view of how knowledge about the world could be generated. It can be defined as an approach to generating

INDUCTION

Statement of observations made

'I have observed that all patients that I have admitted for elective surgery have appeared anxious.'

Generalisation by induction

All patients admitted for elective surgery will be anxious.

DEDUCTION

General theory

Stressors, be they biological, psychological or social, produce specific physiological changes.

Logical deduction

John has stated that he is in constant pain, and he is worried about his wife visiting him after dark.

John is experiencing multiple stressors

John will exhibit specific physiological changes.

Fig. 1.6 Examples to demonstrate inductive and deductive approaches in nursing.

knowledge through the application of reason and was pioneered in the seventeenth century by the French mathematician René Descartes who was concerned with the finding out as to why anything can be said to be true.

Auguste Comte founded positivism in the nineteenth century. Positivism considered that only data which was arrived at by experiment and objective observation was 'positive' truth. Empirical methods for generating knowledge therefore involve 'the collection of "facts" by means of careful observation and experiment and the subsequent derivation of laws and theories from those facts by some logical progression' (Chalmers, 1982).

From the 1920s through to the 1960s philosophy of science has been dominated by 'logical positivism' (later to be renamed logical empiricism). This approach is considered to be an extreme form of empiricism and was postulated by a group of philosophers subsequently named the 'Vienna Circle'. This view is encapsulated by the 'received view' or 'the scientific method'. The focus of this view of science is the 'justification' of discovery and resulted from 'an amalgamation of logic with the goals of empiricism in the development of scientific theories' (Meleis, 1985). The key features of logical positivism are

- Only statements confirmed by sensory data, through sensory experience are valid
- True statements are only those based on experience and known through experience
- Rejection of abstraction as a method of generating theory, and any ethical considerations
- Science is value-free and scientific method is the only method for generating knowledge
- Scientific method is characterised by 'reductionism, quantifiability, objectivity and operationalization' (Watson, 1981)

The approach outlined above has been criticised because it takes for granted 'cause', and rejects the effects of context on discovery. As a result, the use of the scientific method is no longer seen to be the predominant approach to knowledge generation by many disciplines, although nursing has based much of its early theory building efforts on this approach even though such reductionist ideas are incompatible with the holistic values embodied in nursing models (see Chapters 3 and 8 for further considerations of holism). Problems in developing nursing's knowledge base, according to Meleis (1985), have therefore occurred because nursing has used this outdated approach to develop knowledge about aspects of nursing which 'are neither reducible, quantifiable, nor objective'. Benner (1984) and Rogers (1989) also purport that nursing cannot be separated from the context of care, and suggest that many aspects of nursing cannot therefore be reduced to the minutest detail and examined. It is Meleis's view that nurse theorists have not followed the 'received view', but that they have generated their conceptual frameworks from their experiences, and include ideas that are 'subjective, intuitive, humanistic, integrative and in many instances not based on sense-data'. (Meleis, 1985).

Sir Karl Popper, the British philosopher of science, has, since the 1950s, rejected the doctrine that all knowledge starts from perception and sensation, and proposes instead that it is developed through guesswork and refutation. He suggests that propositions are only valid if they have repeatedly and exhaustably survived attempts to falsify them, although it has been found that it is as difficult to falsify theories as it is to confirm them (Suppe and Jacox, 1985).

Pragmatism is an American school of philosophy which is concerned with the usefulness of knowledge. It was first proposed by Charles Peirce supported by his friend William James but not really acknowledged until later into the twentieth century. Pragmatists consider that truth, and therefore knowledge, is validated by whether it can be put to good use, rather than whether there is evidence to support it.

Figure 1.7 outlines chronologically famous philosophers of science and their main contribution to the understanding of scientific knowledge.

Today, there are constant changes in views as to how philosophy of science describes knowledge and although the positivists have been discredited there is no one view that has displaced it. The main concern in nursing is identified by Suppe and Jacox (1985), who state that nursing literature continues to reflect the discredited ideas of the logical positivists, and that nurses interested in developing and testing

Date	Person/founders	Ideas
384–322 B.C.	Aristotle	**Deductive logic**
1561–1626	Bacon	**Inductive method**
1596–1650	Descartes	**Rationalism**
1632–1704	Locke	**Empiricism**
1798–1857	Comte	**Positivism**
1920s	'The Vienna Circle' of philosophers	**Logical positivism/ logical empiricism**
1930s	Peirce/William James/ Dewey/Kaplan	**Pragmatism**
1950s	Popper	**Falsification**

Fig. 1.7 Important people and their ideas in philosophy of science.

theory must become aware of issues within the philosophy of science.· In their conclusion they state that 'Multiple approaches to theory development and testing should be encouraged', therefore identifying the need for greater diversity and tolerance in theory testing than was previously permitted by the logical empiricist. They finally consider that 'Debates about inductive versus deductive and qualitative versus quantitative approaches to theory development and testing are useful insofar as they make clear that alternatives exist'.

Knowledge and power

What is the relationship between knowledge and power? Power is often considered as being a rather unpleasant characteristic with cynical connotations, and although there may be some grain of truth in such a view, there are in fact many positive aspects as well. The amount of power in society has been described by the sociologist Weber as being constant, and therefore power held by one group implies less power for other groups.

Many sociologists consider the concept of power from a 'macro' perspective, that is one concerned with whole populations and societies, for example the Marxist perspective (see Chapter 9). However, others such as Dahl consider power from a more interpersonal perspective. He considers that power is being exerted when someone's behaviour deviates as a result of influence. Dahl defines power in the following way:

'Power is not an attribute. Power is a particular kind of social relationship.
'Power refers to dependence relationships between people'
(Dahl, cited Potter and Sarre, 1974)

Power and influence go together; the social exchange theory of Homans too would support this idea in that all interactions involve an exchange of something in return for something else. Power may be legitimate in the form of authority (i.e. there is some recognised official backing), for example one's manager has the authority to demand to know what one may be doing. French and Raven (1953) have produced one classification of power types (Fig. 1.8).

Within nursing all these power types can be seen. Many are concerned with knowledge, be that 'know-how' or 'know-that' knowledge. For example in the works of Stein (1968), a psychiatrist who described the Doctor-Nurse relationship, nurses were identified as possessing a great deal of power which they used very subtly and skilfully to influence medical decision-making regarding patient management. This was achieved in the way they provided cues to

PHYSICAL POWER   The threat of abuse or actual abuse

RESOURCE POWER   The power to award something which is desired by the potential recipient

POSITION POWER   Legal and legitimate power associated with a position

EXPERT POWER   An individual may have power because of knowledge possessed, or because they convey the impression that they possess specialised knowledge

PERSONAL POWER   Sometimes called charismatic power as it is the power associated with the person and their personality

NEGATIVE POWER   The power to stop things happening

Fig. 1.8 Types of power (French and Raven, 1953).

medical colleagues hence maintaining medical omnipotence. On analysing this example, all the power types appear present. The physical power source is covert and is not necessarily physical but involves the possible threat of coercion, for example if the doctor repeatedly does not take note of the cues being given by the nurse about the best course of action in a certain situation then the nurse may have little hesitation in telephoning the doctor in the middle of the night about some aspect of care which could have waited until the morning. Regarding resource power the nurse does have the power to reward through her co-operation and general ability to 'make life easier' for the doctor via various initiatives that the nurse can take. Position power resides with the more senior members of the nursing team who are often more permanent than medical staff who pass through. Generally the medical staff rely on senior nursing staff to 'show them the ropes'. Expert and personal power can be exerted through the power of persuasion and skilled interpersonal skills. Negative power too can be exerted very subtly through non co-operation or by filtering information.

How nurses control patients' behaviour through language is another illustration of the use of power. The use of controlling may or may not be deliberate, but often relates to lack of know-how in interpersonal skills, or lack of personal knowledge about how self may effect others. Such behaviour on the nurse's part may also reflect insufficient moral knowledge. Instances of such controlling language are presented in the work of Lanceley (1985); the quotations in Fig. 1.9 illustrate some of her examples.

Thus, according to Dahl, power exists in all relationships between people. As nurses are party to professional relationships with clients and colleagues it is therefore not only essential for nurses to know about types of power but also what methods of influence are used to perpetuate the power source. Handy (1985) considers that methods

'We're just going to stand you up'
'Come on Anne, take your tablets... there's a good girl'
'Now you must stay with us for a while'
'You will have some lunch, won't you?'

Fig. 1.9 Examples of controlling language used by nurses, cited by Lanceley (1985).

of influence fall into two groups, overt and unseen, and these are summarised in Fig. 1.10.

Potter (1975) aptly summarises the benefits of knowing about power and also relates such benefits to practice settings in the following quotation:

'The correct identification of power relationships can be of the greatest practical significance for people attempting to get things done in society'

Therefore if nurses want to be influential in achieving positive change within health care settings, knowledge of power dynamics is an essential prerequisite. Power and influence are fundamental concepts to understand in relation to health promotion (Chapter 3) and politics (Chapter 9).

Knowledge and professionalism

Chinn and Jacobs (1987) define a profession as 'a vocation that requires specialised knowledge, provides a role in society that is valued, and employs some means of internal regulation'.

Rogers (1989) considers that professional practice results from the application of knowledge and that nursing is a learned profession, that it is both an art and a science. She defines science as an abstract body of knowledge that is systematically and logically arrived at. This does not imply that knowledge should be empirical knowledge, but only that the methods used should reflect the process of science.

POWER SOURCE	INFLUENCE	
	Overt	**Unseen**
PHYSICAL	force	ecology (i.e. environment)
RESOURCE	exchange	magnetism
POSITION	rules and procedures	—
EXPERT	rules and procedures	—
PERSONAL	persuasion	—

Fig. 1.10 Methods of influence. (After Handy, 1985.)

Rogers considers that there is a need for an abstract body of knowledge that is concerned with the nature of nursing. She purports that the knowledge base for a profession is different from examining the activity of that profession. Rogers (1989) provides a useful analogy to demonstrate this point in the discipline of biology amongst other examples, where she states that studying what biologists do is not the same as studying biology. Likewise studying what nurses do is not the same as studying nursing. This therefore is how a knowledge base unique to nursing could be explained.

According to Moore (1969) the 'criteria for a profession dictate that there must be a body of knowledge and that this body of knowledge can be communicated by others'. Whether nurses develop knowledge purely for the purpose of aspiring to professional status can sidetrack us away from the purpose of knowledge generation which is, as this author sees it, to improve the care that we can offer to our clients. Professionalism may be a secondary benefit of this purpose. But even professional status in itself can improve the service through the higher status that nursing achieves. The more respected its views are by professionals the more influence it can exert on the health care provision of tomorrow. This can only be achieved through increasing nursing's knowledge (expert power), and making that knowledge evident through nurses' position (position power).

Knowledge and accountability

Whether one considers that nursing is a profession or not, professionalism is linked to accountability. Denyes *et al.* (1989) state that scientific accountability is a characteristic of a profession. Leddy and Pepper (1989) too consider that the 'concept of the professional includes legal and moral accountability for the individual's own actions'. Accountability is therefore inextricably linked to being a professional. It is also associated with autonomy, responsibility and authority. Bergman (1981) considers accountability to include three dimensions:

- personal responsibility
- authority
- reporting

She has developed a model that illustrates the relationship of accountability to knowledge. Knowledge, skill and attitude are considered the most basic pre-requisites for accountability. Responsibility is the next pre-requisite, followed by authority. Responsibility and authority are therefore part of accountability. Responsibility must be given or taken to carry out an action (Bergmann, 1981). Authority is legitimised power, i.e. the formal backing or legal right to carry out the responsibility (Bergmann, 1981). The reporting aspect of accountability relates to answerability. The nurse is answerable to the client first and foremost, but also to professional colleagues for standards of practice, the employer with whom she has a contract and finally the law. One aspect not covered by Bergmann's model is that of autonomy. Autonomy relates to independence of action and 'means that one can perform one's total professional functions on the basis of one's own knowledge and judgement' (Leddy and Pepper, 1989). It is the making of decisions and the acting on them. To be autonomous one must be accountable. Accountability and autonomy both require a sound knowledge basis for practice which further supports the need to clearly establish and continually develop the body of knowledge on which practice is based.

Conclusion

'Nursing thus depends on the scientific knowledge of human behaviour in health and in illness, the aesthetic perception of significant human experiences, a personal understanding of the unique individuality of the self and the capacity to make choices within concrete situations involving particular moral judgements'

(Carper, 1978)

This chapter has contributed some insight into the nature of knowledge and how it is intricately tied up with nursing itself. The nature of knowledge has been considered and a review of specific topics related to knowledge completed, so that the point has now been reached where specific aspects of nursing knowledge, in its various forms, can be considered in forthcoming chapters, with thoughts about the future road to nursing knowledge in the closing chapter.

References

Adam, E. (1985). Toward more clarity in terminology: frameworks, theories and models. *Journal of Nursing Education*, **24(4)**, 151–5.

Barber, P. (1986). The psychiatric nurse's failure therapeutically to nurture. *Nursing Practice*, **1(3)**, 138–41.

Benner, P. (1984). *From Novice to Expert: Excellence and Power in Clinical Nursing Practice*. Addiston-Wesley, Menlo Park.

Bergendel, G.(1983). Higher education and knowledge policies. *Journal of Higher Education*, **54(6)**, 599–628.

Bergmann, R. (1981). Accountability—definition and dimensions. *International Nursing Review*, **28(2)**, 53–9.

Bevis, E. M. (1982). *Curriculum Building in Nursing: a Process*, 3rd edition. Mosby, St. Louis.

Boore, J. (1978). *Prescription for Recovery*. Royal College of Nursing, London.

Burnard, P. (1987). Towards an epistemological basis for experiential learning in nurse education. *Journal of Advanced Nursing*, **12(2)**, 189–93.

Burnard, P. (1988). Emotional release. *Journal of District Nursing*, **6(11)**, 6, 9.

Carper, B. A. (1978). Fundamental patterns of knowing in nursing. *Advances in Nursing Science*, **1(1)**, 13–23.

Chalmers, A. F. (1982).What is This Thing Called Science? 2nd edition. Open University Press, Milton Keynes.

Chinn, P. L. and Jacobs, M. K. (1987). *Theory and Nursing*, 2nd edition. Mosby, St. Louis.

Concise Oxford Dictionary (1976). 6th edition. Oxford University, Press, Oxford.

Creed,F. (1981). Life events and appendectomy. *The Lancet*, **1(8235)**, 1381–5.

Dahl, R. A. (1974). Power. In *Dimensions of Society*, D. Potter and P. Sarre (Eds), pp 446–5. Hodder & Stoughton, Sevenoaks.

Denyes, M. J., Connor, N. A., Oakley, D. and Ferguson, S. (1989). Integrating nursing theory, practice and research through collaborative research. *Journal of Advanced Nursing*, **14(2)**, 141–5.

Dickoff, J. and James, P. (1968). A theory of theories: A position paper. *Nursing Research*, **17(3)**, 197–203.

Dickoff, J., James, P. and Wiedenback, E. (1968). Theory in a practice discipline. Part 1. Practice oriented theory. *Nursing Research*, **17(5)**, 415–35.

Engel, G. (1962). *Psychological Development in Health and Disease*. Saunders, Philadelphia.

Fawcett, J. (1978). The relationship between theory and research: a double helix. *Advances in Nursing Science*, **1(1)**, 49–62.

Fawcett, J. (1984). *Analysis and Evaluation of Conceptual Models of Nursing*. Davis, Philadelphia.

Fitzpatrick, J. (1989). The empirical approach to the development of nursing science. In *Conceptual Models of Nursing*, 2nd edition, J. Fitzpatrick and A. Whall (Eds). Appleton & Lange, Norwalk.

French, J. and Raven, B. (1953). The bases of social power. In *Group Dynamics*, D. Cartwright and A. Lander (Eds), pp 259–69. Tavistock, London.

Gilligan, C. (1982). *In a Different Voice*. Harvard University Press, Cambridge, Mass.

Goldberger, L. (1966). Experimental isolation: an overview. *American Journal of Psychiatry*, **122**, 774–82.

Gordon, M. (1982). *Nursing Diagnosis: Process and Application*. McGraw-Hill, New York.

Handy, C. B. (1985). *Understanding Organizations*, 3rd edition. Penguin, Harmondsworth.

Hayward, J. (1975). *Information – a Prescription Against Pain*. Royal College of Nursing, London.

Henderson, V. (1966). *The Nature of Nursing: a Definition and its Implications for Practice Research and Education*. Macmillan, New York.

Heron, J. (1981). Philosophical basis for a new paradigm. In *Human Inquiry: a Sourcebook of New Paradigm Research*, P. Reason and J. Rowan (Eds), pp. 19–35. Wiley, Chichester.

Johnson, D. (1968). Professional practice and specialization in nursing. *Image* **2** (3), 2–7.

Johnson, D. (1974). Development of theory: a requisite for nursing as a primary health care profession. *Nursing Research*, **23(5)**, 372–7.

King, I. M. (1981). *A Theory for Nursing*. Wiley, New York.

Kohlberg, L. (1981). *The Philosophy of Moral Development: Moral Stages and the Idea of Justice*. Harper & Row, San Francisco.

Kübler-Ross, E. (1970). *On Death and Dying*. Tavistock, London.

Kuhn, T. (1970). *The Structure of Scientific Revolutions*, 2nd edition. University of Chicago Press, Chicago.

Lanceley, A. (1985). Use of controlling language in the rehabilitation of the elderly. *Journal of Advanced Nursing*, **10(2)**, 125–35.

Leddy, S. and Pepper, J. (1989). *Conceptual Bases of Professional Nursing*, 2nd edition. Lippincott, Philadelphia.

Levine, M. (1988). Antecedents from adjunctive disciplines: creation of nursing theory. *Nursing Science Quarterly*, **1(1)**, 16–25.

Manley, K. (1989). *Primary Nursing in Intensive Care*. Scutari, Harrow.

Meleis, A. (1985). *Theoretical Nursing: Development and Progress*. Lippincott, Philadelphia.

Merton, R. K. (1967). *On Theoretical Sociology*. Free Press, New York.

Moore, M. A. (1969). The professional practice of nursing: the knowledge and how it is used. *Nursing Forum*, **8(4)**, 361–73.

Orem, D. (1985). *Nursing: Concepts of Practice*, 3rd edition. McGraw-Hill, New York.

Orlando, I. J. (1961). *The Dynamic Nurse-Patient Relationship*. Putnam, New York.

Parkes, C. M. (1986). *Bereavement: Studies of Grief in Adult Life*, 2nd edition. Penguin, Harmondsworth.

Parkes, C. M., Benjamin, B. and Fitzgerald, R. (1969). Broken heart: a statistical study of increased mortality among widowers. *British Medical Journal*, **1**, 740–3.

Peplau, H. E. (1952). *Interpersonal Relations in Nursing*, Putnam,

New York.

Petrosino, B., Becker, H. and Christian, B. (1988). Infection rates in central venous catheter dressings. *Oncology Nursing Forum*, **15(6)**, 709–17.

Polit, D. and Hungler, P. (1987). *Nursing Research: Principles and Methods*, 3rd edition. Lippincott, Philadelphia.

Polanyi, M. (1958). *Personal Knowledge*. University of Chicago Press, Chicago.

Potter, D. (1975). Power, conflict and integration: a study guide. In *Power*, Open University, pp 7–51. Open University Press, Milton Keynes. (Social sciences: a foundation course: Making sense of society, D101 Block 8 Units 25–28).

Potter, D. and Sarre, P. (Eds) (1974). *Dimensions of Society: A reader*. Hodder and Stoughton/Open University Press, Sevenoaks.

Riehl, S. and Roy, C. (1980). *Adaptation Level Theory*. Harper and Row, New York.

Riehl-Sisca, J. P. (1989). *Conceptual Models for Nursing Practice*, 3rd edition. Appleton & Lange, Norwalk.

Rogers, M. E. (1970). *An Introduction to the Theoretical Basis of Nursing*. Davis, Philadelphia.

Rogers, M. E. (1989). Nursing: a science of unitary human beings. In *Conceptual Models for Nursing Practice*, J. P. Riehl-Sisca (Ed.), pp. 181–95. Appleton & Lange, Norwalk.

Roy, C. (1984). *Introduction to Nursing: an Adaptation Model*, 2nd edition. Prentice-Hall, Englewood Cliffs.

Runkle, G. (1985). *Theory and Practice: an Introduction to Philosophy*. Holt, Rinehart and Winston, New York.

Ryle, G. (1949). *The Concept of Mind*. Penguin, Harmondsworth.

Sarter, B. (1988). Philosophical sources of nursing theory. *Nursing Science Quarterly*, **1(2)**, 52–9.

Stein, L. (1968). The doctor-nurse game. *American Journal of Nursing*, **68(1)**, 101–5.

Strong, P. and Robinson, J. (1988). *New Model Management: Griffiths and the NHS*. Nursing Policy Studies Centre, University of Warwick, Coventry.

Suppe, F. and Jacox, A. K. (1985). Philosophy of science and the development of nursing theory. *Annual Review of Nursing Research*, **3**, 241–67.

Visintainer, M. (1986). The nature of knowledge and theory in nursing. *Image*, **18(2)**, 32–8.

Walker, L. O. and Avant, K. C. (1988). *Strategies for Theory Construction in Nursing*, 2nd edition. Appleton & Lange, Norwalk.

Watson, J. (1981). Nursing's scientific quest. *Nursing Outlook*, **29(7)**, 413–16.

Wiedenbach, E. (1964). *Clinical Nursing: a Helping Art*. Springer, New York.

2 Research – What it is and what it is not

Introduction

This chapter will introduce the reader to the function and potential of research in nursing. It will address some of the fundamental questions raised by those new to the subject. In a single chapter it is obviously impossible to provide a comprehensive overview of the topic, but it is hoped that many of the major issues will be addressed and discussed and that further investigation of the topic will be stimulated.

The chapter is divided into sections, each of which will address one of the following questions:

- The place of nursing research – why bother with the subject?
- What is nursing research? – definitions and parameters
- What it is not – limitations of research
- Applications and implementation – how can research findings be used in practice?
- The art and value of critique – is this a skill worth developing?

A short summary reflects on the main themes of the chapter and reviews some of the broad issues facing nurses when considering nursing research.

The place of nursing research (or why bother with the subject?)

Hunt (1981) identified that nurses are becoming increasingly more conscious of the need to be able to demonstrate a rational basis for the care they give. In recent years increasing pressures on qualified staff to pay more than lip service to the concept of accountability for practice has further fuelled this need.

This chapter will explore the relationship between research and nursing practice and demonstrate that sympathy and understanding for the former can provide the basis for identifying the rationale for, and lead to improvements in, the latter. In common with many others in this book this chapter will make use of Henderson's (1969) definition of nursing:

'In a broad sense nursing care is derived from what has been called the unique function of the nurse . . . to assist the individual, sick or well, in the performance of those activities contributing to health or its recovery (or to a peaceful death) that he would perform unaided if he had the necessary strength, will or knowledge. And to do this in such a way as to help him to gain independence as rapidly as possible. This aspect of her work, this part of her function she initiates and controls; of this she is the master.'

Assisting patients to achieve goals is accomplished by a variety of nursing care actions – some relatively routine and others requiring specific individualised planning based on information available and the use of professional judgement. How does a nurse determine which are the appropriate nursing actions to undertake for the benefit of the patient?

Tradition and custom dictate much of what nurses do. Henderson (1969) summarises tradition and custom as 'what we all know to be true . . . nursing develops by role modelling, being handed down, usually going unchallenged because we have always done it that way . . .'. In this situation the applicability or usefulness of the action is not generally questioned. The taking of temperatures four hourly, or the starving of patients from twelve midnight for operation during the morning session, which may be any time from seven in the morning to twelve midday, are examples of such practice. This source of decision making is often coupled with authority, either from the Ward Sister, for example 'Sister likes us to use this particular treatment for wounds', 'Sister likes the beds made in this way'; or from higher up the management structure through policies and procedures, such as medicine administration policies and catheterisation routines. In these cases because someone else has made the decision as to the course of action to take there is, perhaps, no need to understand, or even explore, the rationale for the practice.

Trial and error can also be the source of decision making for practice. When faced with an unfamiliar situation the care delivered can often be the result of trial and error, which is generally unsystematic and haphazard, but may be successful in solving individual problems. By working through a random scheme of trying method (a) then (b) and then (c) and so on the 'right' treatment might eventually be found, or the patient may recover despite the treatment offered. This is analogous to trying to find a way to stop a baby crying in the middle of the night by adopting a succession of different strategies such as rocking, feeding, ignoring, and so on. When success is achieved the situation is not generally analysed and lessons learned for next time; the triumphant person tends just to creep away relieved. The consequence of this route of decision making is that whilst success may ultimately be achieved, the reason why (the rationale) is obscure and therefore one is not in a position to be able to predict with confidence whether the same method would work again in the future.

It must be said that in certain situations both these decision making pathways are acceptable, however research as an aid for decision making offers certain features not to be found in these other methods. Research, when properly conducted, can provide unbiased, objective evidence on which to base a decision. It can supply a description of the 'reality' of the current situation for example, rather than a 'rose tinted' picture of what is thought to be happening. It can provide predictive information in which an analysis of past events can be used to accurately predict future trends such as recruitment and retention issues, outbreak of certain infectious diseases, or uptake of further education courses. Research can provide objective evaluation of two methods of treatment, or choices of nursing action, and this evidence can be used to make a professional judgement in the clinical situation, thus tradition, custom, authority and trial and error can be superceded by the delivery of nursing care based on sound scientific evidence of its efficacy.

To illustrate the contribution that research has to make to nursing three situations will be described.

Research can provide scientifically defensible reasons for nursing actions. Perhaps it is not possible to provide a firm theoretical basis for all nursing actions, however many clinical practices have now been examined under research conditions and effective, and efficient, courses of action have been scientifically identified. For example research conducted by Norton *et al.* (1962), Barton and Barton (1981) and others has determined appropriate action to be taken if pressure sores are to be avoided (regular relief of pressure, the use of pressure reducing beds and mattresses and so on). Hayward (1975) and Boore (1978) have conducted widely accepted research which demonstrates that the provision of pre-operative information is a beneficial aid to post-operative recovery.

Research can increase cost effectiveness of nursing activities. Nurses, in common with other health care professionals, are being put under ever increasing pressure to provide a value for money service, whilst at the same time having to make cuts in the service to constantly strive to keep within target spending levels. With the advent of ward accounting and the responsibility for ward budgets being increasingly invested in the ward sister research has an important role to play in the provision of sound evidence to help to guide the most prudent use of available funds. Reliance on systematically collected research findings can, where available, save wards and departments considerable amounts of money by reducing poor 'trial and error' spending. In management circles it is often argued that, at times of economic constraints, research is a luxury which cannot be financially supported. The author would argue that it is at these times that research is most valuable. A simple survey of bath additives conducted by Sleep and Grant (1988) clearly demonstrates the savings that can result from the implementation of research findings. Sleep and Grant conducted an experimental study of bath additives used by post-natal mothers for the first 10 days post delivery. The sample of 1800 mothers were each assigned to one of three groups: one group added salt to the bath water, another added Savlon solution, and the third group did not use any bath additive. The results indicated that all three groups found the baths soothing and helpful in reducing discomfort, and the midwives concerned reported no significant differences in the rates of healing or the incidence of any complications such as infection. Based on the results of this study Health Authorities and individuals can save considerable amounts of money by following a policy of not using any bath additives for this client group. Romney (1982) conducted a similar trial, also focusing on maternity patients. She conducted an experiment to examine the rates of infection amongst groups of women who were shaved pre-delivery and groups who were not. As with Sleep and Grant's study no differences were evident between the outcome measure examined, i.e. the rates of infection in the two groups. The study provided a sound scientific basis for not performing pre-delivery shaves. Nursing time and unnecessary expenditure on razors were saved, to say nothing of the increased satisfaction experienced by the future mothers.

Whilst this chapter draws most of its examples from nursing practice research it is important to outline the potential contribution that research has to make to other areas, for example education and management. In the field of nursing education research studies can provide teachers with research-based evidence on which to select and monitor different teaching strategies and methods. For example Jacka and Lewin (1987) undertook a study to investigate the nature of the learning that occurred in the classroom and that which occurred in the clinical setting. The study also developed ways of measuring the levels of instruction opportunity and integration within the students' training. Knowledge of nursing practice research can equip the teacher with the ability to teach from a research basis which in turn will provide the student with the how and the why of nursing practice and procedures. Davis (1987) has edited a very useful introductory book which examines a range of research projects and developments currently applicable to nurse education.

Research endeavour is often seen to be in conflict with management endeavour. The main reason for this is a result of the different time perspectives which are commonly adopted by the two groups. The cliche 'management want an answer yesterday' could be coupled with one for researchers – 'researchers can only think in terms of having results in 3–5 years time'. There is more than a grain of truth in this. Managers, by the very nature of their position, need to answer current problems immediately. Researchers on the other hand, by following the scientific rigour of the research process, have to allow themselves time to examine problems in depth. In fact, managers and researchers need to develop an interactive relationship. If managers use researchers to examine certain of their problems it may be possible for some future problems to be avoided. For example, in the area of recruitment and retention of staff the manager must concern him or herself with ensuring that sufficient nurses are in post to provide a full range of services, but may be faced with different patterns of employment in different areas of the hospital. A researcher could take an objective look at the situation, conduct interviews with staff, follow up people who leave or fail to take up employment when offered it, and investigate any causal relationships which seem to be apparent, thus providing the manager with evidence on which to base further strategies. The researcher needs the manager to generate the research questions worthy of investigation, whilst the manager needs someone to take a look at the overall situation, whilst he or she provides the day to day management, and then produces the evidence (or answers) to overcome the problems.

This section has shown that nursing and research should have an interactive relationship. Nursing cannot develop without research to provide scientific knowledge on which to base practice (and education and management), and by the same token research cannot develop without nursing practice to generate the questions which warrant investigation and to implement or utilise the results. The nature of this relationship is summarised in Fig. 2.1.

The following section focuses on how research can fulfil this role.

What is research – definitions and parameters

Research means different things to different people. To some it is a way of life – it is an attitude to problem solving (by being research-minded) which can be applied to almost every area of professional and indeed non-professional problems. In essence, being research-minded means that the individual develops the following attributes:

- An enquiring attitude of mind
- A logical approach to problems
- An awareness of the existence of research reports
- A willingness and ability to read, evaluate, select and make use of research findings

To others research is an activity pursued by academic nurses in ivory towers remote from reality. No researcher, to my knowledge,

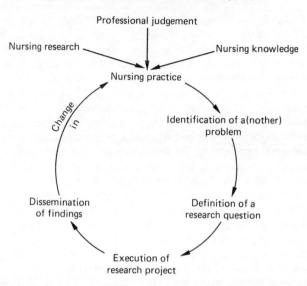

Fig. 2.1 Inter-relationship between nursing practice and nursing research.

has anything approaching an ivory tower; the lucky few may find a quiet corner, possibly a desk and, for the really fortunate ones, possibly a part share in a computer. Practitioners often describe researchers as people who provide complicated pieces of information illustrated by incomprehensible tables and graphs and littered with unintelligible statistical tests, few of which seem directly translatable to practice but may be used by management or other such groups, and of no use to themselves.

This section will seek to demonstrate that research is not separate from nursing but something which must form an integral part of every nurse's professional life. In many situations research is the most appropriate way to solve problems. Research can be defined as:

'an attempt to increase the body of knowledge (i.e. what is currently known about nursing) by discovery of new facts and relationships through a process of systematic scientific enquiry'
(MacLeod Clark and Hockey, 1979)

This definition specifies a 'process' and, in essence, this is what research is; it offers a method (the research process) of problem solving which has many characteristics to commend it over other problem solving methods. It is scientific, systematic and objective. In the previous section other sources of nursing knowledge were discussed, including tradition, custom, authority, and trial and error learning. One way of beginning to understand the value of research is to examine the qualities of research as a basis for problem solving and decision making compared with these other sources of knowledge.

Research can provide evidence on which to base selection of appropriate treatment/course of action whereas tradition and trial and error can, at best, provide experience. Research can provide information to explain why a method, a treatment or a course of action actually works (research based rationales). Tradition and trial and error are not generally concerned with rationales. If rationales are provided they tend to be subjective and judgmental rather than objective and scientific. Research, through the use of inferential statistics, can provide parameters as to how far the available evidence may be confidently generalised to a wider population. Experiential evidence cannot, with the same reliability, be used in this way.

How does a researcher set out to discover this evidence or nursing knowledge? Research always starts with a question. Of this rather obvious point Lancaster (1975) said that research '. . . needs people who ask questions, who have "hunches", who want to find a better way of doing things, who refuse to be put off by platitudinous replies to their questions. Without such people research would never get started.' A topic for research may come from practical experience, from reading, through discussion with colleagues, or just as a 'flash of inspiration'. Whatever the source of the problem the same series of steps must be systematically followed if reliable and objective scientific evidence concerning the problem is to be revealed. These steps, referred to as the research process, are listed below.

(*i*)   The topic of study is identified and the research question posed.

(*ii*) A search of relevant literature is undertaken.

(*iii*) The research question is refined (and, if appropriate, a hypothesis is formulated).

(*iv*) The investigation is planned and data collection methods developed.

(*v*)   A pilot study is conducted.

(*vi*) The main data set is gathered.

(*vii*) The raw data is sorted and analysed.

(*viii*) Conclusions and generalisations are drawn from the analysed data.

(*ix*) A report containing the findings is prepared.

(*x*)   This information is disseminated to the appropriate people.

(*xi*) The findings are utilised/implemented as appropriate.

It is not within the scope of this chapter to present more than a brief introduction to the main considerations and components of these steps.

Posing the question

Posing the question follows directly from identification of a particular problem that you wish to solve, or from an idea or vague hunch you want to explore. There are three main sources of research questions; they can be generated from experience, from other research or from theory.

Experience may lead to the identification of a specific problem, or perhaps just a 'hunch' as to a way in which care could be improved, or maybe a desire to understand the rationale for the success of a particular course of action. Research questions can be developed from all such suggestions. Investigating the question in a scientific way by following the research process may produce evidence which will help to explain the situation and may indicate a proposed change in practice.

Reading reports of completed research can also be a rich source of research questions. Speculation as to whether the evidence generated by a particular study would apply in the reader's own sitution may prompt a desire to repeat the study in a different location to test the validity and the reliability of the original study, and also perhaps to lead to a wider implementation of the recommendation based on the findings.

A third source of research questions is directly from theory. A nursing theory is a set of assumptions put forward to explain events. The explanation is, or should be, the best available summary of the current knowledge on a specific subject. Research questions can be developed by logical deduction from theories. An hypothesis can be generated to test the theory, and if the hypothesis is confirmed then the theory can be supported.

In reality the nature of the investigation which is undertaken and the actual research question(s) which form the focus of the investigation are determined by a range of external constraining or self limiting factors. These include:

- time available to be devoted to the problem
- the levels of knowledge and experience of research within the research team
- the availability of financial and other resources such as access to expert statistical advice and computing facilities.

In the context of all these external constraints the final definition of the research question to be addressed and the methods to be adopted is generally made following the second stage of the research process, i.e. the literature search.

Searching the literature

Searching the literature can be an exciting and illuminating experience or a frustrating and disappointing journey leading nowhere. Keys to successful literature searching include the following.

- A helpful, skilled librarian.
- Familiarity with the layout of the libraries to be used, e.g. how far back do the journals on the shelves go to, is there another location for older journals?
- Knowledge of the principles of literature searching, familiarity with indexes, bibliographies, methods for computer search (use librarians if needed).
- Conscientious indexing of sources investigated – an unrecorded reference source may take many hours to retrace. Index cards or a computerised index of sources examined, including full reference, and comments to remind you of the content should be kept and frequently updated throughout the project.

What should the literature be searched for? In broad terms a literature search is a search for material which provides information on the following aspects of the problem under investigation – the size of the problem; any commentators identifying the problem; have other research studies investigated the problem; or does it seem to be unique? If the problem has been previously identified can the history of the problem be traced?

The aim of the literature search is to develop a theoretical framework which encompasses the above factors and provides a justification for and the investigation method to be adopted for the project. In practice the following steps may prove useful.

(*i*)   Define the topic in terms of keywords and synonyms which will guide the search through indexes and abstracts.

(*ii*) Decide how widely you wish to search. For example, are you going to include just United Kingdom research or research from other countries as well? How far is it reasonable to go back to look for material? (The smaller the amount of literature on a topic generally the farther back the search needs to go.) Are any foreign language papers to be considered? If so, can translation be arranged?

(*iii*) Is it appropriate to search outside recognised nursing literature? For example, should medical, dietetic, or physiotherapy literature be included in the search? The topic and the range of reference obtained from the initial investigation of available nursing literature may guide this decision.

A literature search should not be conducted in isolation but should be coupled with discussion of findings with colleagues, experts, mentors, in fact anyone who is interested in the same problem. A final hint for a student new to the art of literature searching is that time spent discovering the material available from different sources is time well spent. It is useful, for example, to understand what indexes, abstracts, bibliographies, on-line searches and so on can offer. Time spent with a librarian or working through a guided study exercise may prove very useful in terms of developing an ability to search the literature efficiently and effectively in the future. Further consideration is given to the art and value of critical reading on pp. 44–5.

Refinement of the research question

Following the literature search the researcher is in a position to decide exactly what the purpose of the study is to be. This involves developing the initial question or idea into a form that is suitable for investigation by the research process. This stage generally consists of defining precisely what you are interested in and narrowing the original question down into a very specific question for which a clear cut answer is obtainable. For example a general hunch that some nurses assess wounds in rather different ways can be developed into several widely different research studies. Amongst many alternatives it could lead to:

(*i*) a study of documented records of wounds kept by nurses;
(*ii*) a descriptive account of the criteria used by nurses when deciding how to manage a wound; or
(*iii*) an observational study of whether nurses change their practice following a wound care study day.

In each case the researcher has focused from the initial topic into a particular, more specific direction. But in each situation further clear definition of the specific aspects to be studied is required before the research can proceed. The research question should contain a single idea and not several. The final format of the research focus can be in the form of a statement or a hypothesis. A hypothesis is a specific form of research question that states a predicted relationship between variables, in such a way that it can be directly tested.

Planning the investigation

At this stage the research method selected is developed into a reality for the topic of study. In essence this involves choosing the appropriate research method, seeking permission and, where appropriate, ethical approval for carrying out the investigation, the development of the data collection method(s) to be used, the planning and preparation necessary for calculating, identifying and incorporating the sample to be studied, and the training of data collectors where appropriate.

Within the context of this chapter it is not possible to discuss all the aspects of the range of research methods available. The following brief description of some of the main methods and terms used will, it is hoped, allay some of the confusion often encountered at the early stages of becoming familiar with research and stimulate further study of a range of these methods.

Descriptive method

In a descriptive study the researcher does not change any aspect of the area or subjects being studied. The study aims to describe the current situation. The area to be investigated is generally presented in the form of a research question. Many descriptive studies take the form of surveys, for example David *et al.*(1983) surveyed current treatments across England for patients with established pressure sores. A total of 737 wards in 20 health districts were surveyed, and a total of 961 patients with one or more pressure sores, seen by the research team. Descriptive information relating to the (then) current practice of nursing care of patients with pressure sores was collected.

It may be thought that descriptive information of this nature cannot have a direct effect on practice, however a summary of some of the uses the pressure sore data was put to may quell such an idea. The findings were used to formulate and focus future research ventures, and have enabled managers and others to rationalise and review resource allocation. The research prompted pharmacists and wound care experts to examine the efficacy of the huge range of products found to be in use for the treatment of sores. A total of 98 products were identified during the survey. In addition, the survey findings provided valuable education material which in many instances encouraged ward managers and others to review local practices in respect of pressure sore management.

Experimental method

In an experimental study an attempt is made to reveal the existence of a relationship beween two or more factors (variables). In its simplest form this might be establishing whether a particular form of treatment is better than no treatment. The experiment would proceed by giving the treatment to one group of patients and no treatment to another similar group. The effect of the treatment or no treatment would be measured for both groups and the results compared. For example Romney (1982), in addition to conducting a trial of pre-delivery shaving (see p. 31) conducted a similar trial on the value, if any, of pre-delivery enemas. Her hypothesis was that there would be no difference in the rates of faecal contamination, duration of labour, and incidence of infection between mothers who did and did not receive an enema prior to delivery. The research evidence generated supported this hypothesis and widespread changes in maternity practice resulted.

Quantitative and Qualitative Research

Quantitative research refers to research which involves measurements that can be directly recorded and quantified. In essence, quantitative research is concerned with the measurement of 'facts', for example physiological measurements of fluid balance and temperature, tests of knowledge under examination conditions, rates of admission and discharge, rates of recruitment and wastage.

Qualitative research refers to studies which attempt to measure concepts which do not lend themselves to direct measurement, such as pain, anxiety, attitudes, and opinions. Indicators to represent the concepts need to be developed and therefore this approach is more subjective than quantitative research. However it is important to recognise the need for both types of research in nursing, which is concerned with both physiological and psychological dimensions. There is often an inappropriate distinction drawn between these two approaches which supports the belief that quantitative is scientific and reliable in a way that qualitative research can never be. Goodwin and Goodwin (1984) argue that the methods should be seen as opposite ends of the same spectrum and not mutually exclusive methods. They point out that they are in fact just two different approaches to data collection and analysis and not two different philosophies of life. In nursing research it is often appropriate to use both quantitative and qualitative data collection methods in order to obtain a realistic picture of the true situation. For example Boore (1978), when looking at the relationship between the amount of pre-operative information received and the rate of post-operative recovery, collected both physiological (quantitative) and psychological (qualitative) data in order to demonstrate a positive effect between the provision of pre-operative information and the promotion of recovery.

Action research

Action research, a term first used by Kurt Lewin (1948), is a type of applied social research. The main feature of action research is that the researcher and the practitioners collaborate throughout, unlike the majority of other methods where the researcher adopts a 'fly on the wall' role. As evidence becomes available to indicate a possible positive change to practice, practice will be changed during the course of the study. The study continues by investigating the consequences of the change. The advantages of this method for local problem solving are considerable. However, because of the on-going developmental nature of the changes in practice there are limitations to the general application of the findings. Further useful discussions on the method can be found in Greenwood (1984), Topwell (1979) and Lathlean and Farnish (1984).

Data collection methods

Data can be collected using a variety of methods which can be grouped together into four major categories: data collection by observation; by questioning; by looking things up; and by concurrent recording. A variety of instruments can be used for each of these approaches. For example, observation data can be recorded on video film or directly on to a simple chart, such as that used for recording observed temperature and blood pressure measurements or on a carefully devised recording sheet which allows a data collector to record a variety of events observed. Data can be obtained by questioning either by the use of a questionnaire which is completed in the absence of the researcher, or by interview when a researcher asks questions face to face. The schedule used needs to be appropriate to the method and to the questions being asked. For example it is possible to offer clarification in a face to face interview but not possible to do this in a postal questionnaire and questions need to be formulated to take account of this. Data can be collected from a wide variety of records which may be patients' care records or management information which is routinely collected. Data may also be collected by asking participants in the study to compile information relating to an aspect of their work/life, for example in the form of an activities or food diary.

Pilot study

A pilot study is a small scale trial of the main data collection methods to be used. During the planning stage many pre-pilot studies may be carried out, but a final 'dry run' should be carried out to ensure that no insoluble problems will be encountered during main data collection. For example the pilot study may reveal problems with recruiting suitable subjects, or may reveal that superfluous data is being generated. Steps can be taken to sort out these problems prior to the collection of the main data set. If major modifications are required then a further pilot study may be necessary. In the event of poor reliability, validity or logistical problems, changes should be made to the data collecting methods prior to collecting the main data set.

A data collection instrument is said to be reliable *if* it is used on two separate occasions and the same results are obtained, providing that the 'who' or 'what' being measured has not changed. For example a ruler made of elastic is clearly not reliable, nor is the following question included on a questionnaire: 'Please list qualifications obtained whilst at school'. This may be interpreted as passes obtained in the General Certificate of Education or the General Certificate of Secondary Education examinations, but is open to interpretation to include for example all ballet, swimming and piano qualifications obtained whilst between the ages of five years and leaving school. The reliability of obtaining the required information can be improved if the question states exactly which type of qualifications are being referred to.

A data collection instrument is valid if it actually measures what it is intended to measure. The researcher must ensure that an abstract concept such as pain is validly reflected in the range of information collected which may include patient report of pain using a numerical indicator (a pain thermometer), timing and nature of analgesia received, reports of previous pain experiences, factors which relate to anxiety status, outcome of definition of the pain (if pain is reported to be low then is discharge an option, if pain is reported to be high does the respondent run the risk of further surgery or painful treatment?). Generally a single question or observation can only be a valid data collection method when collecting information relating to a simple construct for example age, sex, height or current weight. In order to be valid a more complex construct should be operationally defined in such a way as to cover all relevant aspects of the construct.

Problems of reliability and validity must be addressed prior to collecting the main data set.

Collection of the main data set

This is the most tedious part of any project as it involves the performance of many repetitive tasks. Data must be collected from the subjects in a consistent way and researchers must not allow themselves to 'drift' into asking new questions, or applying new knowledge gathered as the project evolves.

Analysis of data

Once data has been collected it needs to be sorted, analysed and presented in such a way that interpretation of the findings is possible.

Plans for analysis should be made throughout all preceding stages. The nature of the analysis that can be undertaken depends on the nature of the data collected. Data can be grouped, classified and coded to enable a picture to be built up. Features of the data can be counted and frequencies of responses calculated. Beyond this, more detailed and sophisticated pictures can be established using statistical methods. Expert statistical advice may be required for this.

Conclusions

Once data has been analysed and presented in an easily assimilated form, for example using tables, graphs and histograms, conclusions can be drawn. Conclusions should summarise all that has been learned from the data set and all the inferences and generalisations that can be drawn.

Report

A report should summarise all the stages of the research project. Readers of the report should be able to follow the research process through and to understand how the conclusions were arrived at. The findings then need disseminating by publication, presentation of the report to appropriate groups, and through education channels via seminars, study days and conferences.

Implementation

The final stage of the research process, implementation, is discussed on pp. 46–9.

What it is not – limitations of nursing research

Broadly speaking, limitations of nursing research can be divided into three main groups:

(*i*)   those limitations which are a consequence of the problem being unsuitable for investigation by the research methods;

(*ii*)   those limitations which result from attempting to 'measure the unmeasurable'; and

(*iii*)   those which result from the failure, for whatever reason, to adhere to the research process.

One of the first hurdles faced by a student of research method is that of learning to pose a 'researchable question'. Not all nursing problems are directly, or indeed indirectly, researchable. Scientific research cannot be used to answer questions of a moral or ethical nature – many of which are faced by nurses throughout their professional lives. Such problems include how do you determine which patient should be offered a kidney transplant when only a limited number of transplants are possible? Is it appropriate to carry out HIV testing in certain circumstances without the patient's consent? Should nurses be allowed to withdraw from certain medical procedures, such as termination of pregnancy, on moral or religious grounds?

Secondly, there are limitations which result from the problems of conducting qualitative research; for example research which seeks to investigate phenomena which cannot be directly measured, such as pain, anxiety, or aggression. If you adopt the maxim that pain is what the patient says it is, then it is impossible, at present, to measure pain in a purely quantitative way. It is therefore necessary to get the patient to attempt to interpret his or her feeling of pain into a measurable form. Hayward (1975) developed a pain thermometer which the patient could use to indicate the intensity of the pain being experienced. This is a qualitative measurement of pain and, as people are not consistent both in the way they feel pain and in the way they describe pain, it is not possible to use this measurement to accurately determine how much analgesia is required in all cases.

Thirdly, research has limitations in that the value of evidence produced will be influenced by the way the problem was investigated. Polit and Hungler (1985) point out that 'virtually every research study contains some flaw'. All studies are bound by certain constraints of time, financial resources, personnel to conduct the research, and the skills and knowledge of such personnel, both of the topic under investigation and of research methodology. From the outset the problem under investigation can be approached in a variety of ways, and at each stage of the research process decisions and compromises must be made. For example, which variables can be controlled? Which can be left to random variation? How should the sample be selected? How large a sample should be taken? What is the most appropriate and most feasible method(s) for data collection? How many revisions of the data collection can be allowed for and when must main data collection be started? How much time is there for the training of data collectors? What support from a competent statistician is available, at both the design and the data handling and analysis stage? What material is to be included in the final report? How widely is the report to be circulated? At each stage decisions have to be made and limitations of the methods are faced. Flaws of design, or the introduction of certain biases either knowingly or unknowingly, can alter the whole value of the research and may lead to inappropriate conclusions being drawn.

It must be remembered by any reader of research that, whilst the researcher may have tried his or her hardest to conduct an objective and unbiased study, certain compromises will have been made and the resultant product must be examined with care to weigh up the value of the evidence produced to support the claims made in the report. The following discussion on critical reading examines these ideas in more depth.

Art and value of critique

Critique is 'a judgement of merit of works of literature, and expression (statement) and exposition (interpretation) of such judgement' (Concise Oxford Dictionary, 1984). By no means does the word only refer to negative criticism – it is the overall judgement of the good, the bad, the value and not least the applicability of the work being reviewed.

The art of critique

The art of critique is not as mystical and intangible as it sounds. It is an acquired skill which will develop with practice and, it has been argued, should be part of the basic mental equipment of every practicing nurse (Committee on Nursing, 1972) and not just a skill confined to nurse researchers and graduate nurses. A research report cannot benefit nursing care unless its contents are carefully examined, its conclusions considered, lessons learned and nursing practice changed where appropriate.

The development of the art of critique lies in the maxim of practice makes perfect, and the following are a few guiding principles. The adoption of a questioning approach to one's reading may or may not come easily; to many it does not. The presentation, in print, of a plausible set of conclusions, coupled with some incomprehensible statistics and an author with several letters after his or her name may lead to an unquestioning acceptance of the correctness of the claims made. In research, as has been previously stated, all that is produced is evidence and this evidence *must* be carefully scrutinised before changes in practice can confidently be made. A basic understanding of the research process provides the key to the development of a questioning approach. In the early stages of developing this skill a check list, such as that produced by Hawthorn (1983), can be very helpful. A further principle to aid success is the adoption of a rigorous note-taking habit, either on index cards, in a note book, or using a word processor. A note of the author, title, full reference, and brief summary of content of all useful articles read (and a note of location of the volume if using several libraries), will do much to enhance the review of the material covered and may avoid hours of frustration.

In essence, a research report should provide sufficient information to enable the reader to weigh up in his or her own mind the nature of the problem/hypothesis under investigation, the background to the problem, the why and wherefore of the methodology adopted, the reliability and validity of the data obtained, the appropriateness of the analysis performed and the conclusions drawn. The reader should guard against making allowances for information not included in the report. The author is in control of the evidence which he or she chooses to provide in order that the reader may assess the conclusions reached, and if the information is incomplete it is undesirable to infer too far. For example, in a study of the effectiveness of pressure sore treatment, McClemont *et al.* (1979) report a marked difference in time taken to de-slough sores for groups of patients receiving different treatments. The clear implication is that the difference is due to the treatment. However it is possible that the difference is due to some other factor which differs between the patient groups, for example that one group is more seriously ill. The authors provide no information on which to decide whether or not this is a possibility. The authors' conclusions lead the reader to believe that the results are not affected by other factors: this is a dangerous assumption.

The critical reader should develop the skills of a detective, backing judgements with other reading and sound professional knowledge and experience. It is an art that develops with practice.

The value of critique

Many values of critique have already been referred to. Research should not be allowed to sit on shelves of libraries and offices, never to be used. It should be published and disseminated to as wide an audience as possible so that it may directly or indirectly improve the quality of patient care. A reader of research should have a specific goal in mind, for example
- reading for general interest
- the development of a theoretical framework for a proposed project or investigation
- completion of an academic exercise
- looking for answers to specific problems

All these may be achieved by critically reading research. The value of critical reading is that it may provide the reader with the answers that he or she is searching for.

Implementation

Nursing research cannot implement itself. Implementation requires that nurses identify the research relevant to their area of work or responsibilities, weigh up the evidence presented and then formulate a plan to best utilise the findings (if appropriate). What is required is truly research minded practitioner nurses who seek out, evaluate, interpret and then utilise the research which is available.

An examination of these four stages of implementation reveals the reality of problems which will be encountered. Finding time to seek out relevant research is not always seen as a priority by many practitioners. Studies such as those conducted by Myco (1980) and Barnett (1981) have shown that nurses tend to read very little in the way of professional material of any kind. In the author's experience, when questioning groups of nurses at the beginning of a research course/lecture as to the professional reading they had undertaken in the preceding week many will admit to having looked at the weekly journals only. On further questioning the respondents tend to identify that, within these journals, the news pages and the job advertisements have received attention and few are able to recount the content or even the subject matter of any research reports contained in the journal. A possible solution to this problem is the establishment of a 'journal club' where a group of nurses agree to review a range of professional journals relevant to their sphere of work. Each member has responsibility to examine just one or two journals to identify any papers which may be relevant to the group. As many professional journals are issued only monthly or bi-monthly the journal club should meet about six times a year. At the meeting each member should report the content of any relevant findings to the group who can together reflect on possible implications of the study; for instance, is it just interesting or does it warrant further consideration, or possible implementation? This can be a very successful venture and many other research related activities may be able to be carried out by and through the group, for example arranging seminars and developing proposals for small scale studies.

Where should nurses be looking for material? In the United Kingdom there are two refereed general journals where researchers may choose to publish their report – the *Journal of Advanced Nursing* and *The International Journal of Nursing Studies*, both of which cover research on all aspects of nursing practice, education and management from the United Kingdom and abroad. Several nursing research journals are produced in the United States of America, including *Nursing Research*, *Research in Nursing and Health*, and *Western Journal of Nursing Research*.

In addition, most nursing specialities are served by specialist journals, and it is appropriate for many nurses to seek information from journals that are not specifically nursing but are from related disciplines. These journals are not generally found at railway stations or in the newsagents alongside the weekly publications and their price is too prohibitive to recommend the purchase of individual copies. Hence the visiting of professional libraries will be required in order that the available material can be reviewed. Knowing about relevant research demands an interest and a willingness to seek out the information. The feeling that 'somebody else' will keep one up to date does not bode well for progress. Teaching from a research-based curriculum which encourages questioning and examination of available evidence for the theories and practices being taught may go some way to alleviate the apathy and encourage individuals to see that keeping up to date with relevant research is the responsibility of all practitioner nurses.

The second step towards successful implementation is an ability to weigh up the evidence in an informed way. Hunt (1981) argues that one of the inhibitory factors to successful implementation is that nurses do not believe research findings. It could be argued that, in order not to believe research findings, such findings need to have been critically read and understood, and the evidence weighed up in such a way as to be in a position not to believe findings. In reality this is not often the case. Unwillingness to accept research findings which directly challenge traditionally held beliefs and practices is not uncommon. The disbelief of the findings is a defence for the accepted practice. For example a traditional approach to wound care was to keep the wound clean and dry and therefore nurses may be unwilling to accept research findings which support the idea that a moist wound environment will encourage more rapid healing than a dry wound environment.

One way of overcoming this scepticism is to encourage nurses to accept research for what it is, namely evidence, and to ask them to be prepared to objectively weigh up the strengths and weaknesses of the evidence, as they would if in a position of jury member in a court of law. Nurses need to decide if the results and conclusions appear to be reasonable, formulated from an appropriate sample, and of sufficient statistical significance. At the same time, nurses need to learn to re-examine practices for which they are unable to provide a sound rationale or research basis, and be prepared to examine new evidence, as it becomes available, which may indicate a possible change in practice.

A further component in the process of implementing research findings is the need to understand them. The ability to understand research findings occurs as a result of a sound understanding of the subject under study, a basic knowledge of research theory and methods, a modicum of statistical appreciation and a willingness to read carefully and thoroughly and exercise a professional judgement whilst reading. Understanding does not come easily at first, but, with wide reading, more and more research methods are met and basic knowledge and skills will develop over time. The novice may well be advised to seek more experienced help, for example from a nurse researcher or a statistician.

Only when these stages have been successfully negotiated can action plans for implementation be drawn up. It is perhaps pertinent to be reminded that not all research is directly implementable, for a variety of reasons previously discussed. Lelean (1982), when writing about the implementation of research, suggests that there would be fewer problems if the word 'implementation' was replaced with 'utilisation'. Lelean illustrates this point with a quotation from MacLeod Clark and Hockey (1979) – a quotation which still holds true:

'To make use of research does not necessarily mean to implement findings – the use of research implies the reading of research reports with insight and comprehension in the first place – sometimes it will encourage the reader to pursue some of the references – sometimes, the reader will be motivated to replicate the research in his or her own area of practice – on occasions, the reader may simply be directed to situations which warrant special attention.'

Thus by using research rather than thinking that research is only useful if it can be directly implemented can stimulate the reader to
- deepen his or her knowledge of the subject by further reading
- examine his or her practice with a view to possible modification
- consider whether replication of the study is warranted/necessary/ desirable, and if so by whom?
- be made aware of an aspect of care which may warrant a closer look
- consideration of implementation.

If implementation is contemplated, the following steps should be observed.

(*i*)   The weight of the evidence for the conclusions of the study should be carefully considered.

(*ii*) The feasibility and resource implications of the proposed implementation should be identified.

(*iii*) The desirability and cost effectiveness of the proposed change should be considered, and the reassurance of quality of care as a result of the proposed change – does the proposed implementation have a direct positive effect on the quality of patient care or is it something that just makes for an easier life for the nurses?

(*iv*) A strategy for implementation needs to be developed which pays particular attention to the education and training needs of the staff who will be involved.

(*v*) Finally, a review programme should be established to formally evaluate the effectiveness of the change.

Summary

This chapter has provided an overview of research in nursing, and has outlined the methods by which researchers explore problems to generate evidence which will increase the body of nursing knowledge. In summary it is appropriate to reiterate some of the major points raised and to reflect on the overall potential contribution research can make to nursing.

Nurses need research to enable them to identify and demonstrate a rational basis for the care that they give. There must be a move away from tradition and custom as the basis for what nurses do and a striving to develop scientific knowledge for practice. This will serve to improve the care delivered to patients and clients and strengthen the knowledge base on which the profession of nursing is based.

With the increasing pressures on nurses, in common with other health care professionals, to establish quality assurance programmes research has a vital role to play. Quality assurance has, inherent in it, the concept of the delivery of care at predetermined levels. This presupposes that levels can be set, and that it is possible to measure care delivered in the work place to determine whether the level is attained. It is not appropriate to dwell on the complex issues surrounding quality assurance. However, it is appropriate to spell out what should by now be obvious. Research based knowledge and its application provides a vital key to the success of quality assurance. It holds the route to the scientific and objective basis for the selection of appropriate courses of action and also provides the methods for objective measurement, such as by audit, questionnaire, structured observation or systematic integration of written records.

In order that nurses can make the best use of research there is a need to develop research mindedness. It is not appropriate nor indeed desirable for all nurses to be able to carry out research, but it is important that they can use the research findings generated by others. To achieve this state of affairs a serious examination of nurse education both at basic and post basic levels needs to occur. The advent of Project 2000 provides a clear opportunity. But nursing will not become a research minded profession over night. Many of the skills will only develop with practice; for example developing the art of critique (see p.45). Thus it must be the responsibility of each individual, both nurse teacher and nurse practitioner, to develop his or her own research skills and to share this developing expertise with others.

Research needs to be read and used. It has already been stated that not all research is suitable for instant implementation in a clinical setting but if research is to fulfil its potential for nursing it must be tried, tested, challenged, developed, and, when appropriate, rejected. This will only come about if nurse practitioners, nurse researchers and nurse managers each have sympathy for the role the others have to play, and each realise that together they can interact to the benefit of patients and clients. Nurse practitioners can identify problems which are appropriate for study, nurse researchers can systematically study the problem and generate scientifically based recommendations and nurse managers have the potential of acting on the recommendations. Together these three branches of the profession can work together to the benefit of patients and clients.

References

Barnett, D. E. (1981). Do nurses read? *Nursing Times*, **77(50)**, 2131–3.

Barton, A. and Barton, N. (1981). *The Management and Prevention of Pressure Sores*. Faber and Faber, London.

Boore, J. (1978). *Prescription for Recovery*. Royal College of Nursing, London.

Committee on Nursing (1972). *Report*. H.M.S.O., London. (Chairman, A. Briggs)

David, J. A., Chapman, R. G., Chapman, E. J., and Lockett, B. (1983). *An Investigation of the Current Methods Used in Nursing for the Care of Patients with Established Pressure Sores*. Nursing Practice Research Unit, Northwick Park Hospital and Clinical Research Centre, Harrow.

Davis, B. (Ed.) (1987). *Nursing Education: Research and Developments*. Croom Helm, London.

Goodwin, L. D. and Goodwin, W. L. (1984). Qualitative vs. quantitative research or qualitative and quantitative research. *Nursing Research*, **33(6)**, 378–80.

Greenwood, J. (1984). Nursing research: a position paper. *Journal of Advanced Nursing*, **9(1)**, 77–82.

Hawthorn, P. J. (1983). Occasional paper. Principles of research: a checklist. *Nursing Times*, **79(35)**, 41–3.

Hayward, J. (1975). *Information – a Prescription against Pain*. Royal College of Nursing, London.

Henderson, V. (1969). *Basic Principles of Nursing Care*. Revised edition. Karger, Basel.

Hunt, J. (1981). Indicators for nursing practice: the use of research findings. *Journal of Advanced Nursing*, **6(3)**, 189–94.

Jacka, K. and Lewin, D. (1987). *The Clinical Learning of Student Nurses*. Nursing Education Research Unit, University of London, London. (NERU report no. 6.)

Lancaster, A. (1975). *Guidelines to Research in Nursing. No. 1: Nursing, Nurses and Research*, 2nd edition. King Edward's Hospital Fund, London.

Lathlean, J. and Farnish, S. (1984). *The Ward Sister Training Project: an Evaluation of a Training Scheme for Ward Sisters*. Nursing Education Research Unit, Department of Nursing Studies, King's College, University of London, London.

Lelean, S. R. (1982). The implementation of research findings into nursing practice. *International Journal of Nursing Studies*, **19(4)**, 223–30.

Lewin, K. (1948). *Resolving Social Conflict*. Harper & Row, New York.

McClemont, E. J. W., Shand, I. G. and Ramsay, B. (1979). Pressure sores: a new method of treatment. *British Journal of Clinical Practice*, **33(1)**, 21–5.

Macleod Clark, J. and Hockey, L. (1979). *Research for the Enquiring Nurse*. HM+M, London.

Myco, F. (1980). Nursing research information: are nurse educators and practitioners seeking it out? *Journal of Advanced Nursing*, **5(6)**, 637–46.

Norton, D., McLaren, R., and Exton-Smith, A. N. (1962). *An Investigation of Geriatric Nursing Problems in Hospital*. National Corporation for the Care of Old People, London.

Polit, D. F., and Hungler, B. P. (1985). *Essentials of Nursing Research: Methods and Applications*. Lippincott, Philadelphia.

Romney, M. L. (1982). Nursing research in obstetrics and gynaecology. *International Journal of Nursing Studies*, **19(4)**, 193–203.

Sleep, J. and Grant, A. (1988). Occasional paper. Effects of salt and savlon bath concentrate post-partum. *Nursing Times and Nursing Mirror*, **84(21)**, 55–7.

Towell, D. (1979). A 'social systems' approach to research and change in nursing care. *International Journal of Nursing Studies*, **16(1)**, 111–21.

3 Health and health promotion – consensus and conflict

'We use the words 'normal' and 'healthy' when we talk about people, and we probably know what we mean. From time to time we may profit from trying to state what we mean, at risk of saying what is obvious and at risk of finding out we do not know the answer.'

(Winnicott, 1986)

Health is one of the most frequently used words in our vocabulary. Yet it is something prone to assumption, preconception and misconception. Amazingly under-researched, health is a vital tenet of all nursing models. This chapter will expose the reader to a broad range of ideas about health which may otherwise take many months of study. *Health promotion* is currently an over-used and abused term about which there is much confusion. It is timely to clarify the meaning and implications of this term which represents the most important and one of the most rapidly expanding areas of health care.

The literature of the last ten years suggests criticism is more in order than congratulation (Rodmell and Watt, 1986). However this chapter should be viewed more as a signpost than as a map. Table 3.1 summarises the major areas of contention and consensus which will be discussed in the text.

What is truth?

'Put yourself on the margins but don't be endlessly naming them ... choose ... but be prepared to be flexible here'

(Riley, 1985)

Beattie (1986) wrote of a modern, sophisticated phenomenon which allows 'selective presentation of scientific evidence to support an official position'. His concern was that the government had publicly asserted that it is acceptable to be 'economical with the truth'. Anxious that people should be allowed to make 'reasoned choices' Seedhouse (1986) argued that this 'can come only from possession of the fullest relevant information'. He believed that health education without a complete explanation becomes indoctrination and propaganda. History is often thought of as fact. Writing in *What is*

Table 3.1 Health promotion and nursing – some areas of consensus and conflict.

Consensus	Conflict
Current nurse role in health education is not valued	Variation in views on health, its measurement and maintainance – among professionals, and between the public and professionals
Nurses have in the past been poor at patient teaching	
The role of nurses in health education and health promotion should expand	Definitions of health promotion
	The relative importance of policy versus individual action and self care versus social care
A disease centred approach is limited: education for, and promotion of, health is needed	
	The role of various approaches: high gloss, individualistic, shock techniques, authoritarian
Education and promotion roles are for all nurses not just those in the community	
	The importance of positive and negative role modelling: parents, professionals and media
Individual behaviour changes may be impossible or ineffective without politico-economic and socio-ecological changes	
	The use of a risk or epidemiological approach
The value of facilitation, discussion and consultation	The significance of the Health Belief Model

History?, Carr (1964) added to this discussion of truth: 'It used to be said that facts speak for themselves. This is, of course, untrue.' He reasoned that the historian selects which facts will speak and decides the order and context of presentation. Facts then speak only through the *interpretation* of the author.

Farrant and Russell (1986) give a lengthy exposition of their deep concerns about the basis of truth in health information offered to the public on heart disease. Evidence is accumulating that the conventional individual risk factors such as diet and smoking cannot alone explain the incidence of heart disease. What is needed is an hypothesis which includes:

(*i*)   a large emphasis on chronic psychosocial stress; and

(*ii*)   the role played by the food, agricultural and tobacco industries.

If the 'do-it-yourself lifestyle' stance is the only one taken to the prevention of heart disease, then these two additional factors have not been reflected honestly. Farrant and Russell described health information as a politically defined compromise rather than based on scientific evidence. One should question the usefulness of giving only clear, simple, perhaps simplistic guidelines which avoid conflict while there are still areas of inconclusiveness, uncertainty and contention that exist within the scientific literature on heart disease.

Most Britons believe stress to be the major cause of heart disease (Health Education News, 1981). This is used by 'experts' as evidence of an inadequate understanding. However, Manicom suggests it may be that the public 'have a more sophisticated understanding . . . than the medical profession' (Farrant and Russell, 1986). The World Health Organisation (WHO) believe health professionals have a role in making facts better known to the public: 'People have the right to be informed' (WHO, 1985). However, one must proceed with caution if Williams (1984) is correct: 'there are relatively few cases where there is unequivocal evidence that certain courses of action will lead to health'.

Seedhouse (1986) quoted the President of the British Cardiac Society, Professor Oliver, as saying he rejected the currently favoured idea that low fat diets can save people from heart attacks. In 1982 Oliver wrote: 'Much as we like to think otherwise, it is not yet possible to prevent Coronary Heart Disease in the community, let alone in an individual'. Compare this to advice from the Health Education Council in 1984: 'Another way to beat heart disease is to watch what you eat . . . . The best thing to do is to cut down on the total amount of fat you eat by up to a quarter'.

What is health?

The importance of health beliefs

To be admitted to the United Kingdom register of nurses requires competence both in 'advising on the promotion of health and the prevention of illness' and the recognition of 'situations that may be detrimental to the health and well-being of the individual' (Statutory Instrument, 1983). Although the nine competencies are not necessarily prioritised, interestingly these points are the first two on the list.

Promotion, prevention, health, illness and well-being are concepts which need detailed examination, thought and discussion. Familiarity with these terms is not enough – intimacy and commitment is required. The word 'competent' comes from the Latin meaning 'to seek, to strive after, to strive together' (Kirkpatrick, 1983). How much of a new Project 2000 curriculum should be given over to understanding these concepts? It is not simply a case of time allocation or degree of emphasis. What is required is a radical reform

(Fig. 3.1) to match the paradigm shift currently occurring in health care (Seedhouse, 1988). As Bradshaw (1986) put it – for nurses 'to be convinced that the determinants of better health lie outside the NHS' the 'pathogenic orientation of nurse training' must become a 'healthy orientation to nurse education'.

It is important to be aware of different views on health, before giving health advice, for the same reason as the nursing model chosen will inform and underpin planning and the giving of care. The following example will demonstrate this. The nurse who believes it is healthy to be slim, physically fit and normotensive would expect to do health teaching about stress and salt reduction, diet and exercise. The client or patient being approached about these subjects may believe health to be concerned with coping, adopting and having a strong network of support. Health teaching about therapy or counselling, self-esteem and self-help groups would be more appropriate than an overture on lifestyle. In *any* nurse-patient interaction which is centred on promoting health, an assessment of health beliefs is vital. The writer believes that an amazing paradox frequently exists; in carrying out health advice from a medical, disease-oriented paradigm the nurse is taking a professional stance in direct conflict with her own internal lay belief system. Preliminary work on folk health beliefs of health professionals supports this view (Roberson, 1987).

Objective versus subjective health

'It is arguably enough to feel better now rather than to concentrate on . . . disease prevention.'

(Tannahill, 1984)

Despite having had a National *Health* Service for over 40 years, and *Health Visitors* for even longer, little is known about the health beliefs that the public hold. Even less information exists about the health beliefs of professionals. The most researched area of health is the absence of it. For many professionals, particularly epidemiologists, health is defined in terms of morbidity and mortality statistics. This is epitomised in the following quotes from Blaxter (1987): 'the first British health survey, the Survey of Sickness' and 'Traditionally, the measure of health used is mortality'. Most documentation of professional views is about an objective, measurable state – the absence of clinical abnormality, ailment and disease. Research on lay views clearly shows an anomaly. Unlike the 'experts', the public usually rely on subjective estimates of health.

Blaxter's (1987) separation of terms related to ill-health may help here:

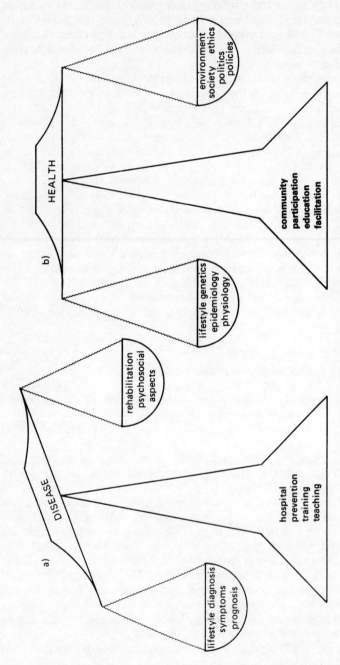

Fig. 3.1 Imbalance and balance in nursing education: (a) pathogenic orientation; (b) healthy orientation.

'*disease*' biological or clinical abnormality
'*illness*' the subjective experience of symptoms of ill-health
'*sickness*' the functional consequences of disease or illness
     (causing a change in lifestyle)
'*disability*' a permanent change in lifestyle.

Blaxter (1987) wrote 'it is obviously possible to have disease without illness, and to have illness without disease'. An example of disease without illness would be a woman with early cervical cancer. Illness without disease could be observed in a person with gross physical symptoms due to AIDS-paranoia. The former would be objectively unhealthy but subjectively may feel well, while the reverse is true for the person with symptoms of AIDS.

It is critical that one distinguishes between these views when talking of promoting health. Is the role of the nurse to pursue measurable health, that is the absence of disease, or subjective health? Obviously the answer has to be that both goals are important. However, the second area has been much neglected in the past. Yet it is the goal that can have most impact on the *quality* of people's lives. The aims of Health For All by the year 2000 (HFA) are only partly about measurably reducing preventable ill-health, i.e. adding years to life. These aims also include improving the lived experience or subjective health of people: 'adding life to years' and 'health to life'. The essence of this relatively recent movement on quality rather than quantity is embodied in the book title 'To live until we say goodbye' (Kubler-Ross, 1978) and in the phrase 'living with AIDS' rather than 'dying with AIDS'.

Defining health?

It has been suggested that if health cannot be defined then health professionals cannot evaluate their work (Noack, 1987). It also becomes difficult even to use the term professionals of *health* care. What does the 'health' in health care worker and Health For All 2000 mean? The former stems from the setting up of the National Health Service. The theory was that by detecting, curing and preventing disease people would be made healthy. So health and disease were placed at opposite ends of a continuum (Fig. 3.2). Being disease-free equated with health in the minds of planners and politicians. Al-

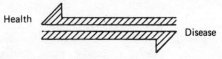

Fig. 3.2 A health-disease continuum.

though there has been a reduction in some diseases prevalent in 1948, new problems have arisen, for example, auto-immunity, diseases of affluence and AIDS, while menstruation and the menopause have been medicalised. 'Health' in HFA 2000 relates to a very different philosophy than the one involved in setting up the NHS. It is actually about a 'sense of health' (WHO, 1985). Also it is about people not the nation, and communities not populations. It is more about access, equity, participation and opportunity than medical treatment per se.

To *define* health would be to deny its breadth as an issue. Robinson (1983) suggested an *analysis* would be more appropriate than definitions – 'discovering the general principles' (Kirkpatrick, 1983). Moreover, what is needed is a resolution of the many and varied dissertations on health into a framework which can be used to improve the planning and evaluation of health care (Noack, 1987).

Analysing beliefs about health

It is important to realise just how high health is on the agenda of most people in this country. Health is one of the most talked about subjects, apart from the weather. 'How are you' is a common greeting and on departing we often say 'Keep well' or 'Take care' (Richman, 1987). It is uncommon to talk of hailing someone now. However, the greeting 'Hail' comes from the Old English hāl meaning whole. 'Good health' is a welcome toast for all occasions and *health* is also derived from hāl.

Newman (1986) wrote that 'we have become idolatrous of health'. This worship goes on in health farms, health gyms and health food stores. Beauticians wear white coats symbolising their 'medical' power to heal while chemist shops (with white coated assistants) commonly have signs inside and outside declaring 'health and beauty'. We talk of having a healthy bank account, a healthy atmosphere, a healthy outlook and healthy attitudes. 'Sick' is ascribed to the acts of some criminals. It is hard not to be envious of the dangerous but seductive skin tan and comment 'You look healthy'.

Four models of health beliefs

'What does being healthy mean to you?' is the question most studies of beliefs about health seek to answer. The 'lived experience of health' (Parse in Woods *et al.*, 1988) is described by looking at the way people perceive and conceive health. The answers given are the subjective thoughts and feelings of individuals. Smith (1981) has proposed that four models of health consistently emerge from theorists. These four models will be used to give clarity and structure to the following review of what might otherwise appear to be a mêlée of dissimilar lay and professional beliefs.

Clinical model of health

'Health and disease are not symmetrical concepts . . . And, while there are many diseases, there is in a sense only one health.'
(Attributed to Engelhardt, 1975 in Noack, 1987)

Health as the absence of ailments and disease is reflected in the clinical model. Two nurse theorists subscribe to this rather negative view of health. Orlando described health as freedom from discomfort, while Abdellah wrote that health excludes illness (in Marriner, 1986). For Helman (1984) the clinical model was similar to a numerical definition where health is described 'by reference to certain physical and biochemical parameters, such as weight, height, . . . blood count, . . . heart size'. Health, then, is conformity to a range of normal values.

Newman (1986) abhorred the portrayal of dichotomised health and illness where the former is a positive state to be desired and the latter is a negative state. She believed it is a view which 'has pervaded most of our thinking from very early in life'. In being brought up to believe that not only is health a personal responsibility but also within individual control, those who do not have it tend to be viewed as inferior, irresponsible or even repulsive. Newman proposed a synthesised view of health and disease rather than a polarised one. Thus, for her, disease was 'a meaningful aspect of health'. Newman (1986) laid great emphasis on the view of Martha Rogers that 'health and illness are simply expressions of the life process – one no more important than the other'.

Syred (1981) took the polarisation of health and illness one step further by saying that the continuum starts 'with good health at one end of the scale and death at the other' (see Fig. 3.3). Nursing intervention is more about changing the course of disease processes than promoting health. The idea that death is the opposite to health seems shockingly negative. However, before this clinical model of health is deemed worthless by professionals, it is important to consider research which suggests it is a view that many lay people

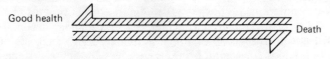

Fig. 3.3 Syred's (1981) health–death continuum.

hold. Noack (1987) wrote 'Worldwide, health is defined in negative terms as the absence of disease'. Although Seedhouse (1986) described the health-disease continuum as the most limited model available, research into lay definitions of health finds positive health an elusive concept.

Health as the absence of disease was a view held by the socially disadvantaged families that Blaxter and Patterson studied. Morgan *et al.* (1985), describing this research, wrote 'There was . . . no evidence of a positive conception of health'. Both Herzlich, studying in France in the 1970s, and Williams, surveying the views of the elderly in Aberdeen in the 1980s, are reported by Morgan *et al.* to have found beliefs about health as the absence of disease. Woods *et al.* (1988), while emphasising the positive views of health held by their large sample of American women, admitted that clinical health was the most frequently cited model and was used by more than 50 per cent of respondents.

Role performance model of health

The emphasis in this model is on health being the ability to perform socially defined roles. Thoughts on this model fall into three categories.

(*i*) The most negative approach and the one which has received most criticism is the functionalist or sociological view of health. In 1951 Parsons wrote that health is the 'state of optimum capacity for an individual for the effective performance of the roles and tasks for which he has been socialised' (cited in Morgan *et al.*, 1985). The central belief here is that people should be well not for their own sakes but because they have role obligations to others and the cost to society is high when they are ill (Richman, 1987). Seedhouse (1986) was heavily critical of this opinion partly because it infers that people with incapacitating disability cannot be healthy. He also felt that the roles and tasks people perform may cause them to become unhealthy as with exposure to coal dust or noise. A worrying implication of this concept is that those no longer fit or able to work due to disability or age may receive a health service in proportion to their reduced value to society (Morgan *et al.*, 1985).

(*ii*) A second approach to this model reflects opinions expressed by the lay population. Dubos (1984) summarised this view of health as 'the ability of the individual to function in a manner acceptable to himself and to the group of which he is part'. This suggests people want to function for what it brings themselves and those close to them rather than as a *duty* and for the good of society generally. Blaxter and Paterson (1982) found that women considered themselves healthy, despite reporting high levels of morbidity, as long as they could carry out their normal roles and the children could continue to go to school. The women were of working class background and it may be that denial of symptoms and continuing to function is a survival strategy (Richman, 1987). That people may feel unhealthy while fulfilling their role as mother or employee is one thing. However it is less satisfactory that people should, while continuing to function, have to *deny* illness to avoid poverty and hunger. The ability to perform roles was low on the list of views about health from the research of Woods *et al.* (1988). It may be that the value of role performance is only realised when threatened by ill-health. Most people, in taking it for granted, may not spontaneously mention it. However, 17 per cent of the 528 respondents mentioned the following points:

> Able to be as active as you want.
> Able to do usual functions.
> Able to get through it.
> Predictably being able to do things.

(*iii*)   The third notion of the role performance model is about people having a *right* to enough health to be able to carry out roles. The philosophy of Health For All 2000 is based on this approach. Health is for people to be able to make full use of their capacities (WHO, 1985). Smith and Jacobson (1988) wrote that people would be healthy if capable of both meeting their obligations *and* 'enjoying the rewards of living in their community'. This is a complete reversal of Parsons' view. Instead of people having a duty to society, society has a duty to people.

Adaptive model of health

Several nurse theorists believe health to be about the ability to adapt or cope: they have written of continuous adaptation to stress (King), adaptive capability (Levine), independence (Adam, Henderson), and coping (Roy) (cited in Marriner,1986).

One of the most widely read critics of modern medicine, Ivan Illich (1976), believed health to be the *process* of adaptation rather than a state. Health for him was about healing when damaged, growing up, ageing, coping with change and autonomy. This is similar to the view of Dubos (1984), that life and health are about independence, free-will, the struggle with danger, finding new solutions and responding positively to life's challenges. Seedhouse (1986) described all these views on health as an ability to adapt as vague with a 'sugar coating of ambiguity'. He condemned the writers for not describing exactly what the ability to adapt is or how it might be created or enhanced.

As there is little support for health as adaptive ability in the literature on lay beliefs, it is possibly a professional conception with unclear relevance to clients. In the study by Woods *et al.* (1988) as few as 14 per cent of the women reported using an adaptive image for health. They used words such as flexibility, putting things in perspective, acceptance of life's situation, ability to take anything mentally and being in control.

At first sight Antonovsky's continuum of ease and dis-ease (Fig. 3.4) appears similar to those described for the clinical model of health (Figs 3.2, 3.3). Believing that well-being (ease) is reduced to a level of being pain free and able to function fully, Noack (1987) was critical of the concept. However, Sullivan (1989) evaluated the model from a nursing perspective and found it to be health-oriented rather than from the pathogenic paradigm. The focus is not on why someone gets a disease but on a new question: Why do some people remain well 'despite omnipresent stressors'? Sullivan (1989). The answer to this question seems to be related to having a strong sense of coherence. Sullivan described this health promoting coherence as feeling that events are under some kind of control (not necessarily one's own), so they are 'comprehensible rather than bewildering'. Thus the stimuli one experiences are predictable, explicable and are to be seen as challenges worth facing, knowing that one has the resources available to meet the demands made.

The focus of this model is not the position at either end of the continuum but the *process of creating health* (salutogenesis). If the movement towards health ceases one does not have a state of disease. There is instead a *potential* for health breakdown. In aiming to promote health in a client the nurse using this model would assess and reinforce their sense of coherence. Exploring the extent of coherence may be carried out using certain issues for discussion, such as the following questions taken from Helman (1981) who was writing about folk models of illness:

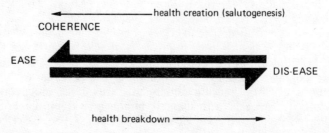

Fig. 3.4 Antonovsky's salutogenic model (Sullivan, 1989).

What has happened?
Why has it happened?
Why to me?
Why now?
What would happen if nothing was done about it?
What should I do about it?

Littlewood (1989) wrote that 'To date nursing models have not incorporated the importance of the patient's own model of illness causation'. She believed that psychological models root problems in an individual's personality, whereas in using an anthropological model one is looking more at an individual's understanding and the meanings they ascribe to events. Sullivan (1989) described the sense of coherence, the individual's understanding, as the *link* between personality and health.

Closely associated with the ideas of health as an ability to adapt are those around the concept of health as a strength or internal reserve. Dubos (1984) defined this in Darwinian terms as a fixity of the internal environment which controls and maintains an individual despite a need to adapt to changes in the external environment. Research suggests that views about a reserve of health or inner strength are an important tenet in lay beliefs. Some people believe a *lack* of internal strength makes one susceptible to AIDS (Aggleton *et al.*, 1989). Thus it is not a virus *per se* which causes AIDS but an inherent weakness with which one is born or which develops by adopting certain lifestyles.

Nurses are frequently heard to say that they tend not to deal adequately with patients' spiritual needs. Seedhouse (1986) reported on the work of Oliver Sacks during the Viennese sleeping sickness epidemic of 1916. He wrote that 'He was frequently overwhelmed by the impression of a tremendous inner strength . . . . He makes a case that this spirit is . . . a quality . . . which drives people to continue to develop in the face of apparently insurmountable odds'. It may be that spiritual strength could be tapped by nurses in developing a salutogenic sense of coherence.

Physical strength is commonly found as a lay belief about health. Williams (1983) found in his research with elderly Aberdonians that weakness was seen as the opposite of health but this was not in itself disease, more a proneness to be ill. Similarly of the three dimensions of lay beliefs found by Herzlich (1960) one was a combination of physical strength and a potential for resistance to illness. Many of the people who are learning to live with AIDS are working from a similar belief about health. Improvements in health status and quality of living are being produced by an *immuno-supportive* lifestyle, viz getting plenty of sleep, eating well, cutting down on caffeine, nicotine and alcohol, encouraging plenty of social contact and maintaining a positive self image.

Eudaemonistic model of health

Woods *et al.* (1988) wrote that this model has connotations of exuberant well being. Although the term 'eudaemonistic' is not one familiar to most nurses, the model has proved useful in nursing research. The word comes from the Greek meaning a well or happy spirit (Kirkpatrick, 1983). The results of the research into women's health beliefs by Woods *et al.* (1988) showed an overwhelming response to this model. The women used nine subdivisions of the model and 88 per cent of all health images given were eudaemonistic. Some examples of phrases given within each category of the model are shown in Table 3.2. Positive affect was cited by 49 per cent of respondents, fitness by 44 per cent, healthy lifestyle by 24 per cent and harmony by 24 per cent.

The positive concepts of health embodied in the eudaemonistic model are extremely attractive but it must be remembered that there are still relatively few studies of lay beliefs and, in these, there is only limited evidence for a positive view of health. Morgan *et al.* (1985), commenting on Blaxter and Patterson's work of the early 1980s, wrote of the high levels of ill-health present in the lower working classes which might explain the 'lack of a positive conception of health'.

Writing in 1989, Clarke and Lowe reviewed the literature and found no accepted methods for researching beliefs about positive health. They followed a suggestion by Blaxter and asked:

Who is the healthiest person you know?
How do you know they are healthy?
What do people do to keep healthy?

The responses they got, mainly from young people, fitted well some of the categories of Woods *et al.* (1988). Comments were mostly about appearance (body image) particularly of the eyes and face, physical activity (fitness) and diet (healthy lifestyle). However, areas of dissimilarity were the use of local folklore escape clauses about alcohol intake and smoking, and infrequent comment on obesity.

Common themes in the eudaemonistic model are independence, interdependence (family, friends, community) and control. Responses may depend on whether or not those interviewed *feel* healthy, and thus 'in control', at the *time* of the research. Too few studies mention current health status. Van Maanen (1988) compared the views of healthy American elderly with a British elderly group whom she defined as unhealthy because of their temporary residence in a community hospital. The American group had a positive eudaemonistic opinion on health as a state of mind (positive affect), healthy lifestyle and social involvement. The British elderly held a eudae-

Table 3.2 Some examples of phrases used for each of the categories within the eudaemonistic model of health (after Woods *et al.*, 1988).

Positive affect	**Fitness**
happy	stamina
exhilarating	strength
affectionate	energetic
feel good	rested
positive mental attitude	in good shape
sense of well being	able to be active
Healthy lifestyle	**Harmony**
taking care of self	spiritually whole
good eating habits	sense of purpose
not smoking	relaxed
moderate intake of alcohol	peace of mind
exercising	satisfied
eat balanced diet	balance
Social involvement	**Cognitive function**
liked by others	think rationally
involved in the community	creative
able to love and care	alert
feel good about relationships	having many interests
able to enjoy family	inquisitive
Body image	**Positive self concept**
ideal weight	self confident
look good	high self esteem
good feelings re body	sense of self worth
Self fulfilled	
able to achieve goals	
reaching optimum	
productive	
self aware	

monistic outlook in relation to the *past* when talking of a state of well being and independence (positive affect), hard work and accomplishments (positive self concept). However, *currently* their social involvement was reduced to giving the staff sweets and health was seen primarily as the absence of disease.

Looking at a group of middle aged working class women, Blaxter (1984) found 'control' to be striking in its absence. The women were talking of how they believed disease is caused, from which beliefs about health can be inferred. They believed ill-health to be caused by such things as infections, poisons in the environment, poverty and childbirth. Individual behaviour and responsibility for oneself were rarely mentioned, which denotes an almost total absence of belief about power and control to enhance health. The research findings of Calnan (1987) reinforced those of Blaxter. Women in social classes I and II held eudaemonistic views of health but those of women in classes IV and V were overwhelmingly about not being ill and 'getting through the day'.

Cognitive function was cited as a health image by only 10 per cent of the women in the study by Woods *et al.* (1988). Dubos (1984) wrote of the Greek goddess, Hygeia: 'She was the guardian of health who symbolised beliefs that remaining well depended on wisdom and reason – having a healthy mind would give one a healthy body.' Dubos also described how the sister of Hygeia, Panakeia, from whom we get the word 'panacea', became more powerful, representing healing through drugs. We are perhaps now seeing a reversal of their status and power.

Beliefs about health as harmony, balance or equilibrium are mentioned by many authors such as Dubos, Herzlich and Calnan. This is also a common theme with nurse theorists. Parse wrote of health as energy interchange; Rogers used the word symphony; Neuman used harmony while Johnson described health as dynamic and when minimal energy is required for maintenance (Marriner, 1986).

Health as self-fulfilment is frequently cited in the literature. In *Dibs – In Search of Self*, Axline (1966) gives this description of what it means to be a complete person: 'I guess Dibs only wanted what we all want on a world-wide scale. A chance to feel worth while. A chance to be a person wanted, respected, accepted as a human being worthy of dignity'. It seems that this category of the eudaemonistic model is one of the areas of health beliefs most favoured by nurse theorists. The following are all taken from Marriner (1986):

Nurse theorist	*Health definition*
Parse	growth, increasing complexity
Peplau	creation, construction, production, maturation
Wiedenbach	self direction
Fitzpatrick	heightened awareness of the meaningfulness of life
Newman	expanded consciousness

Exogenous health beliefs – a fifth dimension

There are several other rather disparate conceptions of health which merit attention. They do not fit Smith's four models but have the unifying link of being very much external to the individual or 'exogenous'. The clinical, role performance, adaptive and eudaemonistic models are all endogenous beliefs. There are four main exogenous beliefs: health as an ideal, a commodity, a moral condition and as luck. The first two views are held mainly by professionals and the media while the second two are mainly lay beliefs.

Health as an ideal

This is reflected in a description of health by Abdellah as a state with no unmet needs (Marriner, 1986). The oft quoted, oft criticised, World Health Organisation definition of health (1946) is very similar: 'a state of complete physical, mental and social well-being and not merely the absence of disease or infirmity'. Dubos (1984) likens this state of perfect health to a mirage or an illusion. In earlier work of 1959 Dubos condemned contemporary dreamers who try to draw people to a Utopia, which by definition is imaginary, so that the health we supposedly once held in some past 'golden age' could be reclaimed. Those who set up perfect health as the objective are usually trying to sell something. Dubos believed the health service was 'selling' magic bullets of medicine or miracle cures that do not really exist. The fashion trade, cosmetic and food industries also set up through advertising an ideal that few can attain even if they buy the products. One of the hallmarks of our current era is the philosophy of 'wanner be' (I want to be) – a dissatisfaction with what one has because the media make it seem that most people have more. Consider the following statement, written by Sally Brampton of the Observer, found on the dust cover of a book by Walker and Cannon (1984):

'We have lost touch with what is naturally good for us to such an extent that few of us remember what the boundless energy and optimism engendered by good health actually feels like.'

If self-esteem is one of the more important elements of health (Dickson, 1982), nurses must be cautious in promoting a view of *health for tomorrow* that by definition *devalues* what someone has *today*.

Health as a commodity

Phrases like 'clean bill of health' and 'healthy, wealthy and wise' epitomise this view of health as a commodity which is very closely linked by advertisers to health as an ideal. There is a very broad range of purchases which will supposedly help individuals achieve perfect health. These include vitamins, membership of a gym, ionisers, water filters, track suits, books about diet, beds, bracelets, eye lotions, herbal products and anything which is organic or preservative free! The aim of the manufacturers is profit not health. Thus arguments to buy are very persuasive and often omit the drawbacks such as high fat and sugar content in some high fibre cereal bars and the risks of food poisoning when preservatives are omitted. Crisps can now be bought with the following information on the packet:

Jacket potatoes. Higher in *fibre* than traditional crisps. *Free from artificial colours*, flavours and preservatives. *Natural* vinegar flavour. *Nutritious* snack.

The average low fat yoghurt is likely to contain ten times less fat than a packet of crisps. 'Low fat' crisps now have to be described 'lower fat' as they still contain 60 per cent of the usual fat level of crisps. With hardly any fat, and no salt, a medium sized banana has twice as much fibre as high fibre crisps.

Patients are now 'clients' and *consumers* of health care. Talk is of buying in expertise and the right to private health care for those who can afford it. Seedhouse (1986), in his critique of this model, said that health as a commodity means that it is outside the responsibility of the individual. Thus health can be bought, sold, given, taken and lost, but the only personal investment required is money. Losing health might be just bad luck, like losing a wallet.

Health as luck

Helman (1984) wrote of the lay belief that ill-health might be caused by bad luck or fate. Blaxter (1984) found that working class women believed tuberculosis or cancer could occur at random. Comments were made reflecting this fatalistic view: it could happen to anyone; I'm just the type. Looking at beliefs about health and illness in working class Londoners, Cornwell (1984) heard frequent comments about fate, destiny and health being a matter of luck or a lottery. Beliefs about chance and bad luck as a cause of AIDS have been found in young people (Aggleton *et al.*, 1989). The obvious dangers of all these views are that people will be less likely to feel empowered to promote health or avoid illness than if a more rational belief existed.

Health as a moral condition

Lay belief that one is morally responsible for one's own health is common. Health or lack of it is caused not by a *healthy* lifestyle but by being a *good* or *bad* person. The terms 'good health' and 'bad health' reinforce the notion that one may be rewarded according to the kind of person one is. Cornwell (1984) found that being good was about hard work, moderation, virtue, cleanliness and decency. If people were good, she found reports of their ill-health were described as unjust and undeserved. Cornwell also found that people wished to hide illness as if they were ashamed and were prone to making excuses about symptoms. One man with eczema was at pains to explain the cleanliness of the house he lived in and that his eating habits were good. The morality of health hinges on beliefs about ascribing guilt. A current example of this is seen in ideas about some people with HIV being 'innocent' (haemophiliacs and babies) and others being 'guilty' (gay men and drug users) (Aggleton *et al.*, 1989). Guilt inducement is used in some health education campaigns to manipulate people's behaviour. Examples of this are the television advertisement aimed at men who, in risking heart disease, risk the livelihood and comfort of their family and also the poster showing a smoking pregnant woman with the slogan 'Do you want this cigarette more than you want this baby?'. Charles and Kerr (1966) describe how 'good' and 'bad' food are used as issues with women who are caught between salads and quiches or feeding their husbands with 'proper' food because he 'deserves' it.

Implications of this discussion of health beliefs

It should be apparent to anyone reading the first half of this chapter that beliefs about health are very varied and are often defended with passion. Preparing people to be *health* care professionals for the future has to be as complex as these beliefs are diverse. Those who are developing a *health oriented* curriculum for the education of Project 2000 nurses will find in these pages much to digest about the need for the inclusion of a very different knowledge base. This will include ethics, politics, sociology, ethnography, media studies, history, economics, epidemiology, philosophy and, above all, the ability to view health as a multifaceted issue.

Health promotion – imperatives, bandwagon or salesmanship?

'The National Health Service . . . has little control or influence over the determinants of health . . . . Health is gained, maintained or lost in the worlds of work, leisure, home and city life.'
Robbins (1987)

What is health promotion?

It is obviously vital to decide what the term 'health promotion' covers, as it is something all registered nurses must be competent to advise on (Statutory Instrument, 1983). Many people use health promotion synonymously with 'health education'. It is important to clarify the meanings of both these expressions so that we become fully aware of the extent of our role. As Strehlow (1983) was writing of 'the promotion of health', Walt and Constantinides (1983) were writing of 'health promotion'. These authors had very different concepts in mind. Strehlow was in fact talking *only* of health education and even this she would not define. She wrote that it is not bounded by custom or tradition and has a limitless scope which is not popular – 'consumers in general do not consider health education a necessary element'. In 1986 Saan said that health promotion was emerging 'as a new and dominant concept', deriving popularity from its combination of community development, participation and equity. The beliefs Walt and Constantinides held about health promotion are summarised in Fig. 3.5. They described it as being on a continuum, with health education near the opposite end. Health education places the responsibility for health on individuals who, once informed of unhealthy behaviour, are then at fault if they do not act to improve their health. The basis of health promotion is a belief that people do not always have the power to change behaviour. The prerequisite to enable people to change is a transformation of the environment in which they live and work.

Are health education and health promotion *poles apart* as a continuum might suggest? Some writers propose a concept of health promotion which instead *includes* health education (Tannahill, 1985). Health education as *part* of health promotion means the latter

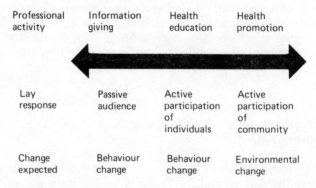

Fig. 3.5 Walt and Constantinides' (1983) view of health education and health promotion.

becomes a broader umbrella expression including *other* activities apart from the communication of health information to the public. Noack (1987) wrote of two forms of health promotion. The personal approach is about individual behaviour change in response to health education. A community approach is described as being very different from the personal one in terms of its goals and strategies. It involves different segments or sectors of society such as housing, pollution control, traffic safety and the production, taxation and sale of products which affect health. Promotion of health by this approach is by seeking changes in policy, legislation and administration to reduce the negative consequences of industrialisation, urbanisation and the distribution of wealth and to improve working conditions.

The priorities

It has been suggested that the appropriate emphasis of health promotion in developing countries would be the community approach whereas in developed countries it should be the individual approach (Noack, 1987; WHO, 1986). However, community-oriented activity is directed at ensuring that the *prerequisites for health* exist as a context within which individual choices about behaviour can be made. After examining a list of health prerequisites it is abundantly clear that the deficits in this country also require a community approach (see Table 3.3).

The World Health Organisation (1986) submitted that changing to a healthy lifestyle in a non-conducive environment is like trying to roll an impossibly heavy ball up a steep incline (Fig. 3.6). Changes in behaviour can only realistically occur if the slope of the incline is reduced by improvements in *sectors* of society such as agriculture, housing, education and employment. An alternative term for community health promotion is the intersectoral or multisectoral approach. In May 1986 the World Health Organisation adopted a resolution defining intersectoral cooperation in national strategies for

Table 3.3 Health prerequisites (after WHO, 1985; pp. 14–21).

Decent food at prices within people's means
Basic education to increase levels of literacy
A continuous supply of safe drinking water
Proper sanitation
Decent housing at a reasonable price
Secure work and a useful role in society providing an adequate income
Freedom from the fear of war (particularly nuclear)

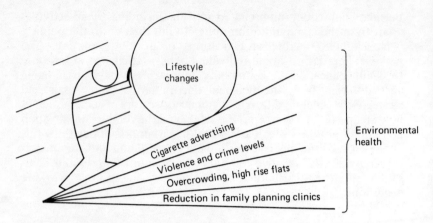

Fig. 3.6   Changing to a healthy lifestyle in a non-conducive environment. (Adapted from WHO, 1986.)

Health for All 2000 as the recognition 'that factors which influence health are found in all sectors of development'.

Nurse education – imperatives

The United Kingdom was called upon, along with other Member States of the World Health Organisation, to

'. . . ensure that the training of health professionals at all levels encompasses an adequate awareness of the relationships between environment, living conditions, lifestyles and local health problems in order to enable them to establish a meaningful collaboration with professionals in other health-related sectors'.

(WHO, 1986)

A recent English National Board document (1989) sought to guide the development of new Project 2000 curricula along these lines. Content to be included in the Common Foundation Programme is an exploration of power and social change and an examination of local, national and international policies. However, social, political and environmental influences are to be only *in addition* to other subjects. Frost and Nunkoosing (1989), in setting out a framework of possible areas to be included in a Common Foundation Programme, mentioned the word health only three times: as a goal of nursing, related to recreation and as 'various health care policies' which sounded like extras rather than core issues.

Australia, Canada and the United States, unlike the United Kingdom, have listed national priorities for health promotion and have detailed the responsibilities of health care workers in mediation and advocacy (Epp, 1987; Robbins, 1987; Gott, 1988). The closest this country has come to this has been a consultation document on priorities for health *education* (Health Education Authority, 1988); guidelines on Health for All 2000 for health service managers (Trent region: Faculty of Community Medicine, 1988) and a strategy for the 1990s from an independent committee (Smith and Jacobson, 1988). The latter is excellent but without political approval it is not comparable to the other countries named who have a statement of intent by the Minister for Health (Epp, 1987) or a Presidential Committee for health promotion (Robbins, 1987).

Caution seems advisable as new developments in nurse education emerge. Nearly two decades ago a popular nursing text (Pearce, 1971) highlighted the significance of public health measures. More recently public health as part of the curriculum has been in decline. Educationalists should note the arguments that a 'New Public Health' is needed – a 'restoration of Britain's public health heritage' (Public Health Alliance, 1988). It is only in this way that it will be possible to face new and old challenges such as food poisoning and homelessness. The number of texts for nurses using the term health promotion in the title is increasing (Ewles and Simnett, 1985; Edelman and Mandle, 1986; Murray and Zentner, 1989). However, all of these are about personal health promotion. There does not appear to be any recent text specifically for nurses on health promotion which is community-oriented. Assurance that information on the new public health is available in print can be gained by looking at the relatively new journal Health Promotion, Measurement in health promotion and protection by Abelin *et al.* (1987) and The Nation's Health by Smith and Jacobson (1988). Currently it is unlikely that this literature is either widely read or widely available.

High profile, high gloss

'Major developments in this field must not be cast aside in the heady momentum of the current bandwagon'

(Tannahill, 1987)

Over the past few years many Health *Education* Units have become Health *Promotion* Units. Was this change brought about by an understanding that health cannot be improved by education alone? If so, when the Health Education *Council* demised, why did we see the creation of a Health *Education* Authority (HEA), not a Health *Promotion* Authority? What do the words mean? Council means deliberation, discussion and advice (Kirkpatrick, 1983). Is the HEA *in* authority or *an* authority, that is in control or a knowledgeable expert? Perhaps the answers lie in what these new beings *do* that is different from the old. A major difference between the HEA and the HEC is the present vogue of a much higher level of expensive mass media advertising to attempt to get health messages across to the public. However, Aggleton and Homans (1987) argued that mass media campaigns generally show just short term increases in knowledge and only a slight shift in attitudes. Health Education Units were like Alladin's Caves. A visit could produce a wealth of free material to use with groups of any age, on any subject from poisonous toadstools to safety on the beach. Now you may have to pay for posters and leaflets from your Health Promotion Unit. Also it is likely that help will be confined to a limited number of key areas identified as priorities for policy, namely heart disease, smoking, alcohol and drug misuse, stress, exercise, cervical and breast cancer, dental health and, of course, the ubiquitous AIDS. Tannahill (1987) claimed that having diseases or behaviours as topics does not make sense. A far more holistic and positive programme would use key community settings such as schools, the workplace and deprived communities as well as key groups like the elderly, the unemployed and ethnic minorities.

If Health Promotion Units are working around a group of disease topics, and focusing on the behaviour and responsibility of the individual, their use of the word promotion does not fit the broad community-oriented concepts outlined above. Williams (1984) made a strong case for promotion in the Health Promotion Unit sense to mean hard sell and salesmanship. This technique, she believed, may trade on our fears and insecurities as well as our eternal optimism for health. Williams advised caution in continuing to sell ideas for health. When people purchase goods there is usually tangible evidence of the outlay. However, if we 'buy' healthy lifestyles the immediate effects may be only pain and effort. Caution is also advisable in manipulating lives to improve statistics. Dental health may improve if sweets are cut out but, if children eat more nuts and crisps instead, cholesterol levels increase. Williams advocated a more appropriate style of health promotion in activities like lobbying to have sugar and salt removed from canned foods.

Call for action and clarification

'Official support for different approaches to health promotion is given in inverse relation to their effectiveness'

(Stone, 1989)

1. Rather than using the term health promotion 'loosely without clarification of underlying assumptions or interpretations', it is suggeted that 'all planning documents . . . include a definition' (Tannahill, 1987).

2. Clarification is also required as to the goals being aimed for. Butterworth (1989) described the five year strategic plan of the HEA (1988) as well fitting the targets of Health For All 2000 and Project 2000 itself as a 'child of Health For All'. However, recently some of the HEA strategies have been criticised by the government and the organisation has been told to 'fall in line' (Butterworth, 1989). The HEA has recently said that they have 'to establish realistic priorities and many targets are not within its scope to achieve' (HEA, 1989).

3. It is necessary to be 'more explicit about where responsibilities for health rest as well as about what those responsibilites are' (Smith and Jacobson, 1988). Since the publication of *Prevention and health: everybody's business* (Department of Health and Social Security, 1976), the conclusion has been that this responsibility lies with the individual. However, the most important health determinants have been shown to relate to socio-environmental engineering of public health aspects by legislation and taxation (McKeown, 1979); see point A in Fig. 3.7. While attempts to change individual behaviour receive high levels of support from professionals, these methods are relatively ineffective (point C, Fig. 3.7). Immunisation and monophasic screening, such as cervical smears, have proven value (point B, Fig. 3.7), but multiphasic screening such as work done in a well man clinic has not been shown to have significant effects despite trials lasting many years (Stone, 1987). Care needs to be taken that, because so much time is spent pulling drowning individuals out of the river, no-one remembers to look upstream to see who is pushing them in or why they fall in (McKinley, 1975 in Tones, 1981).

4. 'How can statutory services best be allocated to respond to today's public health challenge?'

(Public Health Alliance, 1988)

Robbins has suggested that health promotion as a specialisation *must* be shared between professional groups if it is to give the public maximum control over their health. Roles for nurses have been described by various authors. Edelman and Mandle (1986) suggested roles of advocate, facilitator, consultant and educator. Skills in leadership, creativity, health assessment and mediation will be required (Edelman and Mandle, 1986; Gott, 1988; Morton, 1989). Above all, nurses must first become whole themselves (Chinn,

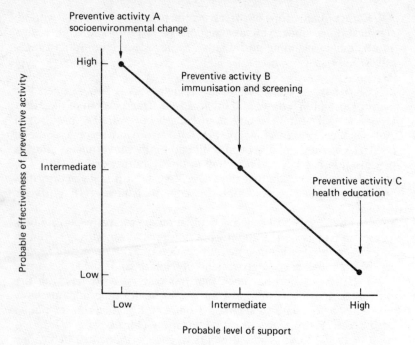

Fig. 3.7 The inverse relationship between different approaches to health promotion and their effectiveness. (From Stone, 1989.)

1988)so that they release the power they have to promote healing in others.

5. As professionals nurses have to decide for themselves the health messages people need. Rodmell and Watt (1986) wrote that *choice* had been *reified*, that is described as a real and almost concrete object instead of an abstract potential. Tannahill (1984) suggested free rational choice is 'illusory'. The present government seems to believe that individuals do have freedom, control, power and choice. The previous government had similar beliefs about people's health (DHSS, 1976). Milio (1983, in Draper, 1986) makes it clear that nurses are moving along a continuum which has love and caring at one end with power and coercion at the other. Nurse theorists make much of the special therapeutic relationships that nurses can create. Presumably health messages should spring from this philosophy of therapy and care, mutual support and social trust, otherwise 'we are tattering the social fabric that sustains us, and in the process the most disadvantaged among us are the first to topple into uncertainty, want and illness' (Milio, 1983).

A universal model of health promotion?

The model presented here (Fig. 3.8) is a combination of Tannahill's (1985) model of three overlapping spheres of activity and a model proposed by the World Health Organization (1984). Tannahill (1987) sees health education as the key sphere while Stone (1989) argues for health protection being the most effective area for effort (see also Fig. 3.7). These three lines of approach give a subtle, useful and dynamic view of health promotion which is a long way from the idea that it is something different to, or simply the same as, health education.

Some key issues in health education

'Health education has developed somewhat untraditionally with problem solving and application preceding theory'
(Dwore and Mazarazzo, 1981)

The risk approach

'You can do something to reduce the *risk* . . . the older you are, the greater the *risk* of having a heart attack . . . men are more at *risk*

Tannahill (1985)

1) *Health education*
Educational activity aimed at positively enhancing well being and the use of preventive and non-preventive health services

2) *Prevention*
Preventive procedures such as immunisation and screening

3) *Health protection*
Decisions by local, national and international government or other influential bodies in industry and commerce which promote health

WHO (1984)

Promotion of self help and self care
What people *do* themselves to promote their own health

Extended opportunites, more accessible services
Actions which make it *easier* for people to promote their health by providing cycle tracks, family planning facilities, immunisation, safe play areas etc.

Creation of a healthier environment
Improving the environment without necessarily requiring individual effort – reducing lead levels, imposing speed limits, improving housing etc.

Fig. 3.8 A universal model of health promotion.

from heart disease than women . . . you might be taking a life-and-death *risk* every day . . . By smoking, eating too much of the wrong food and not getting exercise and relaxation you could be gambling . . . This booklet has shown the *risk* of heart disease can be reduced.'
Health Education Council (1984), Beating Heart Disease

Insurance companies and the military have been using the concept of susceptibility to risk since the turn of the century (Alexander, 1988). Although the concept of risk is not new, it should be remembered that its application in the health service is recent (Backett *et al.*, 1984). Use of the risk approach in health education has only been subjected to research processes in the last two decades and is not yet thoroughly underpinned by theory. In 1976 the DHSS wrote of risk factors that 'we have little real evidence as yet to show that getting rid of these attributes reduces the statistical risk'. Reducing risk factors may be a plausible means of decreasing morbidity but it is not yet proven.

Backett *et al.* (1984) described the situation thus: 'The hypothesis on which the risk approach rests, therefore, is that the more accurate these measures of risk are, the more readily will the need for help be understood and the better . . . will be the response'. The assumptions in this hypothesis and the use of the high risk strategy have been questioned by many authors. Rose (1981) disputed the value of using the risk approach with *individuals*. He advocated a mass approach to dealing with risk such as reducing salt intake. He suggested that the individual approach may be much more limited than was at first realised. Large benefits are conferred on only a few people with high risk factors while in fact a major part of the morbidity and mortality figures are comprised of large numbers of people exposed to only a low risk. Rose continued: 'The mass approach is inherently the only ultimate answer to the problem of a mass disease'. He argued that the downward shifting of diastolic blood pressure by a mere 2–3 Hg might equal all the life-saving benefits of current antihypertensive treatment. Alexander (1988) questioned the ascendancy of the risk factors notion which ignores the issue of disease causation links with socio-economic status. On this point Farrant and Russell (1986) argued for the lessening of the effects of chronic psychosocial stress to be considered in reducing coronary heart disease. Seedhouse (1986) suggested a need to assess the degree of risk of the *intervention*. Drug treatment for hyperlipidaemia is apparently relatively safe but Rose (1981) estimated one death per 1000 patients treated.

Another problem with the concept of medical and educative intervention after screening for high risk factors is that the largest recent trial to demonstrate the effectiveness of this measure was inconclusive (Oliver, 1982). This American trial lasted seven years and involved nearly 13 000 participants. It may be that social pressure to conform could be more effective in reducing levels of risk factors such as obesity and smoking than advice to change for medical reasons (Rose, 1981). Morgan *et al.* (1985) wrote that campaigns which aim to reduce the chances of getting disease use an epidemiological model. This explanation of disease causation used by experts was not found in the constructs of any lay beliefs examined by Calnan and Johnson (1983). People either had general fears of diseases that they did not feel personally vulnerable to or believed they were vulnerable because a disease was in the family. This theory of inheritance presumably indicated a fatalistic view with little chance of being able to alter the risk by changing behaviour.

The Oxford Prevention of Heart Attack and Stroke Project has used nurse facilitators to encourage a systematic case finding approach to hypertension, smoking and obesity (Fullard, 1989). So far this has only shown an increase in *recording* of these indices in patients' notes. Tudor-Hart (1985) argued that half the people who are known to have hypertension are not being treated and of those being treated half are not well controlled. On the smoking front the work of Macleod Clark *et al.* (1987) suggested health care workers would need additional training to assist a move away from a prescriptive form of health education if their interventions are to be successful. However, heightened susceptibility to disease will not necessarily be associated with intentions to act (Hill and Shugg, 1989). Additionally it may be the perceived or real *difficulty* of changing which has more impact on behaviour than potential benefits (Sennot-Miller and Miller, 1987). So simply identifying people with risk factors does not mean they will necessarily get the treatment they need or an effective form of health education and they may focus more on the real problems of new behaviour than on the more abstract advantages of reducing risk. Reducing difficulty and increasing social pressure may facilitate change better than an individual risk approach. The targets of Heartbeat Wales are those of a mass strategy and include 'restricting smoking in public places, better food labelling, price incentives, increasing availability of 'healthy' foods in shops, workplace canteens and restaurants . . .' (Catford and Parish, 1989).

With question marks hanging over the risk reduction approach it may be useful to differentiate between health protecting behaviours which are risk and disease prevention oriented and the more positive concept of a health *promoting* lifestyle. This is attributed to research by Belloc and Breslow (1972) and is discussed by McKeown (1979), Edelman and Mandle (1986) and Walker *et al.* (1988). They describe seven habits for good health:

> sleeping 7 to 8 hours per night
> eating breakfast

avoiding snacks between meals
maintaining near optimal weight
exercise daily
consuming alcohol moderately
avoiding smoking.

Research in America showed that following six or seven of these habits halved mortality rates as compared to people who followed zero to three habits. Health for elderly people following most of the habits was said to be as good as health for people thirty to forty years younger who followed only a few. However, uptake of all seven habits was thought to be as low as 10 to 20 per cent of the population. It has not yet been clarified why health promoting lifestyles should be more successful than health protecting behaviours. It may be that risk reduction is attempted too late after much damage has already been done, while health promoting lifestyles may have been ongoing for many years thus preventing damage. There are, however, many unanswered questions. What is the role of sleep? Why is a general approach to health good at reducing many diseases while a specific approach to one disease – cardiovascular – shows mixed results? While awaiting answers it is important that we note the implications of being over prescriptive and even dogmatic about risk factors in the absence of more assurance.

Individualism

Naidoo (1986) wrote that individualism is 'the dominant ideology underlying modern health education'. She argued that there are three main criticisms of this approach:
  (*i*)   the denial of social effects on health;
  (*ii*) the assumption that people have free choice; and
  (*iii*) its general ineffectiveness.
Rodmell and Watt (1986) suggested that as 'lifestylism' it involves the pathologisation of typical conduct and in causing a sense of moral failure and inadequacy it is unhealthy and unhelpful.

Arguing for a new focus for strategies to improve health, Chapman (1987) compared health education to a *host directed* approach like the giving of antimalaria drugs. He advocated *vector* and *environment* directed strategies, in smoking for instance, aimed at the tobacco industry and the sociocultural and political climate. In the case of malaria this would mean the reduction or eradiction of mosquitoes. If ill-health is directly attributed to individual behaviour alone, then it becomes easy to blame people as they have supposedly inflicted damage on themselves (Naidoo, 1986). Examples of this kind of guilt inducing victim-blaming are common: smoking during pregnancy, obesity, HIV and AIDS, and almost all conditions directly or indirectly related to stress from gastric ulcers to arthritis. Even hypothermia in the elderly has been suggested as due to them leaving bedroom windows open at night and not wearing enough clothes (Guardian, 1988)! Ewles and Simnett(1985) offer further criticisms of the individualistic or behaviour change approach to health education:

(*i*)   it assumes experts know best and that lay people believe this;
(*ii*)   it often means imposing middle class values on working class people; and
(*iii*) rebelliousness may occur, causing behaviour opposite to that intended.

A powerful argument was offered by French and Adams (1986). They wrote that, so far, there is no convincing evidence that changes in behaviour facilitated by health education have improved levels of health. Robbins believed that individualism, or 'healthism' as he called it, is a narrow approach which treats health as a goal and not as a resource. The focus of education then is searching and striving for something ideal which one does not have rather than enhancing what one already has.

The health belief model

First described in the 1950s (Mikhail, 1981), and attributed to Becker and Rosenstock (Becker and Maiman, 1975), the health belief model (HBM) is an attempt to explain 'the large-scale discrepancies which generally exist between what care givers think their clients should do, and what the clients actually do' (Shillitoe and Christie, 1989). The HBM *implies* that knowledge of a client's health beliefs may help a health worker influence health-related behaviour in the 'right' direction. However, Mikhail advises caution in applying any theory uncritically to nursing especially as, in this case, the HBM is only partially developed and in need of some refinement. Although individual elements of the model have much empirical support, most studies have been conducted restrospectively and depend on self reported information. Hence what people *say* at one point in time causes their behaviour change may not be what actually caused it some time before. Additionally, Mikhail warns that research has still not determined the conditions under which health beliefs are acquired and altered or how stable such beliefs are. Shillitoe and Christie (1989) summarised the model thus: 'it presupposes that what someone does will depend partly upon the expected outcome of that action, and partly on the value that is attached to that outcome'. In Fig. 3.9 it can be seen that the model combines subjective beliefs about illness in terms of vulnerability to, and the severity of, disease

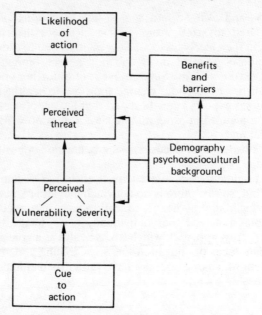

Fig. 3.9 The health belief model (after Becker and Maiman, 1975).

with a weighing up of the advantages and disadvantages of changing behaviour. An example of the model in action is given in Fig. 3.10.

The points on the model where a health worker might expect to have most effect are the initial stimulus or 'cue to action' and in affecting beliefs about the perceived threat and the cost implications of both benefits and difficulties.

The HBM is a more detailed version of that known as the KAP model (Knowledge, Attitude, Practice) which was popular in the 1950s and 1960s (Walt and Constantinides, 1983) and may still be found underlying modern health education. The assumption was that once someone had a certain knowledge, attitudes would change and the outcome would be a new healthier behaviour. This is a form of individualism and can lead to victim blaming. The KAP model suggests that people smoke cigarettes because they do not know the damage this can cause. If they are informed of the danger, they will stop smoking. This approach is obviously simplistic and naive. It denies the probability that the links between knowledge, attitudes and behaviour are neither consistent nor unidirectional (Coutts and Hardy, 1985).

Shillitoe and Christie (1989) give several major criticisms of the HBM.

– It assumes the relationship between threat and action is linear, whereas it is likely to be curvilinear. At maximum levels of threat, action is likely to be inhibited not enhanced.

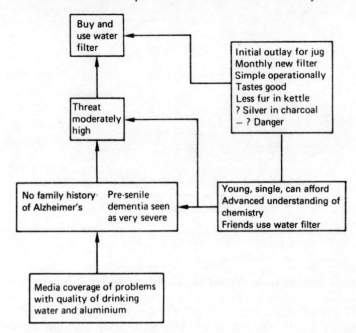

Fig. 3.10 The health belief model in action – to drink or not to drink?

- Health behaviour is seen only as an avoidance of negative or unpleasant experiences while it seems probable that society's perceptions of healthy behaviour are changing and may now also be about reinforcing positive feelings.
- *Past* behaviour may be more powerful than *beliefs* in predicting behaviour.
- Despite nearly forty years elapsing since the construction of the HBM, there is a 'relative absence of data on the efficacy of modifying different dimensions of the model to achieve desired health behaviour'.

Hunt and Macleod (1987) added to the controversy on the HBM. They wrote that contrary to the idea that people change to health-related behaviour directly after a cue to action, for reasons of *health*, it seems much more likely that other factors such as financial worries, a new job or a new relationship may trigger the change, sometimes a long while after the initial cue. They proposed a useful model of stages of behaviour change based on work by Prochaska and Di Climente in 1983 (Fig. 3.11). Nursing interventions may prove valuable at any stage of the model but again, like the HBM, there are no conclusive research studies to assist the development of nursing theory here.

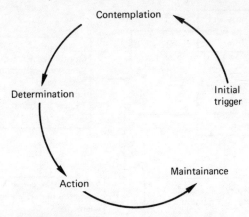

Fig. 3.11 A model of behaviour change stages (after Prochaska and Ci Clemente, 1983. In Hunt and Macleod, 1987).

Health promotion: What is it? What will it become?

The heading for this last section is the title of an article by Green and Raeburn (1988). The writer will follow the lead these authors have given in offering a need for an integration of views which are still commonly debated as polarities. The time for arguing about definitions of health promotion is over. Ewles and Simnett (1985) and Evans (1988) have represented ideas about health promotion on opposing axes forming a map to guide theory and practice. Figure 3.12 shows on a similar map that nursing activity has traditionally focused on the education side (Wilson-Barnett, 1988) rather than on changes in society and policy. Green and Raeburn asserted that halting the 'retreat into separate ideological camps' would be a triumph. They proposed that the integrative focus should be *the community* and that the central concept of health promotion should be *enabling* (Fig. 3.13). Green and Raeburn define enabling as 'a matter of power over the distribution of resources and the setting of priorities'. It is vital for a transformation of the health of this nation and the service offered that new initiatives in education under the aegis of Project 2000 place *nursing* in the centre of Figure 3.13 alongside Health For All 2000, with the emphasis similarly on the community and skills of enabling.

Some remaining concerns

Rootman (1989) believed that there is now much knowledge on health promotion but that it is not understandable or accessible to the

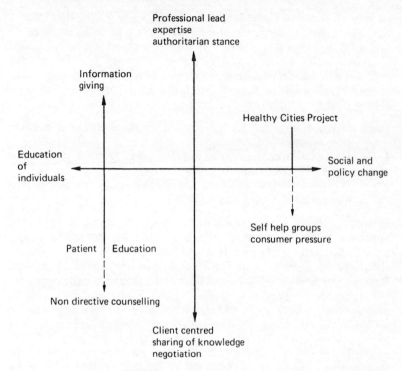

Fig. 3.12   A map of health promotion polarities (after Ewles and
Simnett, 1985; Wilson-Barnett, 1988 and Evans, 1988).

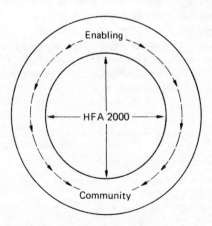

Fig. 3.13   An integrated view of health promotion (after Green and
Raeburn, 1988).

people who need it. However, Milio (1988), while feeling that there is no dispute over *health goals*, argued that there is virtually no research and little experience to draw on as to means of *reaching* these goals.

Unless health messages can be framed correctly 'a society of risk aversive individuals' may be created (McLeroy, 1989) who will ignore conflicting information through confusion or irritation. Wilson *et al.* (1988) discussed three ways of framing messages of health:

Gain   If you change to this new behaviour there will be a positive consequence.

Loss   If you fail to change to this new behaviour you will not receive a positive consequence.

Fear   If you continue to engage in the old behaviour you will receive a negative consequence.

However, there are no indications from research as to which approach might prove most effective with different client health beliefs. Mikhail (1981) and Hill and Shugg (1989) believed nurses should provide clients with information on the *benefits* of change. Research by Sennott-Miller and Miller (1987) suggested the opposite. What health workers have failed to do in the past is to frame messages in a fourth way – to help clients focus on and *overcome the difficulties* of new lifestyles. They often know what the consequences of behaviours are but need help with the means of change.

In 1985 Dr Mahler, then Director General of the World Health Organisation, argued that HFA 2000 would only be possible with the collaboration of all levels of nurses. He believed nurses were more ready for change than any other professional group and could lead the way powerfully through a better understanding of Primary Health Care (in Mussallem, 1988). At any given time about 5 per cent of the population is in acute care, with about 90 per cent of nurses caring for them. During preparation for practice most of these nurses are likely to have had a very limited experience in community care, little emphasis on health education and almost no input on health promotion. There is, in Project 2000, a rich opportunity to redress this imbalance.

References

Abelin, T., Brzezinski, Z. J. and Carstairs, V. D. (Eds) (1987). *Measurement in Health Promotion and Protection*. World Health Organization, Copenhagen.

Aggleton, P. and Homans, H. (1987). *Educating About AIDS*. NHS Training Authority, Bristol.

Aggleton, P., Homans, H., Mojsa, J., Watson, S. and Watney, S. (1989). *AIDS: Scientific and Social Issues*. Churchill Livingstone,

Edinburgh.
Alexander, J. (1988). The ideological construction of risk: an analysis of corporate health programs in the 1980s. *Social Science and Medicine*, 26(5), 559-67.
Axline, V. M. (1966). *Dibs – In Search of Self*. Penguin, Harmondsworth.
Backett, E. M., Davies, A. M. and Petros-Barvazian, A. (1984). *The Risk Approach in Health Care*. World Health Organization, Geneva.
Beattie, A. (1986). Foreword. In *The Politics of Health Information*, W. Farrant and J. Russell (Eds), pp. 7–8. Institute of Education, London.
Becker, M. H. and Maiman, B. A. (1975). Sociobehavioural determinants of compliance with health and medical care recommendations. *Medical Care*, 13(1), 10–24.
Blaxter, M. (1984). The causes of disease: women talking. In *Health and Disease*, N. Black, D. Boswell, A. Gray, S. Murphy, and J. Popay (Eds), pp. 34–43. Open University Press, Milton Keynes.
Blaxter, M. (1987). Self reported health. In *The Health and Lifestyle Survey*, B. D. Cox, M. Blaxter, A. L. J. Buckle, N. P. Fenner, J. F. Golding, M. Gore, F. A. Huppert, J. Nickson, M. Roth, J. Stark, M. E. J. Wadsworth and W. Whichelow, pp. 5–16. Health Promotion Research Trust, London.
Blaxter, M. and Paterson, E. (1982). *Mothers and Daughters*. Heinemann, London.
Bradshaw, P. (1986). Agents of positive health. *Senior Nurse*, 4(2), 8–9.
Butterworth, T. (1989). Of public concern. *Nursing Times and Nursing Mirror*, 85(22).
Calnan, M. (1987). *Health and Illness: the Lay Perspective*. Tavistock, London.
Calnan, M. and Johnson, B. (1983). Influencing health behaviour: how significant is the general practitioner? *Health Education Journal*, 42(2), 34–45.
Carr, E. H. (1964). *What is History?* Penguin, Harmondsworth.
Catford, J. and Parish, R. (1989). 'Heartbeat Wales': new horizons for health promotion in the community – the philosophy and practice of Heartbeat Wales. In *Changing Ideas in Health Care*, D. Seedhouse and A. Cribb (Eds), pp. 127–42. Wiley, Chichester.
Chapman, S. (1987). Small fish in big ponds. In *Health Education, Youth and Community: a Review of Research and Developments*, G. Campbell (Ed.), pp.24–8. Palmer, London.
Charles, N. and Kerr, M. (1986). Issues of responsibility and control in the feeding of families. In *The Politics of Health Education*, S. Rodmell and A. Watt (Eds), pp. 57–76. Routledge & Kegan Paul, London.

Chinn, P. L. (1988). Promoting health. *Advances in Nursing Science*, **11(1)**, vi.

Clarke, R. and Lowe, F. (1989). Positive health – some lay perspectives. *Health Promotion*, **3(4)**, 401–6.

Cornwell, J. (1984). *Hard-earned Lives*. Tavistock, London.

Coutts, L. C. and Hardy L. K. (1985). *Teaching for Health*. Churchill Livingstone, Edinburgh.

Department of Health and Social Security (1976). *Prevention and Health: Everybody's Business*. H.M.S.O., London.

Dickson, A. (1982). *A Woman in Your Own Right*. Quartet, London.

Draper, P. (1986). Nancy Milio's work and its importance for the development of health promotion. *Health Promotion*, **1(1)**, 101–6.

Dubos, R. (1984). Mirage of health. In *Health and Disease*, N. Black, D. Boswell, A. Gray, S. Murphy, and J. Popay (Eds), pp. 4–9. Open University Press, Milton Keynes.

Dwore, R. and Matarazzo, J. (1981). The behavioural sciences and health education. *Health Education*, May/June, pp. 4–7.

Edelman, C. and Mandle, C. L. (1986). *Health Promotion throughout the Lifespan*. Mosby, St. Louis.

English National Board for Nursing, Midwifery and Health Visiting (1989). *Project 2000 – 'A New Preparation for Practice'; Guidelines and Criteria for Course Development and the Formulation of Collaborative Links Between Approved Training Institutions within the National Health Service and Centres of Higher Education*. E.N.B., London.

Epp, J. (1987). Achieving health for all: a framework for health promotion. *Canadian Nurse*, **83(11)**, Supplement, 1–13.

Evans, I. (1988). *Development of a Facilitation Role for Health Education in Nursing Practice*. M.A. thesis, University of London.

Ewles, L. and Simnett, I. (1985). *Promoting Health*. Wiley, Chichester.

Faculty of Community Medicine (1988). *Health for All: a Management Agenda*. Institute of Health Services Management, London.

Farrant, W. and Russell, J. (1986). *The Policies of Health Information*. Institute of Education, London.

French, J. and Adams, L. (1986). From analysis to synthesis: theories of health education. *Health Education Journal*, **45(2)**, 71–4.

Frost, S. and Nunkoosing, K. (1989). Quest. Building a strong foundation. *Nursing Times and Nursing Mirror*, **85(1)**, 59–60.

Fullard, E. (1989). The facilitator of prevention in primary care: the birth of a new professional. In *Changing Ideas in Health Care*, D. Seedhouse and A. Cribb (Eds), pp. 195–210. Wiley, Chichester.

Gott, M. (1988). *Nursing, Distance Learning, and Health Promotion in Western Canada*. Unpublished report. Winston Churchill Trust.

Green, L. W. and Raeburn, J. M. (1988). Health promotion. What is it? What will it become? *Health Promotion*, **3(2)**, 151–9.

Guardian(1988). Currie reaffirms responsibility of individual in preventive medicine. The *Guardian*, 29th October, 4.
Health Education Authority (1988). *Working for Health. The New Health Education Authority. A Consultation Document.* H.E.A., London.
Health Education Authority (1989). *Working for Health. Responses to the Health Education Authority Consultation Exercise.* H.E.A., London.
Health Education Council (1984). *Beating Heart Disease.* H.E.C., London.
Helman, C. G. (1981). Disease versus illness in general practice. *Journal of the Royal College of General Practitioners*, **31**, 548–52.
Helman, C. (1984). *Culture, Health and Illness.* Wright, Bristol.
Herzlich, C. (1960). *Health and Illness.* Academic Press, London.
Hill, D. J. and Shugg, D. (1989). Breast self-examination practices and attitudes among breast cancer, benign breast disease and general practice patients. *Health Education Research*, **4(2)**, 193–203.
Hunt, S. M. and Macleod, M. (1987). Health and behavioural change: some lay perspectives. *Community Medicine*, **9(1)**, 68–76.
Illich, I. (1976). *Limits to Medicine. Medical Nemesis: the Expropriation of Health.* Marion Boyars, London.
Kirkpatrick, E. M. (Ed.) (1983). *Chambers Twentieth Century Dictionary.* Chambers, Edinburgh.
Kubler-Ross, E. (1978). *To Live Until We Say Goodbye.* Prentice-Hall, London.
Littlewood, J. (1989). A model for nursing using anthropological literature. *International Journal of Nursing Studies*, **26(3)**, 221–9.
Macleod Clark, J., Haverty, S. and Kendall, S. (1987). *Helping Patients and Clients to Stop Smoking. Phase 2: Assessing the Effectiveness of the Nurse's Role: Final Report.* University of London, Department of Nursing Studies, London.
Marriner, A. (1986). *Nursing Theorists and Their Work.* Mosby, St. Louis.
McKeown, T. (1979). *The Role of Medicine: Dream, Mirage or Nemesis?* Blackwell, Oxford.
McLeroy, K. R. (1989). Issues in risk communication. *Health Education Research*, **4(2)**, 169–70.
Mikhail, B. (1981). The health belief model: a review and critical evaluation of the model, research, and practice. *Advances in Nursing Science*, **4(1)**, 65–82.
Milio, N. (1983). Redefining today's health problem. *Health Affairs*, **2**, 28–44.
Milio, N. (1988). Strategies for health-promoting policy: a study of four national case studies. *Health Promotion*, **3(3)**, 307–11.
Morgan, M., Calnan, M. and Manning, N. (1985). *Sociological*

Approaches to Health and Medicine. Croom Helm, London.

Morton, P. G. (1989). *Health Assessment in Nursing*. Springhouse, Springhouse.

Murray, R. B. and Zentner, J. P. (1989). *Nursing Concepts for Health Promotion*. Prentice-Hall, Hemel Hempstead.

Mussallem, H. K. (1985). Prevention and patterns of disease: prospects and research directions in nursing for the future. In *Prevention and Nursing*, L. E. Willis and M. E. Linwood (Eds), pp. 147–62. Churchill Livingstone, Edinburgh.

Naidoo, J. (1986). Limits to individualism. In *The Politics of Health Education*. S. Rodmell and A. Watt (Eds), pp. 17–37. Routledge & Kegan Paul, London.

Newman, M. A. (1986). *Health as Expanding Consciousness*. Mosby, St. Louis.

Noack, H. (1987). Concepts of health promotion. In *Measurement in Health Promotion and Protection*, T. Abelin, Z. J. Brzezinski and V. D. Carstairs (Eds), pp. 5–28. World Health Organization, Copenhagen.

Oliver, N. F. (1982). Does control of risk factors prevent coronary heart disease? *British Medical Journal*, **285**, 1065–6.

Pearce, E. (1971). *A General Textbook of Nursing*. Faber & Faber, London.

Public Health Alliance (1988). *Beyond Acheson: An Agenda for the New Public Health*. Public Health Alliance, Birmingham.

Richman, J. (1987). *Medicine and Health*. Longman, London.

Riley, D. (1985). *Dry Air*. Virago, London.

Robbins, C. (Ed.) (1987). *Health Promotion in North America: Implications for the U.K.* Health Education Council and King Edward's Hospital Fund, London.

Roberson, M. H. B. (1987). Folk health beliefs of health professionals. *Western Journal of Nursing Research*, **9(2)**, 257–63.

Robinson, K. (1983). What is health? In *Community Health*, J. Clark and J. Henderson (Eds), pp. 11–18. Churchill Livingstone, Edinburgh.

Rodmell, S. and Watt, A. (1986). Conventional health education: problems and possibilities. In *The Politics of Health Education*, S. Rodmell and A. Watt (Eds), pp. 1–16. Routledge Kegan Paul, London.

Rootman, I. (1989). Knowledge for health promotion: a summary of Canadian literature reviews. *Health Promotion*, **4(1)**, 67–72.

Rose, G. (1981). Strategy of prevention: lessons from cardiovascular disease. *British Medical Journal*, **282**, 1847–51.

Saan, H.. (1986). Health promotion and health education: living with a dominant concept. *Health Promotion*, **1(3)**, 253–5.

Seedhouse, D. (1986). *Health: the Foundations of Achievement*. Wiley, Chichester.

Seedhouse, D. (1988). *Ethics: the Heart of Health Care.* Wiley, Chichester.
Sennott-Miller, L. and Miller, J. L. L.(1987). Difficulty: a neglected factor in health promotion.*Nursing Research*, **36(5)**, 268–72.
Shillitoe, R. W. and Christie, M. J.(1989). Determinants of self-care: the health belief model. *Holistic Medicine*, **4(1)**, 3–17.
Smith, A. and Jacobson, B. (1988). *The nation's health. A strategy for the 1990s: a report from an Independent Multidisciplinary Committee.* King Edward's Hospital Fund, London (Chairman A. Smith).
Smith, J. A. (1981). The idea of health: a philosophical inquiry. *Advances in Nursing Science*, **3(3)**, 43–50.
Statutory Instrument (1983). *Nurses, Midwives and Health Visitors Rules Approval Order.* H.M.S.O., London. (SI no. 873).
Stone, I.(1987). Screen fantasy. *New Society*, **82(1302)**, 12–13.
Stone, I. (1989) Upside down prevention. *Health Service Journal*, **99**, 890–1.
Strehlow, M. S. (1983). *Education for Health.* Harper & Row, London.
Sullivan, G. C. (1989). Evaluating Antonovsky's Salutogenic model for its adaptability to nursing. *Journal of Advanced Nursing*, **14(4)**, 336–42.
Syred, M. E. J. (1981). The abdication of the role of health education by hospital nurses. *Journal of Advanced Nursing*, **6(1)**, 27–33.
Tannahill, A. (1984). Health promotion – caring concern. *Journal of Medical Ethics*, **10(4)**, 196–8.
Tannahill, A. (1985). What is health promotion? *Health Education Journal*, **44(4)**, 167–8.
Tannahill, A. (1987). Regional health promotion planning and monitoring. *Health Education Journal*, **46(3)**, 125–7.
Tones, E. K. (1981). Health education: prevention or subversion? *Journal of the Royal Society of Health*, **101(3)**, 413–16.
Tudor-Hart, J. (1985). When practice is not perfect. *Nursing Times*, **81(39)**, 28–9.
Van Maanen, H. M. T. (1988). Being old does not always mean being sick: perspectives on conditions of health as perceived by British and American elderly. *Journal of Advanced Nursing*, **13(6)**, 701–9.
Walker, C. and Cannon, G. (1984). *The Food Scandal.* Century, London.
Walker, S. N., Volkan, K., Sechrist, K. R. and Pender, N. J. (1988). Health-promoting life styles of older adults: comparisons with young and middle-aged adults, correlates and patterns. *Advances in Nursing Science*, **11(1)**, 76–90.
Walt, G. and Constantinides, P. (1983). *Community Health Education in Commonwealth Countries.* Commonwealth Secretariat, London..
Williams, G. (1984). Health promotion – caring concern or slick

salesmanship? *Journal of Medical Ethics*, **10(4)**, 191–5.
Wilson, E. K., Purdon, S. E. and Wallston, K. A. (1988). Compliance to health recommendations: a theoretical overview of message framing. *Health Education Research*, **3(2)**, 161–71.
Wilson-Barnett, J. (1988). Patient teaching or patient counselling? *Journal of Advanced Nursing*, **13(2)**, 215–22.
Winnicott, D. (1986). *Home is Where we Start From – Essays by a Psychoanalyst*. Penguin, Harmondsworth.
Woods, N. F., Laffrey, S., Duffy, M., Lentz, M. J., Mitchell, E. S., Taylor, D. and Cowan, K. A. (1988). Being healthy. *Advances in Nursing Science*, **11(1)**, 36–46.
World Health Organization (1946). *Constitution of the World Health Organization*. W.H.O., Geneva.
World Health Organization (1984). *Health Promotion: a Discussion Document on the Concept and Principles*. W.H.O., Copenhagen.
World Health Organization (1985). *Targets for Health for All 2000*. W.H.O., Copenhagen.
World Health Organization (1986). *Intersectoral Action for Health*. W.H.O., Geneva.

4 Curriculum pathways to Project 2000

Introduction

This chapter focuses on key issues in curriculum development and innovation in the context of Project 2000. The long sought-after major reforms are underway with quite significant implications for the way courses in nursing education are developed and managed. Demonstration centres have already started their programmes while others are no doubt currently 'working up' Project 2000 courses with fairly tight deadlines for submission. Therefore it seems appropriate to discuss some of the key issues with reference to the process of curriculum innovation over time. Adaptation of the Further Education Curriculum Review Unit's (1982) phases of curriculum innovation will be used as a temporal and conceptual framework to discuss the main issues. They will serve as a conceptual map or 'route guide' along the pathways to Project 2000. The four phases are the initiation, development, implementation and evaluation phases, and to some extent they overlap. However, each will be considered in turn.

1. Initiation phase During this phase curriculum development groups need to identify and articulate priorities for course development. The broad educational intentions of new courses are normally identified during this phase, although their translation into more precise statements of intent is not usually undertaken at this juncture. In addition, general decisions about curriculum development are taken as part of the initiation phase. It is highly probable that every nurse training institution is addressing or has recently worked through this phase by conceptualising and planning Common Foundation and Branch Programmes in nursing.

2. Development phase This is the phase during which the new curriculum is developed and at the end of which the new 'curriculum package', with all the materials required for the implementation of the curriculum, is available for adoption and implementation (Further Education Curriculum Review and Development Unit, 1982). Important decisions made during this phase are concerned with the precise educational intentions of the course, the selection/

rejection of content for the scheme of study, the modes of teaching/ learning and the scheme of assessment. In nursing education this phase is characterised by curriculum development groups producing quality submission documents which are forwarded to the appropriate Statutory Body, for example the English National Board, for consideration by the Approvals Committee. In most cases, and this is likely to be on the increase, documents are also sent to the Council for National Awards (CNAA) or other body, for example a local university, for conjoint validation. It is acknowledged that this is probably the most difficult phase of curriculum innovation, since teaching and secretarial staff are normally working under intense pressure to meet deadlines for submission.

3. Implementation phase   Implementation refers to the curriculum and use of associated materials in action. However, the curriculum 'in action' may differ significantly from the 'formal' curriculum, i.e. the one outlined in the submission document. This situation is most likely to occur if curriculum developers and curriculum users are different groups of people and if a power-coercive or empirical rational change strategy is adopted. There is likely to be a higher degree of congruity between the formal curriculum and the curriculum in action in nursing education if both education and practice-based staff work together in a collegial manner.

4. Evaluation phase   It is recognised that evaluation should be ongoing since it is a judgemental process in which people attempt to ascribe a degree of worth or value to a curriculum. The demands for more rigorous approaches to curriculum evaluation have grown in recent years in both general and nursing education. This academic rigour is likely to be sustained, and rightly so, as nurse training institutions seek and gain conjoint validation for their respective courses.

Having outlined the four phases of curriculum innovation in the context of Project 2000, the following key issues will be addressed with reference to those phases:

- Philosophy
- Educational intentions
- Schemes of study
- Modes of teaching/learning
- Schemes of assessment
- Course evaluation/validation

Philosophy

It is suggested that it is only during the last decade that philosophy has assumed a more prominent feature in course submission documents, and rightly so. In the context of modern philosophy, Schofield (1972) describes three terms which are frequently used in the context of educational philosophy: philosophical analysis, linguistic analysis, and concept analysis. He states that the second and third terms are really more precise expressions of the first. Linguistic analysis examines statements to see if they have any real meaning. For example, the statement 'experiential learning can be interpreted as learning from and/or through experience' makes sense after linguistic analysis. However, concept analysis analyses certain terms (words) which represent ideas or concepts. Analysis of the words 'learning' and 'from/through experience' enable a clearer understanding of the statement to be made. One of the supreme intellects of all time, Leibniz, realised centuries ago that effective communication is often impaired when different people use the same words to mean different things, or different words to mean the same thing (cited Schofield, 1972). He felt that the solution to this problem could be achieved by the development of 'Characteristica Universalis', i.e. a universal symbolism. His concept is mathematical in nature and once established could ensure that philosophical problems could be solved like mathematical problems. If two accountants have a problem regarding a balance of payments, they would 'sit down and calculate'. He asserted that philosophers should behave in the same way. However, the comparison can be challenged in that the accountants would probably be dealing with concrete concepts whereas the philosophers are more likely to be dealing with the abstract. Now, in the absence of a universal symbolism and a dubious analogy, an alternative procedure to conduct philosophical analysis in nursing education is required. An adaptation of Torres and Stanton's (1982) procedure could be used. This comprises the following steps:

1. Identify the key concepts of a course.
2. Conduct a values clarification exercise about those key concepts.
3. Identify relationships and ordering among the concepts.
4. Prepare a draft philosophical statement.
5. Circulate the statement to those who will be involved with the course.
6. Revise the statement following feedback to ensure 'ownership'.

Each step will now be discussed in the context of preparing a Project 2000 course.

Step one can be achieved by using brainstorming or a modified nominal group technique. Brainstorming is a procedure where one person usually writes on a chalkboard or flip-chart the ideas from the group. These ideas should be collected without censure to ensure a free-flow. Some groups may need encouragement to contribute freely and abandon reticence. The nominal group technique could be adapted as follows:

(*i*) group members are asked to write down, in private, the concepts they consider to be key;

(*ii*) ideas are then pooled without discussion so that all group members can see the full list;

(*iii*) open discussion takes place to clarify meaning and produce a final list of key concepts.

Step two is likely to be a fairly lengthy procedure and time should be allowed for the important process of values clarification. In a Project 2000 course it is inevitable that one of the key concepts identified will be *nursing*. In the second open learning package *Managing Change in Nursing Education, Pack 2* (ENB, 1989) the writer suggests that individuals may have attempted to describe the phenomenon called nursing from the perspective of their current specialism, for example adult or mental handicap nursing. However, practice alone can infer a misleading narrowness. On the other hand, 'all embracing' definitions of nursing may also reflect something which could be ascribed to several other vocational occupations. Sladden (1985) captures this point by commenting:

'With nursing roles a particular problem arises in that, if one attempts an exclusive definition (I mean leaving out anything that anyone else can do), nursing disappears altogether. Nursing has to be defined as a particular mix of functions, rather than by one special and exclusive central task, and it is up to nurses themselves to keep hold of the elements in that mix that are important to them.'

In the ENB document (ENB (1989) Pack 2) the writer goes on to suggest that in the quest for conceptual clarity the efforts of Peters (1966) could be considered. Peters proposes that to define the concept '*education*' is in fact problematic. The writer agrees with Peters, for the same reasons why it is problematic to attempt to define nursing. Rather than attempting to define education, Peters instead considers three criteria:

(*i*) education implies the transmission of what is worthwhile to those who become committed to it;

(*ii*) education must involve knowledge and understanding and some sort of 'cognitive perspective' which is not inert; and (*iii*)   education at least rules out some procedures of transmission on the grounds that they lack willingness and voluntariness on the part of the learner.

If Peters' approach is adopted, nursing could be considered in a similar way, by considering its aims rather than trying to define the phenomenon *per se*. For example, Roy (1976) believes that the need for nursing care arises when the client cannot adapt to internal and external environmental demands, e.g. following a cardiac arrest. Levine (1973) identifies four conservation principles of nursing.

(*i*)   Conservation of client energy
(*ii*)   Conservation of structural integrity
(*iii*) Conservation of personal integrity
(*iv*)   Conservation of social integrity

With Levine's approach, one of the aims of nursing is to enable clients to make optimal use of their resources through the nurses' conservation activities. Just as Peters was able to compare what he considered to be the aims of education with other philosophers, such as O'Connor (1957), so too can nurses compare and contrast what they believe to be the aims of nursing, and subsequently nursing education.

It is also likely that learning, notably experiential learning, will be identified as a key concept. Readers are referred back to the earlier discussion (p. 95) regarding linguistic and concept analysis.

For step three of the modified Torres and Stanton procedure, readers are referred to Fig. 4.1 which is how the writer in ENB (1989) Pack 2 depicted the ordering and relationships of the key concepts from a Project 2000 course. The ENB Project 2000 Guidelines (1989) identify five basic concepts which have been extended to include key educational concepts.

Curriculum planners are now in a position to carry out step four of Torres and Stanton's process of formulating a course philosophy. A member of the group with philosophical literary skills can volunteer to write the draft statement! He or she can also carry out steps five and six and enjoy seeing the fruits of rich philosophical debate appear in the course submission document. It is important that there is a relationship between an institution's philosophy and the philosophies of its courses referred to in Fig. 4.2, which is an adaptation of the writer's figure in ENB (1989) Pack 2. It is acknowledged that the realisation of compatibility between the philosophies depicted in Fig. 4.2 is likely to be a challenging process. Amalgamation and linkages are likely to make the process more difficult, but ideally a shared philosophy should be developed. Once a philosophy is established, it should be reflected in all aspects of the curriculum, starting with the educational intentions of a course.

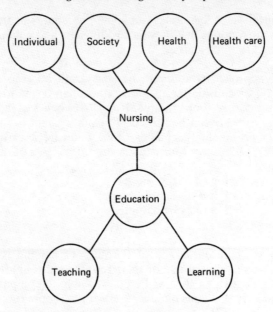

Fig. 4.1 Key concepts for a Project 2000 course.

Educational intentions

As stated in the ENB Project 2000 Guidelines (1989), a Common Foundation Programme provides the basis of a practice-based curriculum from which the four Branch Programmes can be developed. The five aims of a Common Foundation Programme are as follows:

1. Establish the basis for progression to any of the Branch Programmes and subsequent achievement of competent professional practice.
2. Introduce the dynamic nature of nursing and enable students to begin to develop the skills to master their expanding body of knowledge and the challenge of change.
3. Provide experience(s) for students in a variety of settings and with a range of client or patient groups, across the spectrum of primary, secondary and tertiary health care, to enable them to communicate with sensitivity, observe with understanding, reflect with insight, and participate in the delivery of care with knowledge and skill.
4. Provide opportunities for students to develop their intellectual abilities, self-awareness and self-direction.

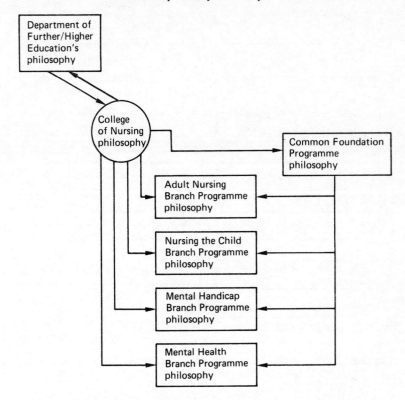

Fig. 4.2   Relationship between institutional and course philosophies.

5.   Enable students to acquire the ability at registration to take responsibiity for their own continued professional development.

Although these general aims provide a frame of reference for Project 2000 curriculum development groups (CDGs), there still remain the practical decisions about formulating more specific learning intentions. Figure 4.3 is a diagrammatic representation of a possible structure for a Project 2000 CDG and associated working groups. The membership of the working groups may be the same people, especially those working groups of the Common Foundation Programme. It is also recommended that there is cross-membership in the Common Foundation and Branch Programme groups. This is likely to help the realisation of the first aim of the Common Foundation group, i.e. to establish the basis of progression to the Branches. Whatever the local arrangements are, it is important to have structures which can develop Common Foundation and Branch Programmes.

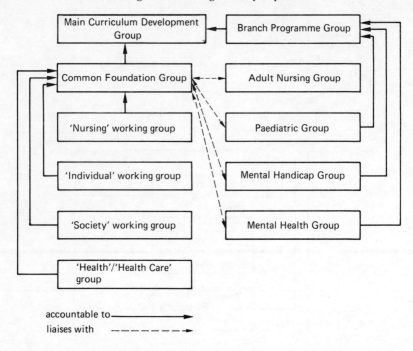

Fig. 4.3 Project 2000 curriculum development/working group structure/relationships.

Schemes of study

The discussion so far has reflected the activities required during the *initiation phase* of curriculum development described earlier (see p. 93). Attention will now be focused on the *development phase* during which important decisions are made about the more specific aspects of the scheme of study and scheme of assessment of a course. This part of the chapter will briefly consider how Bruner's (1966) theory of instruction and Beattie's (1987) fourfold curriculum could be adapted to plan different aspects of a Common Foundation Programme. Bruner (1966), in his social science curriculum project MACOS (Man: A course of study), used a framework which comprised a focus for study; 'springboard' questions to provide direction and a spirit of inquiry, key concepts which are central to the focus and springboard questions, guided discovery learning, and a shift from extrinsic to intrinsic motivation. For example, in the MACOS project the framework is as follows:

Focus: Man's unique adaptation

Springboard questions:
1. What is human about human beings?
2. How did they get that way?
3. How can they be made more so?

Key concepts:
tool making; language; child rearing; social organisation; cosmology

Content:
related to key concepts, e.g. modes of communication for key concept 'language'

Methodology:
inductive approach – study of a nuclear family (Netsilik Eskimo)/ film-based with much use of discussion groups and student diaries

Evaluation:
from student diaries and discussion groups

Applied to a Common Foundation Programme, Bruner's approach could be utilised as follows:

Focus: The nurse as a health educator

Springboard questions:
1. What does it mean to be healthy?
2. What does it mean to be unhealthy?
3. In which ways can nurses actively promote their own health and that of their respective client groups?

Key concepts:
health; altered health states, primary, secondary, tertiary prevention

Content:
related to key concepts, e.g. definitions; determinants; illness

Methodology:
inductive approach by guided discovery learning, e.g. discussion of health of self before moving on to the population at large (methods could include brainstorming, discussion, mini-projects and a range of other experiential methods such as sculpting or guided fantasy)

Evaluation:
to include seminar presentations; health focused care plans; teaching patients aspects of health care; student diaries

It is not within the scope or remit of this chapter to develop the suggestions made regarding the adaptation of Bruner's approach. The intention has been to provide a 'framework for action'. For example, it is up to the reader's imagination on how to use sculpting or guided fantasy with students to address the key concept of health and health care in a Common Foundation Programme, assuming those methods are deemed appropriate.

Bruner's approach is compatible with a philosophy which encourages a problem-solving approach, research-mindedness, and student-centred learning. He has been criticised for emphasising intellectual growth at the expense of effective learning (Jones, 1975), but mindful of this and other criticisms of learning by discovery, nurse teachers can adapt his approach to good effect (Myles, 1987).

An alternative approach to designing a scheme of study will now be discussed. In ENB (1989) Pack 2 the author poses four questions which curriculum planners need to ask of their draft scheme of study. Partially rephrased they read:

1. Have important issued been omitted? If so, which ones?
2. Is there too much content? If so, what could be omitted?
3. Does the scheme of study reflect the course philosophy, and educational intentions of the Common Foundation Programme?
4. Have you kept in mind the problems associated with an eclectic curriculum, e.g. the domination of key subjects and schedules of basic skills over personal and cultural issues?

Beattie's (1987) fourfold curriculum outlined in Fig.4.4 could be used as a 'lens' to focus on the four questions, especially question four. An eclectic curriculum can be dominated by maps of key subjects and schedules of basic skills in lieu of meaningful personal experiences and important cultural issues, such as shifts to community based care.

Beattie proposes that each of the four different approaches to curriculum design has particular strengths and weaknesses, which complement one another. He suggests that the reinstatement of the 'map of subject matter' as a central feature of curriculum planning is mainly due to the need to acquaint students with the rapidly growing and changing fields of knowledge which form the work of nurses. In that context he warns of the potential obsolescence that can befall subject maps, hence the author's previously cited question 2 which is meant to raise issues of validity as well as quantity. Beattie also implies that this approach can lead to what Bernstein (1975) describes as a 'collection code' curriculum reflected by discrete 'packets of knowledge' with strong subject boundary maintenance. Beattie suggests that interdisciplinary themes can ameliorate this problem and foster integration.

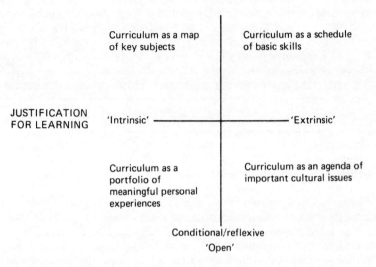

Fig. 4.4 Beattie's (1987) fourfold curriculum.

If the central feature of the curriculum is a schedule of basic skills, it can be criticised as reductionist in nature. Nevertheless, the concept of the Project 2000 nurse as a 'knowledgeable doer' should remind teachers that this approach has a key place in nursing curricula, provided that the schedule is research-based. The attraction of the curriculum as a portfolio of meaningful personal experiences lies in its association with humanistic psychology, andragogy, and experiential learning. This approach may seem even more appropriate for a Project 2000 student whose course should offer more scope and opportunity for negotiated learning. The problems associated with this approach will be discussed under the modes of teaching/learning section of this chapter.

The curriculum as an agenda of important cultural issues has grown in popularity in recent years in both general and nursing education. This is not surprising since the range of dilemmas and debates about health care provision has grown considerably. The shifts in power bases which afford patients/clients more say in the management of their health care, shifts to community-based rather than institution-based care, and the government's recent White Paper 'Working for Patients: The Health Service caring for the carers' provides several starting points for addressing some of the key concepts in a Common Foundation Programme.

Figure 4.5 is an outline of how the principles of the fourfold curriculum could be used to plan how HIV/AIDS might be addressed in an Adult Nursing Branch Programme. It is stressed that Fig. 4.5 is only meant to be illustrative, i.e. a starting point for more detailed planning. This 'multi-model' approach is very appropriate for a Project 2000 curriculum since it can incorporate the benefits of each of the four designs previously described.

Some of the key issues pertaining to the initiation and development phases of curriculum development in the context of Project 2000 have been discussed. Attention will now be turned towards the implementation phase by focusing on modes of teaching/learning.

Modes of teaching/learning

Much has been written about teaching methods in nursing education over the past few years (Ewan and White, 1984; ENB, 1987; Quinn, 1988; ENB, 1989; Kenworthy and Nicklin, 1989). It is not the intention of this chapter to reproduce well-documented material but rather to draw attention to the premise that nurse teachers need to be

MAP OF KEY SUBJECTS	SCHEDULE OF BASIC SKILLS
details of HIV/AIDS AIDS related complex Kaposi's sarcoma AIDS related dementia opportunistic infections immunological aspects epidemiological aspects infection control	safely manage a patient's potentially bio-hazardous secretions with reference to hospital policy formulate an appropriate individualised care plan for a person with AIDS
PORTFOLIO OF MEANINGFUL PERSONAL EXPERIENCES	AGENDA OF IMPORTANT CULTURAL ISSUES
critical incidents from experience in practice settings, personal responses to health education campaigns fears about HIV/AIDS, attitudes to 'safer sex' attitudes of partner.	ethical issues arising from testing for HIV without consent, prejudices regarding sexual orientation, e.g. homosexuality victim blaming, e.g. a drug abuser (rather than drug user) is a victim blaming term, arguments re: 'innocent' and 'guilty' sufferers.

Fig. 4.5 Planning the HIV/AIDS input for an Adult Nursing Branch Programme with reference to the fourfold curriculum.

skilled in the use of a wide range of teaching methods if they are to provide stimulating and challenging experiences for their students. In ENB (1989) Pack 2 the author suggests that experiential learning is likely to be a major feature of Common Foundation and Branch Programmes. In the ENB Project 2000 Guidelines (1989), it is suggested that the nature and implications of client empowerment are addressed. Steinaker and Bell's (1979) experiential learning taxonomy could be adapted as shown in Table 4.1.

It is interesting to note how the role of the teacher alters commensurate with the changing role of the student as the taxonomy is ascended. This conceptual framework has much to recommend it since there is scope for the use of a diverse range of teaching methods which are predominantly student-centred, which may be in the form of a learning contract. A learning contract can be defined as a teaching/learning strategy where a student (or students) negotiates with his or her facilitator the objectives, methods for achieving the objectives, and criteria for evaluating his or her achievement of those objectives. Contracts can range from informal verbal to formal written agreements, and it is suggested that each type is appropriate for Common Foundation and Branch Programmes, the latter format appropriate if linked to competency statements. Before discussing examples and the practical aspects of implementing learning contracts, justification for their increased use will be made with reference to the concept of social need defined by Bradshaw (1972). According

Table 4.1 Experiential learning taxonomy, adapted from Steinaker and Bell (1979).

Level	Role of teacher	Role of student
Exposure	Motivator	Learns about populist models of health
Participation	Catalyst	Involves a client under his or her care in conjoint care planning under supervision
Identification	Moderator	Develops confidence in fostering client self-help
Internalisation	Sustainer	Promoting client empowerment (when appropriate) is a characteristic of his or her nursing care
Dissemination	Critic/evaluator	Teaches other students ways of fostering client empowerment

to Bradshaw, social service is based on need, and in that context he identifies four types: normative, felt, expressed, and comparative. In ENB (1989) Pack 2 the author describes each type.

Normative need is what the expert or professional defines as need in any given context. The pre-registration learning outcomes outlined in the ENB (1989) Pack 2 Project 2000 Guidelines can be regarded as normative in that they suggest the 'desirable standard' to be reached by students to enable them to be admitted to the UKCC's register and to assume the responsibilities and accountability that nursing registration confers. Teacher-designed curriculum objectives can also be regarded as normative in that they are based on professional expertise.

Normative needs change as the body of knowledge increases through research and as societal values change. With reference to the fourfold curriculum discussed previously, maps of key subjects and schedules of basic skills can be further defended on *normative* grounds in that their selection is usually based on professional expertise and research. However, the potential problems of a teaching session based predominantly on normative need are those of paternalism and parochialism, i.e. a 'we know what's best for you' approach.

Felt need is equated with wants and is influenced by individual perceptions. An example of felt need in the context of a Common Foundation Programme might be a student who wished to develop his or her assertion skills. In terms of the fourfold curriculum, portfolios of meaningful experiences are likely to generate *felt* need. The main advantage of teaching sessions based on felt need lies in its student-centredness. One disadvantage for teachers is that they may not feel properly prepared for sessions. Felt need may also be deemed an inadequate measure of 'real' need in that vital curricular areas could be overlooked.

Expressed need is felt need turned into action. The merit of expressed need is the realisation of felt need and this can be achieved by a learning contract.

Comparative need is a measure of need found by studying the characteristics of those in receipt of a service. For example, if the learning contracts of students on an Adult Nursing Branch Programme were based mainly on felt need, whereas the contracts of students on other Branch Programmes were based on normative need, it could be said that the latter groups are 'in need' of learning contracts based on felt need. One of the advantages of teaching sessions based on comparative need is that perspectives can be broadened by consid-

ering what happens with other groups. However, a disadv
Project 2000 context could be that cross-curricular norms
ished and ritualised. This could stifle creativity at both tl
level of curriculum development and at the more 'micro
teaching/learning.

Figure 4.6 illustrates the balance of social need which could
underpin two different learning contracts and asks readers to consider the philosophy which may underpin each respectively. Learning
contract (a) is strongly based on professional judgement and on what
happens on other Branch Programmes with little acknowledgement
of the students' felt and expressed needs. In terms of the fourfold
curriculum it appears to be dominated by a map of key subjects and a
schedule of basic skills. It is likely to be based on an empirical-
rational strategy for changing the student's behaviour. Conversely,
contract (b) is more student-centred and dialectical, i.e. each 'qua-
drant' of the fourfold curriculum may be reflected. It is also based on
a normative re-educative approach to facilitating learning.

With reference to social need, readers are asked to reflect on the
appropriateness of 'concave' and 'convex' learning contracts (contracts (a) and (b) respectively). It is suggested that 'convex' learning
contracts reflect the notion of the curriculum as a 'trading post' on the
cultural boundary between students and teachers, to which ideas and
artefacts are brought, exchanged, and taken away (Jenkins and
Shipman 1976). They should enable the felt needs that students bring
to the 'trading post' to be articulated as expressed needs and
subsequently realised through the learning contract. They can also be
used to articulate and achieve normative needs, therefore 'concave'
contracts do have their place.

Knowles (1984) identifies eight stages of a learning contract which
can be condensed to five as follows:

(*i*)   assess learning needs with reference to a competency scale;

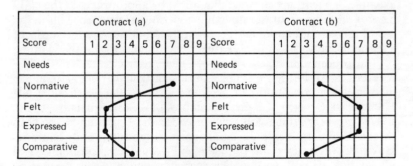

Fig. 4.6 Social need and learning contracts.

(*ii*) formulate appropriate objectives;
(*iii*) identify resources available with related actions and time frames;
(*iv*) carry out contract;
(*v*)   evaluate learning outcomes against objectives of contract.

One of the pre-registration learning outcomes of a Project 2000 course is that students will be able to 'use relevant literature and research to inform the practice of nursing'. A student in the early period of a Common Foundation Programme is unlikely to be familiar with a range of literature on nursing practice and research. However, as the student progresses through the course, it would be expected that he or she always bases his or her care on appropriate research findings if they are available. Therefore, a competency scale for that nurse might be scored as follows:

Absent	Low (awareness)		Moderate (understanding)		High (expert)
0	1	2	3	4	5
	(P)		(R)		

'P' represents the student's present competency and 'R' represents the required competency. As the student progresses through the course his or her competency scale should change as follows:

Absent	Low (awareness)		Moderate (understanding)		High (expert)
0	1	2	3	4	5
			(P)		(R)

The next stage of the process is to formulate more specific objectives which, if achieved, will reduce the 'P–R' interval. Figure 4.7 is an example of a learning contract that might be appropriate, in the early days of the course, for the student who wishes to develop skills in the use of relevant literature and research. It also illustrates the stages of a learning contract identified earlier. The framework for the learning contract outlined in Fig. 4.7 has been adapted from one described by Keyzer (1985). Further examples of this particular framework in use in continuing education can be found in Keyzer (1985) and ENB (1989) Pack 2 which also gives examples of other formats.

The use of learning contracts provides the opportunity for both teachers and students to individualise teaching and learning. However their use can, initially, be very time consuming and demanding for both parties. Once teachers and students are used to

For: Student Nurse Davies
Focus: Use of literature and research findings
Facilitators: Personal tutor
            Common Foundation librarian
            Ward sister (male surgery)
The following objectives, actions, time frames and criteria for
evaluation are agreed.

Signatories _____   Date _____

Objectives	Resources	Actions	Time frames	Criteria for evaluation
1. I wish to develop my information retrieval skills	1. Library 2. Librarian 3. Personal tutor	1. I will contact the librarian to undertake a supervised literature search on 3 topics	3 days	1. I will produce a book and journal list for the 3 selected topics
2. I would like to understand more about how to use research findings on my current ward allocation	1. Ward Sister 2. Personal tutor 3. Librarian 4. Journal Club	1. I will look up 3 research publications related to pre-operative preparation	7 days	1. I will present a brief resume of each research publication/ article to my personal tutor during the next study day 2. I will discuss the articles with my ward sister to review current practice in the light of the findings

Fig. 4.7 Framework for a learning contract (adapted from Keyzer, 1985).

the process, the time constraints become less of a concern. It is worth stressing that often the outcomes of a contract are different from those which were originally envisaged. This situation has to be judged by all parties on individual merit. After all, Peters (1966) did suggest that education is not so much about reaching a destination, but more about travelling with a different point of view!

Following this discussion about the use of Steinaker and Bell's experiential taxonomy and the theory and practice of learning contracts, attention will now be turned to some of the issues pertaining to student assessment in the context of Project 2000.

Schemes of assessment

Schemes of assessment should reflect the students' respective schemes of study. This is sound educational practice since incongruity is illogical and unfair on the students. In ENB (1989) Pack 2 the following seven assumptions are made regarding the nature of assessment:

1. Curriculum development towards Project 2000 should be based on a model where students are encouraged to take an active part in their own learning and their assessment.
2. There is a recognised need on the part of nurse educators to proceed towards an integrated pattern of continuous assessment.
3. The assessment process should follow a multi-method approach, incorporating a diverse range of appropriate methods, without over-assessing the students.
4. Each of the methods should carry a strong formative component yielding some summative data.
5. Teachers and students will both benefit from the interactive nature of teaching and assessing.
6. Common Foundation and Branch Programmes will normally be one continuous educational process incorporating an assessment strategy based on the continuous assessment of theory and practice.
7. Staff in the practice settings need to be supported while they develop the skills necessary for the continuous assessment of theory and practice.

Some of the assumptions merit further comment. For example, earlier in the chapter, it was asserted that the philosophy of a course should be reflected in *all* its aspects. This point is illustrated quite well in the first assumption. With regard to assumption three, the problems of over-assessment cannot be over-emphasised. It can cause unnecessary stress and verity to the analogy of the 'examination tail wagging the curriculum dog'! The responsibility for ensuring comparability across the country lies with the English National Board.

Assumption five has particular appeal since it implies that teachers and their students can enjoy a collegial relationship, each deriving benefit from their exchanges at the educational 'trading post'.

Finally, as outlined in assumption seven, it is imperative that staff in the practice settings receive the support and education that they need to develop their skills. One way of achieving this is the provision of sufficient ENB 998 or other appropriate courses that address the principles of teaching and assessing. As more and more schools offer Common Foundation and Branch Programmes, the demand for such courses is likely to increase, placing extra pressure on departments of continuing education.

As the author stated in ENB (1989) Pack 2, it is first necessary to articulate a philosophy of assessment. This can be achieved by using the adopted Torres and Stanton procedure described earlier in this chapter (p. 95). A values clarification exercise could form part of the process by considering how members of the group feel about the seven assumptions previously cited. The draft statement that emerges from that debate could be similar to the following:

Philosophy of assessment

The philosophy of assessment for the Common Foundation Programme is based on Peters' (1966) three criteria for education. First, assessment will ensure that students meet the entry critieria to proceed to a Branch Programme. It will also ensure that students are able to contribute under supervision to the care required by a range of clients and patients and, in particular, demonstrate observational, communication and caring skills. It is suggested that Peters' first criterion of worthwhileness is fulfilled if those two outcomes are achieved. Second, Peters suggests that knowledge must not be 'inert' and should involve a wider cognitive perspective. Therefore, the scheme of assessment will ensure that students are able to explore and analyse the relevance of the core subjects and their relationship to a range of health care settings. Peters' third and final criterion centres around the mutual acceptability of methods. In this respect, the scheme of assessment will be based on an adult model where students are encouraged to take an active part in the process. It is firmly believed that both students and their assessors will benefit from this negotiation, and that the process of self and peer assessment will be enhanced.

It is worth pointing out that the above statement is only a working draft and would need to be circulated to all those involved with the course for comment and subsequent amendment.

The next stage in the process is to decide exactly what is going to be assessed. Since the scheme should reflect the scheme of study, account must be taken of the learning intentions of the course, which, in a Project 2000 course, should address the pre-registration learning outcomes.

The next step could involve the development of an assessment grid as shown in Fig. 4.8. The assessment methods stated are only there to serve as examples. Members of assessment boards will need to choose a balance of different methods which score highly on the criteria of validity and reliability in the context of what it is they are assessing. For example, an essay is perhaps not the most reliable and valid method to assess whether a student can involve a patient in their own care planning with reference to a particular nursing model. The

Key concept: Nursing Focus: Nursing models	Assessment methods				
	Essay	Objective test	Research critique	Care plan	Problem-solving case study
cognitive aspects: * * practical aspects: * * affective aspects: * *					

Fig. 4.8 An Assessment Grid for a Common Foundation Programme.

ability to develop a negotiated care plan or present a problem-solving case study is probably more appropriate.

External examiners have an important role to play in the development of valid and reliable schemes of assessment. In ENB (1989) Pack 2 the author reports on an interview with an external examiner who, when asked what she was looking for, replied:

'I am looking for reliability. I am of course concerned with the products of assessment, but my main focus is now on the process. By that I mean the structure of the School's Examination Board, their assessment tools and when they are used throughout the course.'

(ENB, 1989; Pack 2)

She went on to say that her reports included reference to the perceived effectiveness of the curriculum, and the elements of the learning environment which support or undermine the curricular aims. She also included a critical appraisal of the inter-marker reliability across different aspects of the theoretical and practical curriculum, and the balance between formative and summative assessment. Statistical data about marks and results are also included. In summary, her reports describe the relationship between the course philosophy, the course aims, the teaching/learning strategies and the mode of assessment (as a matter of interest, five from the six themes chosen for this chapter). This penultimate section of the chapter will conclude by publishing the assertion that if external examiners are afforded open access to people and resources associated with the curriculum, both internal and external assessors should derive greater benefit from this process of peer review. In turn, and of perhaps more significance, students may profit. The concept of peer review is also a feature of the final section of this chapter, course evaluation.

Course evaluation/validation

So far issues apposite to the initiation, development and implementation phases of curriculum development have been addressed. The final part of this chapter will address issues of central concern to the evaluation phase, particularly internal and external validation. Practical guidelines for those involved in curriculum evaluation will be suggested following a clarification of some of the related terminology.

Evaluation is a judgemental process in which people attempt to ascribe a degree of worth or value to a curriculum (Wells, 1987). *Validation* is the process whereby judgement is reached by a group including external peers as to whether a course designed to lead to an award meets the requirements of that award (Council for National Academic Awards, 1988). *Professional accreditation* is given for the recognition that a course properly prepares participants for their professional roles.

Validation and accreditation are two processes which are carried out by duly authorised bodies, for example the CNAA and the ENB, often conjointly. This is certain to be a major feature of Project 2000 courses as more collaborative links are formed between colleges of nursing and midwifery and higher education establishments, since the minimum criteria relating to those links must be at the level of conjoint validation.

The term 'quality assurance' is much in use in nursing education and nursing practice today. It can be regarded as a generic term which encompasses validation. Validation is concerned with 'threshold adequacy' which is based on criterion rather than norm referencing. In other words, if a course falls below threshold adequacy, it will not be validated.

Nixon (1989) considers how styles of validation have shifted from a 'centre' to 'periphery' approach over the last two and a half decades. From 1964 to the early 1970s validation was based on an inquisitorial/adversarial model. This approach is characterised by intermittent face-to-face encounters with the validators, for example General Nursing Council (GNC) Inspectors, who passed judgement (the optimum 'sentence' being a quinquennial reprieve before they returned). During the latter 1970s and early 1980s, the emphasis shifted to institutional self-monitoring, quality enhancement and quality maintenance. The change from GNC Inspectors to ENB Education Officers was intended to foster more collaborative links between training institutions and the statutory bodies through more frequent contact on both formal and informal levels. The 1980s, particularly the latter part of the decade, has seen further shifts towards institutional self-regulation linked to systems of peer review. The greater the rigour an institution affords to internal validation, the less rigour needs to be undertaken during external validation. It is also suggested that peer group review can be a major stimulant to curricular creativity.

The CNAA currently has two types of relationship with institutions: associated and accredited. *Associated* institutions have an increased responsibility for their academic standards. They have negotiated authority to plan and organise validation exercises and to make certain changes. However, the CNAA retains the responsibility for the final approval of all courses and external examiners for those courses. Members of the CNAA would also visit those institutions from time to time to review their effectiveness.

Accredited institutions have been formally recognised by the CNAA to approve new courses on its behalf. Accredited status is awarded when the institution is considered to have developed academic maturity and stringent mechanisms of internal scrutiny. It is worth stressing that an accredited status can be withdrawn if institutions fail to maintain standards.

Walker (1989) identifies two important aims of external validation:
  (*i*)   to ensure value for the students; and
  (*ii*) to ensure value for the community at large.
Both those aims are appropriate for both pre- and post-Project 2000 courses. Student nurses merit a quality curriculum facilitated by a quality teaching cadre, and the consumers of health care (all of us) would hope to benefit from an enhanced quality of client care. Walker goes on to describe five different types of validation judgement: academic, professional, economic, institutional, and judgements about team performance. A brief account of each type of validation judgement related to nursing education follows.

- *Academic validation* is concerned with the overall coherence of the scheme of study and scheme of assessment. In the context of Project 2000 this would relate to the organisation and relationships between Common Foundation and Branch Programmes.

- *Professional validation* asks the question 'Can course members do the job that the course is supposed to prepare them for?' This type of validation appears to be synonymous with professional accreditation and in the context of Project 2000 would pose questions regarding the 12 pre-registration learning outcomes.

- *Economic validation* is concerned with the management of financial, technical and human resources. In the context of Project 2000 this would be concerned with education budgets, resources such as computers and open learning materials, and staff-student ratios.

- *Institutional validation* is concerned with how a course fits in to an institution's strategic plan. In the context of Project 2000, the relationship between pre- and post-basic education could be probed.

● Validation judgement concerned with *team performance* would, in the context of Project 2000, focus on the teaching cadre and practice-based staff concerned with the education of pre-registration students.

In ENB (1989) Pack 2 the latter four validation judgements are all subsumed under academic validation. Nevertheless, Walker provides a classification which brings the process of external validation more sharply into focus. As previously mentioned, institutions with accredited status have demonstrated their academic maturity through the development of rigorous mechanisms of internal validation.

In the context of Project 2000 the three main aims of internal validation would be as follows:

(*i*)   Enquire into the educational quality of the course proposal in the submission documents for the Common Foundation and the Branch Programmes (academic validation).

(*ii*) Ascertain whether the means are available to support the proposal in action (economic validation).

(*iii*) Determine whether the proposal satisfies the known requirements of external validating or accrediting body (academic and professional validation).

As Adelman and Alexander (1982) point out with regard to general education, the third aim should not preponderate over the first two. As the author identified in ENB (1989) Pack 2, Tyler's (1949) four basic questions could be used by curriculum development groups to evaluate their Project 2000 courses by providing the following framework.

1.   *What educational purposes should the institution seek to attain?*
     (a) Is the course framework clearly described and justified?
     (b) Is the course philosophy clearly articulated with reference to key concepts?
     (c) Is the philosophy reflected throughout each aspect of the course?
     (d) Are the learning intentions/outcomes comprehensive enough to facilitate the development of a competent practitioner?
     (e) Is the course content related to the key concepts and course intentions?
     (f) Is the content appropriately balanced and are there any notable omissions?

2. *What educational experiences can be provided that are likely to attain these purposes?*
    (a) Have you decided on the sequencing of placements in the practice settings, using as your yardstick the educational needs of the students?
    (b) What consideration has been given to the fostering of an effective learning environment in order that achievable learning outcomes may be realised?

3. *How can these experiences be effectively organised?*
    (a) How is integration achieved between theory and practice?
    (b) Does the course structure facilitate a progressive broadening and deepening of the students' knowledge and experience?
    (c) Are teaching methods related to the scheme of study and based on the tenets of adult learning?
    (d) Has the level and quality of qualified supervision been established?

4. *How can we determine whether these purposes are being attained?*
    (a) Is there an appropriate balance beween formative and summative assessment?
    (b) Are the assessment methods of a sufficient variety?
    (c) Are the submission dates for coursework realistic? For example, will the students have had sufficient time to complete assignments?
    (d) Is there an appropriate balance between formative and summative modes of curriculum evaluation, addressing both the processes and the outcomes of the course?
    (e) Is there evidence to suggest that curriculum development arises from curriculum evaluation?

    (Adapted from Pendleton, 1988)

If the above questions can be answered with confidence, validation and professional accreditation should be granted.

Summary

This chapter has focused on several key issues which need to be addressed when developing courses geared towards what is described as 'a new preparation for practice'. The conceptual framework chosen to discuss the issues comprised the initiation, development, implementation and evaluation phases of curriculum development, though it is worth stressing that the evaluation phase pervades throughout.

It is acknowledged that some colleges of nursing and midwifery have the means to respond creatively to the challenge which faces them, whereas others will be looking for more guidance. It is hoped that the manner in which some of the issues have been addressed in this chapter will provide some guidance for those 'wrestling' with curriculum development in the context of Project 2000. If that happens to be the case, the main purpose of this chapter will have been achieved.

References

Adelman, C. and Alexander, R. (1982). *The Self-evaluating Institution*. Methuen, London.

Beattie, A. (1987). Making a curriculum work. In *The Curriculum in Nursing Education*, P. Allan and M. Jolley (Eds), pp. 15–34. Croom Helm, London.

Bernstein, B. (1975). *Class, Codes and Control. Volume 3: Towards a Theory of Educational Transmission*. Routledge & Kegan Paul, London.

Bradshaw, G. (1972). The concept of social need. *New Society*, **19(496)**, 640–3.

Bruner, J. S. (1966). *Towards a Theory of Instruction*. Harvard University Press, Cambridge, Mass.

Council for National Academic Awards (1988). *Handbook*. CNAA, London.

English National Board for Nursing, Midwifery and Health Visiting (1987). *Managing Change in Nursing Education. Pack One: Preparing for Change*. ENB, London.

English National Board for Nursing, Midwifery and Health Visiting (1989). *Managing Change in Nursing Education. Pack Two: Workshop Materials for Action*. ENB, London.

Ewan, C. and White, R. (1984). *Teaching Nursing: a Self-instructional Handbook*. Croom Helm, London.

Further Education Curriculum Review and Development Unit (1982). *Curriculum Styles and Strategies*. The FEU, London.

Jenkins, D. and Shipman, M. (1976). *Curriculum: an introduction*. Open Books, London

Jones, R. M. (1975). Man: a course of study. In *Curriculum Design*, M. Golby, J. Greenwald and R. West (Eds), pp. 456–66. Croom Helm, London.

Kenworthy, N. and Nicklin, P. J. (1989). *Teaching and Assessing in Nursing Practice: an Experiential Approach*. Scutari, Harrow.

Keyzer, D. M. (1985). *Learning Contracts: the Trained Nurse and the Implementation of the Nursing Process*. PhD thesis, Institute of Education, University of London.

Knowles, M. (1984). *The Adult Learner: a Neglected Species*, 3rd edition. Gulf, Houston.

Levine, M. C. (1973). *An Introduction to Clinical Nursing*, 2nd edition. Davis, Philadelphia.

Myles, A. P. (1987). Psychology and the curriculum. In *The Curriculum in Nursing Education*, P. Allan and M. Jolley (Eds), pp. 56–84. Croom Helm, London.

Nixon, N. (1989). Unpublished seminar notes from a conference on validation in nursing held at the South Bank Polytechnic.

O'Connor, D. J. (1957). *An Introduction to the Philosophy of Education*. Routledge & Kegan Paul, London.

Pendleton, S. M. (1988). Unpublished paper on internal validation. Institute of Advanced Nursing Education, London.

Peters, R. S. (1966). *Ethics and Education*. Allen & Unwin, London.

Quinn, F. M. (1988). *The Principles and Practice of Nurse Education*, 2nd edition. Croom Helm, London.

Roy, C. (1976). *An Introduction to Nursing: an Adaptation Model*. Prentice-Hall, Englewood Cliffs.

Schofield, H. (1972). *The Philosophy of Education: an Introduction*. Allen & Unwin, London.

Sladden, S. (1985). The politics of progress. In *Proceedings of the 19th Annual Study of the Nursing Studies Association*, University of Edinburgh.

Steinaker, N. W. and Bell, M. R. (1979). *The Experiential Taxonomy: a New Approach to Teaching and Learning*. Academic Press, New York.

Torres, G. and Stanton, M. (1982). *Curriculum Process in Nursing*. Prentice-Hall, Englewood Cliffs.

Tyler, R. (1949). *Basic Principles of Curriculum and Instruction*. University of Chicago Press, Chicago.

Walker, A. (1989). Unpublished seminar notes from a conference on validation in nursing held at the South Bank Polytechnic.

Wells, J. A. C.(1987). Curriculum evaluation. In *The Curriculum in Nursing Education*, P. Allan and M. Jolley (Eds), pp. 176–208. Croom Helm, London.

5 Physiology – its significance in nursing care

Biological sciences in nursing

A great deal of knowledge, planning and anticipation is required for a nurse to even attempt to meet a patient's or potential patient's needs. People, according to their differing individual physical, mental and emotional capacities, adapt and respond differently to a variety of factors, including ageing, stress, and social and cultural influences. Superimposed on all of these factors are changes which occur in ill-health when there may be a reduction in an individual's ability to meet his or her own needs.

Having sufficient knowledge to anticipate and plan to meet needs requires in depth preparation of nurses whose task is further complicated by rapid advances in technology, and increasingly sophisticated methods of treatment and investigation. Patients turn to their nurses for help in understanding and coping with their experiences, and individualised patient care increases such expectations.

In the past most nursing practice was based on the assumption that 'health' could be defined as 'not being ill', and nursing aims were limited to recovery from illness or disease (Williams, 1989). Current concepts of health reflect a broader view and thus create a wider role for nursing. Indeed, not all 'patients' are ill. The pregnant woman, the developing child, the mentally handicapped adult are not ill in the conventional sense, neither do all ill patients recover.

Nursing knowledge will need to be adequate to define the problems, set appropriate goals and plan to meet them for people, sick or well, who need such help from nurses. So nursing can be said to help people manage their lives so that they achieve their individual optimum. However, there is considerable evidence that nurses lack sufficient understanding of the biological sciences for them to function effectively (Akinsanya, 1985). For example, if the nurse's instructions to a patient regarding a 24 hour urine sample omit the requirement to start the collection with an empty bladder, the period of collection may be greater than 24 hours, thus making a nonsense of the biochemical analysis.

The aim of this chapter is thus to encourage nurses to prescribe holistic care from an informed basis which requires a knowledge of the biological sciences. For example, a Health Visitor in her dealings with a child and its family needs to understand not only the physiology of child development but the influences of sociological and psychological factors. Without the physiological information, how would the Health Visitor know if milestones were being achieved normally?

Homeostasis

For an amoeba living in a pond life is relatively simple; the pond provides food and oxygen and accepts waste. It provides a medium for movement and reproduction but may also be a home for predators. Man (*Homo sapiens*) is not a single cell but a combination of some seventy five million million cells and we carry a 20 litre pond within us. Our cells are warm and metabolise quickly, thus having greater demands for food and oxygen and producing more waste. Our cells are highly specialised and less able to tolerate deficiencies or contamination of their surroundings. In short, the 'pond' is overcrowded and the problems of keeping it fit to live in are enormous, as we are not totally independent of our environment. Indeed, a large number of mechanisms co-operate to maintain the physical properties and chemical composition of the 'pond'. This condition of uniformity or balance is known as homeostasis. The study of human physiology is the study of the mechanisms that maintain homeostasis. Changes do occur but always within relatively narrow limits. To achieve this all body systems must play their part and they, in their turn, are subject to the control of the nervous and endocrine systems. Many of the observations which nurses make, for example recordings of blood pressure, temperature, pulse, respiration and urinary output, are to detect changes in homeostasis. In order to differentiate between normal and abnormal recordings nurses need to be able to use correctly any recording apparatus, and to know what is normal for the patient's gender, age, height and weight, otherwise significant failures of homeostasis may not be recognised. A knowledge as to what is normal is just as important with sophisticated electronic monitoring equipment, often used for critically ill patients, when changes in the patient's condition demand early recognition and intervention if the patient's condition is not to deteriorate irretrievably. It is of little use to record declining central venous pressures if no further action is taken.

The physical properties and chemical composition of 'our pond' may be changed by environmental factors. Drinking polluted water or breathing polluted air may have a considerable effect on normal function. Such environments may be encountered in the workplace and monitoring for possible environmental pollutants is part of the work of the occupational health nurse. Indeed, in addition to a wide knowledge of substances hazardous to health, the occupational health nurse regularly screens workers so that any change in, for example, lung function is detected early.

Respiratory system

Oxygen is required continuously by all body tissues for normal metabolism, during which carbon dioxide is made. As it would take almost three months for oxygen to diffuse from the atmosphere to cells deep within the body, some means of transporting the gases is required. The organs of the respiratory system (Fig. 5.1) include the nasal cavities, the pharynx, the larynx, trachea, bronchi, bronchioles

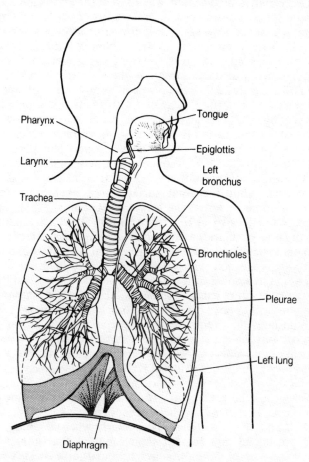

Fig. 5.1 The respiratory system (from Hinchliff *et al.*, 1989; p. 55).

and alveoli. The sites of gaseous exchange are the respiratory bronchioles and alveoli. All the other passages are fairly rigid tubes which warm, moisten, filter and finally conduct air to and then from the exchange sites. The bronchioles are lined with an epithelium which consists of ciliated cells and mucus-secreting goblet cells. Minute particles of dust become trapped in the mucus and are wafted up to the pharynx by the cilia and are then swallowed.

Repeated irritation of the ciliated epithelium, e.g. from atmospheric pollution, or frequent infections, may result in both an increase in and enlargement of (hypertrophy) the goblet cells. This results in an excessive amount of mucus being produced, such as occurs in patients with chronic bronchitis. If such individuals also smoke, cilia are paralysed and then destroyed by the cigarette smoke. Cigarette smoke is also an irritant. The only way to clear the excess mucus is by expectoration, i.e. the smoker's cough! Mucus can provide a breeding ground for bacteria, so affected individuals suffer from repeated chest infections requiring treatment with antibiotics. It can take up to ten years for the lungs to recover from the effects of cigarette smoking; better not to start in the first place!

The walls of the alveoli are composed of a single layer of epithelial cells and the external surface is covered with a network of pulmonary capillaries. Together the alveolar and capillary walls and their basement membranes form the respiratory membrane, which is only 0.5 microns thick, i.e. thinner than a sheet of paper. This allows rapid diffusion of gases. Patients with congested or oedematous lungs have a thickened respiratory membrane and diffusion of gases is slowed.

In a normal adult the total surface area of the respiratory membrane is some seventy square metres (Guyton, 1981). This is equivalent to the floor space of a room 30 ft by 25 ft. The amount of blood in the lung capillaries at any one instant is about 100 mls, so it is easy to understand how diffusion of gases can normally be so rapid. However, lungs clogged with infected mucus as in bronchitis, or exudate, as in pneumonia, will impair gaseous exchange, as diffusion through the layers of mucus or exudate will take longer than normal. Such patients will appear breathless. To achieve adequate gaseous exchange an individual requires 1 sq.metre of lung tissue for every kilogram of body weight (Gould,1989). Loss of respiratory surface, as occurs in emphysema, or obstruction of air passages that lead to the respiratory membranes will also lead to breathlessness.

Consider Joe, aged 56 years. Joe has a wife and two daughters, both married, and he runs a pub. He has smoked heavily for many years and has a persistent cough. A recent cold has left him feeling very unwell and very breathless, particularly when climbing stairs. His wife persuaded him to visit their General Practitioner, who prescribed a course of antibiotics and arranged for a chest X-ray.

- What is the cause of Joe's breathlessness?
- Why has the General Practitioner prescribed antibiotics?

Until about 30 years ago the X-ray was the only means of extracting pictorial information from a living body. Joe was not alarmed at the thought of an X-ray but was perturbed when asked to return to the department two days later for a 'scan'.

- Could you answer Joe's question, 'What is a scan?'

His GP explained that since the 1950s a variety of scanning techniques have become available, ranging from the use of ultra-sound to magnetic resonance imaging (MRI). In computerised axial tomography (CAT) a special type of X-ray equipment is required. The patient is put on to a 'table' which moves slowly through the machine. The X-ray source rotates around the patient sending beams from all directions to a specific predetermined level in the patient's body. Different tissues absorb the X-rays in varying amounts. The machine's computer integrates all the information and produces it as a cross-sectional image of the particular body region that was scanned.

- Joe asks 'Will it hurt?' What is your reply?

MRI uses a different type of radiation. The patient is placed within a machine that produces a strong magnetic field. The hydrogen atoms of water molecules, present in all body tissues, are affected by the magnetic field. The energy released by the movement of the hydrogen atoms is translated by a computer into a visual image.

Joe seemed relieved that he was to have a CAT scan, but unfortunately the presence of a bronchial carcinoma was revealed and his admission to hospital was arranged.

- Why has Joe's breathlessness persisted even though his infection has resolved?

The respiratory system supplies the body with oxygen and rids it of carbon dioxide. For this to happen the lungs must be ventilated with air, and gaseous exchange between the alveoli and blood, and the blood and the tissues must occur. Thus the respiratory and circulatory systems are interdependent, and if either system fails the body's cells will be deprived of oxygen. To aid diffusion in normal alveoli a substance called surfactant is secreted. This acts like a detergent and reduces surface tension, making it easier for alveoli to expand. Premature babies with their immature lungs lack surfactant and thus have to work harder at breathing, and may suffer from 'respiratory distress'.

- How could such babies be helped to breathe?
- What extra problems would be created if a premature baby is nursed in an incubator?

The 'work' of breathing, i.e. pulmonary ventilation, is a completely mechanical process that depends on volume changes occurring within the thorax. Contraction of the diaphragm increases the vertical diameter (height) of the thoracic cavity. Contraction of the intercostal muscles raises the ribs and sternum thereby increasing the diameter of the chest from front to back and from side to side. This is sufficient to increase the volume of the thorax by half a litre. The pressure inside the thorax falls and air rushes in. Volume changes lead to pressure changes (Boyle's Law) which lead to a flow of gases to equalise the pressure (Marieb, 1989). Sitting a patient upright allows the diaphragm to descend even further, as the abdominal contents fall away, thus allowing an even deeper breath. If pulmonary ventilation equals tidal volume × respiratory rate, and the difference in tidal volume (Fig. 5.2) between sitting and lying is some 150 mls, then pulmonary ventilation can be maintained with a decrease in respiratory rate. Hence propping patients upright will reduce the effort of breathing.

Healthy lungs are easily stretched and the ease with which they are distended is known as compliance. Compliance is reduced if fibrous changes occur in the lungs or the rib cage becomes less flexible, which is common in old age. Distending the lungs is important in inspiration.

- What are the effects of reduced compliance?

Elastic recoil is important in expiration. Individuals with emphysema have lungs which are progressively less elastic and more fibrotic. This change hinders both inspiration and expiration. However, loss of elastic recoil means that muscle activity is now required for expiration and breathing becomes more laboured. Indeed, a considerable amount of energy may be required, some 15–20% of the total energy supply instead of the 5% healthy individuals use for breathing (Marieb, 1989). Patients with chronic respiratory disorders may use a large amount of their energy just for breathing. Activities normally taken for granted such as cleaning one's teeth, or washing one's face and hands, may leave these patients gasping for breath and in need of assistance with previously simple tasks.

The amount of air entering and leaving the lungs depends on a variety of factors. Thus a number of different respiratory volumes can be described (Fig. 5.2). As lung volumes and capacities are often abnormal in people with pulmonary diseases a number of devices have been designed for their measurement. Lung function tests may demonstrate the reduction in vital capacity that occurs with restrictive

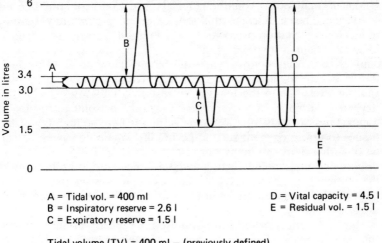

A = Tidal vol. = 400 ml
B = Inspiratory reserve = 2.6 l
C = Expiratory reserve = 1.5 l

D = Vital capacity = 4.5 l
E = Residual vol. = 1.5 l

Tidal volume (TV) = 400 ml – (previously defined)

Inspiratory reserve = 2.6 litres (amount which can be inhaled after a normal, quiet inspiration).

Expiratory reserve = 1.5 litres (amount which can be exhaled after a normal, quiet expiration).

Vital capacity = T.V. + inspiratory reserve + expiratory reserve = 4.5 litres (maximum amount of air that can be inspired after a forced expiration).

Residual volume = 1.5 litres (volume which can never be emptied from the lungs, i.e. all fresh air breathed in mixes with deoxygenated air before gaseous exchange takes place).

Fig. 5.2 Lung volumes.

lung diseases or the difficulty in expiration that occurs in obstructive airways disease.

- What intructions would you give a patient when using a peak flow metre?
- What factors influence peak flow?

Gaseous exchange between the alveoli and blood and between the blood and the tissues, depends on diffusion and the partial pressure gradients of oxygen (O_2) and carbon dioxide (CO_2) that exist on either side of the exchange membrane (see Fig. 5.3). Most oxygen is carried in the blood bound to haemoglobin, a process that is both rapid and reversible.

$$H \cdot Hb + O_2 \underset{tissues}{\overset{lungs}{\rightleftharpoons}} HbO_2$$

reduced haemoglobin   oxyhaemoglobin

Under normal resting conditions a 100 ml of blood contains 19.7 ml of oxygen. Thus a shortage of blood, i.e. haemoglobin, may result in reduced oxygenation (hypoxia), a condition known as anaemic hypoxia. Stagnant hypoxia is the result of impaired circulation, e.g. congestive cardiac failure, when the blood's slow progress through the tissues means much of its oxygen is given up. Interference with gaseous exchange in the lungs as in respiratory diseases, or lack of oxygen to breathe as in carbon monoxide poisoning, results in hypoxic hypoxia. Histotoxic anoxia is the result of an inability of the tissues to utilise oxygen, such as occurs in cyanide poisoning. It can be seen that there are many causes of breathlessness other than lung disease and that one needs to understand the cause in order to meet the patient's need for oxygen. For example, giving oxygen to a patient who is bleeding is akin to shutting the stable door after the horse has bolted.

Some breathless patients are cyanosed. Cyanosis, a bluish tinge to the skin, appears when more than 5 g of haemoglobin per 100 ml of blood is deoxygenated. Thus, by definition, a severely anaemic individual with a haemoglobin level of less than 5 g per 100 ml of blood will not appear cyanosed even when moribund. Carbon monoxide poisoning produces a cherry-red haemoglobin and again, although deficient in oxygen, such patients are not cyanosed. However, chronic lung diseases, such as chronic bronchitis and emphysema, which cause heart failure (cor pulmonale) result in both stagnant and hypoxic hypoxia. This combination is the cause of both severe breathlessness and cyanosis. Patients affected in this way are unable to carry out even the most basic activities of daily living without severe distress.

A considerable number of skills are required by the nurse to minimise the distress and maximise the patient's capabilities.

● With what activities of living will this patient require help?

The control of ventilation is complex. The basic pattern of inspiration followed by expiration is generated by the activity of neurones in the brainstem (medulla oblongata) and midbrain (pons). The pace-setting group of neurones within the medulla is known as the inspiratory centre. Nerve impulses pass from the inspiratory centre via the phrenic (cervical 3, 4 and 5) and intercostal nerves to the diaphragm and intercostal muscles which then contract. High spinal injuries, i.e. in the cervical region, may result not only in quadriplegia but also in respiratory paralysis. Artificial ventilation may be required.

When the discharge of impulses from the inspiratory centre stops, the diaphragm and intercostal muscles relax, the lungs recoil and air is breathed out. Other respiratory centres present in the midbrain, cerebral cortical activity and stretch receptors present in the lungs can all modify the activity of the inspiratory centre. Modifications include talking, laughing and singing or playing a wind instrument. Some modifications are protective, for example coughing. However, medullary activity can be depressed by morphine or suppressed by a barbiturate and/or alcohol overdose. Respiration will be adversely affected or may even stop altogether. The rate and depth of respiration can also be influenced by pulmonary irritant reflexes, for example irritation of the nasal mucosa promotes sneezing. The higher centres, as already mentioned, can modify the inspiratory centre pattern to allow singing or speech, and during swallowing breath control is extremely important if food and/or drink is not to be inhaled. However, these controls are limited and the inspiratory centre will ignore messages from the cerebral cortex if carbon dioxide levels in the blood rise above a critical level. Indeed, chemical factors, i.e. levels of oxygen, carbon dioxide and hydrogen ions, are the most important influences on repiratory rate and depth.

Special receptors, known as chemoreceptors, are present in the medulla oblongata, the aorta and the carotid arteries. Increasing levels of carbon dioxide normally excite the central medullary receptors, which influence the inspiratory centre, and brings about an increase in pulmonary ventilation. However, very high levels of carbon dioxide have a sedative effect on the brain and may even decrease ventilation.

One group of patients who are at risk from carbon dioxide retention are those recovering from anaesthesia. For this reason they should be encouraged to take deep breaths periodically. Cells sensitive to oxygen levels are present in the peripheral (carotid and aortic) chemoreceptors. However, arterial oxygen levels must drop substantially before acting as a stimulus to ventilation. If medullary receptor activity is depressed by anoxia, then the peripheral chemo-receptors act as a back up and ventilation is maintained. Individuals with respiratory diseases, for example chronic bronchitis and/or emphysema, who have permanently elevated levels of carbon dioxide become unresponsive to it as a ventilatory stimulus. It is the low oxygen levels stimulating the peripheral receptors which provide the respiratory or 'anoxic' drive. Giving 100 per cent oxygen to such patients would remove the respiratory stimulus of low oxygen levels and ventilation would cease. It is for this reason that these patients are prescribed a mixture of oxygen with air, i.e. 24, 28 or 32 per cent.

● What are the other hazards of giving oxygen to patients?

Remember Joe – Joe's breathlessness is the result of his lung cancer. Cancer is currently the second major cause of death in the United Kingdom. Unfortunately lung cancer has a low cure rate, as most cases are not diagnosed until they are well advanced. Almost 90 per cent of lung cancer patients, like Joe, were smokers. Not only does the continuous irritation of tobacco smoke promote an increase in mucus and depress the activity of cilia, but there are some 15 carcinogens present in cigarette smoke that may result in a cancerous change.

• What then are the responsibilities of the nurse towards (a) patients, and (b) other individuals who smoke?

The most effective treatment for cancer is removal of the affected tissue, i.e. surgery, but in many cases, as indeed for Joe, radiation and/or chemotherapy may be the only available options. For a patient who is already breathless, the side effects of either radio- or chemotherapy may be even more distressing than usual.

• What are the common side effects of radiotherapy?
• What nursing care will Joe require during this difficult time?

Circulatory system

The respiratory system ensures the blood is oxygenated but the oxygenated blood has to be carried to the tissues, so that the co-operation of the cardiovascular system is vital. Blood leaves the left side of the heart (Fig. 5.3) and then passes into arteries. The arteries branch repeatedly until they become capillaries with walls only one cell thick. It is across the walls of the capillaries that gaseous exchange (tissue respiration) takes place. Oxygen deficient, carbon dioxide rich blood leaves the tissues and travels through progressively larger veins until it reaches the right atrium. From the right side of the heart blood is pumped to the lungs and returns to the left atrium, thus starting its journey again.

Among all the body's tissues, blood is unique because it is a fluid. It accounts for some 8 per cent of the body weight, i.e. 5–6 litres in males and 4–5 in females. Forty-five per cent of blood, i.e. the packed cell volume or haematocrit, is made up of cells and the remaining 55 per cent is plasma. When patients are prescribed packed cells for transfusion, much of the plasma has been removed. Plasma is 90 per cent water and contains many different solutes, for example proteins, nutrients, hormones, waste products, electrolytes and enzymes. Albumin the most abundant of the proteins is made in the liver, and is the major contributor to plasma osmotic pressure. It is this pressure which helps to draw tissue fluid back into the bloodstream. Lack of plasma albumin, as occurs in liver disease, or loss from severe burns, may result in oedema.

• What are the potential problems of a patient with oedema of the sacrum and lower limbs?

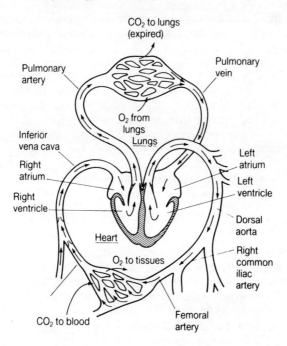

Fig. 5.3 Heart and circulation (from Hinchliff *et al.*, 1989; p. 54).

Red cells or erythrocytes are little more than membrane bags filled with haemoglobin. They have an average life of 120 days and are then destroyed by macrophages in the liver and spleen. This process is known as haemolysis

Excess haemolysis due to faulty 'bags' or abnormal haemoglobin will result in haemolytic anaemia.

● What would be the actual and potential problems of a patient with haemolytic anaemia?

Blood formation, or erythropoiesis, occurs mainly in the red bone marrow of flat bones, for example ribs, sternum or pelvis. The number of red cells in an individual reflects the balance between haemolysis and erythropoiesis. Too many red cells result in a condition known as polycythaemia, too few result in anaemia. The direct stimulus for red cell production is a hormone known as erythropoietin. Hypoxia brings about an increase in the production of erythropoietin by the kidney. Individuals suffering from chronic lung diseases which give rise to hypoxia are likely to develop polycythaemia. The increased number of red cells increases the viscosity of the blood throwing yet further strain onto the heart. Such patients may benefit from frequent 'blood letting'. Individuals with kidney disease may suffer from a lack of erythropoietin and thus develop anaemia (Lote, 1982). This is an added complication to an already distressing condition.

The requirements for normal erythropoiesis include protein, iron, vitamin B_{12} and folic acid. Iron is obtained from the diet and iron absorption from the intestine is carefully controlled. Hence increasing the intake does not necessarily increase the uptake and consequently patients taking oral iron preparations may have black faeces. As 65 per cent of the body's iron is present in haemoglobin, any loss of blood means loss of iron from the body, for example bleeding peptic ulcers, excessive menstrual loss (menorrhagia). Thus iron deficiency anaemia may result from an inadequate intake, malabsorption, or haemorrhagic loss.

- What groups of people are most at risk from developing iron deficiency anaemia?

Vitamin B_{12}, present in green leafy vegetables, is absorbed by the distal part of the small intestine after it has complexed with intrinsic factor secreted by cells in the stomach lining. Lack of intrinsic factor, for example following gastrectomy or following formation of an ileostomy in which the terminal ileum was removed, may result in pernicious anaemia. For these patients vitamin B_{12} is given monthly, by injection, for the rest of their lives.

- How would you explain to a patient why such injections are necessary?

Although white blood cells are less numerous than red cells, they are crucial to the body's defences. There are several types of white cells and they are classified according to the size and complexity of their nucleus, and the type of granules in their cytoplasm (Fig. 5.4). Neutrophils form half of the white cell population, they are active phagocytes and are particularly partial to bacteria. They can leave blood vessels by a process known as diapedesis and move to areas of tissue damage and infection. Indeed, neutrophil numbers increase enormously during acute infections. A collection of tissue fluid, dead and dying white cells and bacteria is known as pus.

- What precautions should a nurse take when dealing with a suppurating wound, i.e. discharging pus?

Basophils are the least numerous of the white cells. Those present in the tissues are known as mast cells. If the basophil/mast cell binds to a particular antibody (immunoglobulin E) granules present in the cytoplasm release histamine and heparin. Histamine causes blood vessels to dilate and become 'leaky', i.e. tissue fluid escapes in large quantities. Heparin prevents clotting. Both chemicals enhance the migration of white cells to an inflamed area. Eosinophils are also

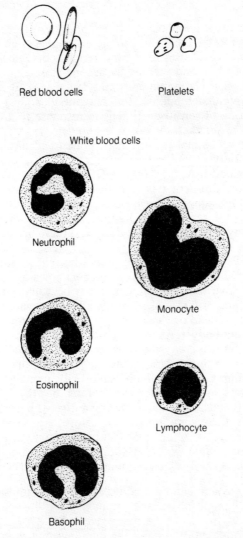

Fig. 5.4 Types of blood cells (from Hinchliff *et al.*, 1989; p. 53).

phagocytic but appear to ingest foreign proteins and immune complexes, rather than bacteria. Granulocytes – neutrophils, basophils and eosinophils – are produced in the bone marrow. Radiation and cytotoxic drugs reduce the number of granulocytes, leaving the patient prey to infection. For their protection such patients are nursed in isolation, i.e. reversed barrier nursing.

- What are the actual and potential problems of a patient nursed in isolation?

Agranulocytes – lymphocytes and monocytes – lack cytoplasmic granules. Monocytes are highly mobile macrophages and are particularly active in chronic infections, for example tuberculosis and certain viral infections. Lymphocytes are the second most common white cell and play a crucial role in immunity. B lymphocytes (B cells) produce antibodies (immunoglobulins). Immunoglobulins (Igs) are secreted by the offspring of sensitised B cells in response to an antigen. As there are large numbers of possible antigens, for example foreign proteins such as animal fur and hair, pollen and dusts, there is an enormous variety of antibodies, but they can be grouped into five classes designated IgA, IgD, IgM, IgG and IgE. To give an analogy, there are many different types of flowers but they can be grouped into classes, for example daisies, heathers, roses, orchids, all of which are obviously different from each other but all are flowers. Similarly there are many different types of daisy and there are many different types of each Ig class.

When B cells encounter an antigen they become plasma cells which start to produce antibodies (Igs), a process known as active humoral immunity. Active humoral immunity can be gained naturally, i.e. during infections, or provoked artificially as in vaccination. Most vaccines contain dead or weakened pathogenic organisms which can provoke an antibody response but not cause the disease. Passive humoral immunity is conferred when an individual receives 'donated' antibodies; for example a foetus via the placenta, or an injection of gamma globulin. Gamma globulin can provide immediate protection against diseases such as rabies and tetanus, but the effect is short-lived. Some B cells, after encountering antigens, become long-lived memory cells. If, at some time in the future, a particular antigen is again encountered, memory cells can bring about the production of antibodies almost immediately. Building up a good supply of memory cells is the purpose of staged immunisation and boosters.

- Whooping cough can kill and occasionally immunisation against whooping cough has caused 'brain damage' in young children. How would you reconcile these facts when giving advice to an anxious young mother about the immunisation of her child?

There are four main types of T lymphocytes (T cells); namely T killer cells, T helper cells, T suppressor cells, and delayed hypersensitivity T cells (Marieb, 1989). Killer cells can directly attack and lyse cells that are cancerous or contain viruses. Helper cells are regulatory and stimulate the proliferation of both T and B cells. Without helper cells there is no immune response. The Human Immunodeficiency Virus (HIV) specifically targets and enters helper cells. The cell is then made to produce more virus particles which then break open the helper cell and seek out others; thus virus particles increase and helper cells are destroyed. This results in a depression of both cell-mediated immunity and humoral immunity, i.e. antibody production. Individuals who develop full-blown AIDS (acquired immune defiency syndrome) do so because they have little or no resistance to infection. Gastrointestinal infections and pneumocystis carinii pneumonia (PCP) are common. Additionally, they are unable to deal with viruses or malignant cells and thus a malignancy of the skin known as Kaposi's sarcoma is also common. Treatment of such individuals is not only aimed at ridding them of infection, for example PCP, but preventing other opportunistic infections occurring. It is for *this* reason that isolation techniques may be required, i.e. to protect the *patient*.

Suppressor cells are also regulatory and, by releasing lymphokines, 'switch off' the immune response when no longer needed. In people with AIDS suppressor cell activity is increased, further limiting T and B cell function.

The immune system protects us from a wide variety of pathogenic organisms and abnormal body cells. Children born without either a T or B cell system suffer from severe combined immune deficiency (SCID). In the past, such children were kept isolated in 'bubbles'. More recently, bone marrow transplants have been carried out to overcome this deficiency. However, unless the marrow is carefully matched to the tissue type of the recipient, the transplanted T cells would mount an attack on their new host (graft versus host disease). New techniques use monoclonal antibodies to remove mature T cells from the donated marrow leaving only the immature marrow stem cells. This makes the donated marrow more compatible.

- What do you understand by the term 'rejection' in the context of organ transplants?
- What drugs may be used to prevent the rejection process?

On occasion the immune system's ability to recognise 'self' as opposed to foreign antigens is lost. The body then produces antibodies and sensitised T cells against tissue no longer recognised as self and destroys it. Such autoimmune diseases include rheumatoid arthritis, Hashimoto's thyroiditis, and possibly multiple sclerosis.

T cell responsiveness is depressed by stress. Indeed, one of the first psychoimmunological studies of humans stemmed from findings that recently bereaved people are far more likely to become ill or die. One study, involving men whose wives had died of breast cancer, demonstrated that T cell responsiveness declined significantly within the month following their wives' deaths, and in some cases remained low for up to a year thereafter (Schleifer *et al.*, 1979, cited Atkinson *et al.*, 1987). One of the interesting findings from animal experiments is that psychological stress does not always have detrimental effects; sometimes it actually increases an animal's resistance to disease. Why this should happen remains unclear but one factor that appears to be important is the extent to which an individual can control the stress by behaving differently. For instance rats that cannot turn off electric shocks develop stomach ulcers at three times the rate of rats that can turn off shocks (Martin, 1987). Further, only 27 per cent of rats subjected to shocks that could not be turned off, rejected implanted tumour cells, but 63 per cent of rats who could turn off shocks rejected implanted tumour cells (Martin, 1987). As the responsiveness of T cells is reduced in rats which have no adrenal glands, it cannot just be the effects of corticosteroids. Thus stressful events resulted in suppressed immune responses in rats, particularly those rats which were unable to control their level of stress. This is also true of humans; for example people who experienced many negative life events, but did not react adversely to them, had high levels of T cells. People who did not 'cope' had a low T cell activity, particularly T killer cells (Martin, 1987).

● In the context of the above information, which individuals may be most at risk from the harmful effects of stress?

● How may a nurse advise or assist in the management of stress?

Interactions between the brain and the immune system are very complex, but the study of psychoimmunology is developing rapidly. In future it may be possible for people to 'manage' their stress better and thus to avoid many of the stress related diseases. Community nurses may need to include advice on stress management as part of health screening.

The third 'cell' type present in blood is a thrombocyte (platelet). Thrombocytes are fragments of a large cell known as a megakaryocyte. Platelets have a major role in haemostasis (a) by forming a plug that temporarily seals the broken vessel; and (b) by orchestrating events that lead to the formation of a clot. If a blood vessel is damaged and the underlying collagen exposed, platelets swell, become sticky and adhere to the area. Once attached, chemicals such as 5 hydroxytryptamine (5.HT) and thromboxane A2, a prostaglandin derivative, are released. These chemicals cause vascular spasm that, together with the platelet plug, seals the vessel. Aspirin inhibits prostaglandin release and thus reduces clot formation. Small daily doses of aspirin may be prescribed for certain individuals to reduce the risk of cerebral thrombolic episodes.

For blood to clot successfully a complex known as prothrombin activator must be formed. If any of the factors, such as factor VIII (antihaemophiliac globulin), required for the production of prothrombin activator are not available, then the production of a clot is impossible. Prothrombin activator, once formed, acts on a plasma protein, i.e. prothrombin, changing it to thrombin. Thrombin then catalyses the change of another plasma protein i.e. fibrinogen to fibrin. It is the fibrin meshwork which is the basis of a clot. Smoking is known to increase platelet stickiness which may increase the risk of thrombus formation. It is for this reason that many cardiac surgeons expect their patients to give up smoking.

The blood is circulated through the body by the pumping action of the heart. Approximately the size of a human fist and weighing less than a pound, the heart lies within the mediastinum. It is enclosed in a double sac of serous membrane known as the pericardium. The myocardium, composed mainly of cardiac muscle, forms the bulk of the heart, whilst the endocardium lines the heart. Valves between the atria and ventricles, and ventricles and great vessels, ensure that blood only travels in one direction. The heart, like any pump, can function with 'leaky' valves provided the malfunction is not too great. Severe valve deformities increase the workload of the heart and may cause it to fail.

The blood supply of the heart is provided by the coronary arteries. Blockage of a coronary artery by atheroma and/or thrombus will deprive the heart muscle, supplied by the artery, of oxygen. In some individuals insufficient oxygen may be available to the heart muscle during exercise, giving rise to the ischaemic pain of angina pectoris. Such individuals may benefit from coronary artery vasodilating drugs such as glyceryl trinitrate to improve oxygenation and thus relieve pain. Coronary by-pass surgery in effect provides new channels for blood to reach the myocardium, i.e. the obstruction is by-passed.

The ability of cardiac muscle to depolarise and contract is inherent. The conduction system consists of specialised cardiac cells that initiate and distribute impulses through the heart, causing the myocardium to depolarise and contract in a sequential manner from atria to ventricles (Fig. 5.5). External nerve stimulation is not required for cardiac contraction but the autonomic nervous system slows or accelerates the heart as necessary. For some patients external nerve stimulation, i.e. a 'pacemaker', is fitted because the normal conducting pathways have been damaged by disease processes.

Body fluids are good conductors of electricity so the electrical currents (depolarisation/repolarisation) generated and transmitted through the heart, also spread through the body. The electrical currents can be monitored, amplified and recorded by the electrocardiograph (ECG).

Consider Henry. Henry is 48-years-old and lives with his wife and two daughters in a London suburb. He is the managing director of a small firm with offices in London and Manchester. He has been fit and well, although slightly overweight, and drinks and smokes moderately. One evening, after entertaining an important client,

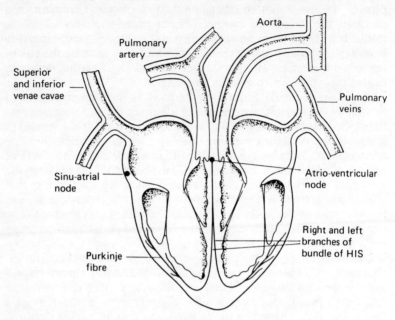

Diagram to show specialized conduction system of the heart

Fig. 5.5 Conduction system of the heart.

Henry collapsed. On arrival at hospital Henry had severe chest pain radiating down his left arm. A myocardial infarction was diagnosed and Henry was transferred to the coronary care unit.

Currently some 25 per cent of all deaths in England and Wales are due to coronary heart disease. Atheromatous plaques form in the coronary vessels which become progressively narrowed. The flow of blood through such vessels is impaired and may even cease if clot formation occurs, i.e. a coronary thrombosis. Atheroma formation is accelerated by inactivity, stress and smoking. Diet is also implicated and there is some agreement that a reduction of animal fats and salt in the diet lessens the risk (COMA, 1984). If the heart is seriously weakened or damaged, such as after an infarction, the cardiac output may be maintained by an increase in heart rate. Thus to avoid throwing even further strain on to the damaged heart, patients like Henry are initially nursed at rest, and the heart's activity monitored.

- With which activities of living will Henry need help in order to provide him (and his heart) with as much rest as possible?
- What psychological support will Henry and his wife and family need?
- What are the possible complications of myocardial infarction, and how may the nurse minimise the risk of their occurrence?

The key to prevention of death from myocardial infarction is to identify those at risk. However, as with Henry, often a heart attack is the first sign of disease. If used early enough, i.e. within six hours, enzymes such as streptokinase, a thrombolytic agent, can be used to dissolve thromboses. Blocking the sympathetic nervous system stimulation of the heart with drugs such as beta adrenergic blockers, for example propanolol, can reduce the strain on a damaged heart by reducing tachycardia. For individuals who have suffered a massive myocardial infarction, a heart transplant may hold out some hope. However, as yet such surgery and the use of artificial hearts has not been very successful. In the USA 'autotransplants' involving use of the patient's own skeletal muscle to 'patch up' the heart have met with some success. A pace-maker is attached to the muscle patch causing it to contract in synchrony with the cardiac muscle.

Such heroics were not necessary for Henry who made an uneventful recovery and returned home six days after his admission. At present the best course of action seems to be preventative, i.e. to practise healthy eating, avoid smoking and to exercise regularly, and Henry decided, with his wife's approval, to give up smoking. Given the warning that his attack had provided and heeding the advice of his nurses and doctors, Henry vowed to change his lifestyle.

- Given the short hospital stay, how may patients like Henry be educated effectively with regard to their health?

Gastro-intestinal system

Food provides the body's energy which is produced during tissue respiration. The digestive system takes in food, changes it to a form the body can use and then gets rid of the indigestible remains. During digestion foods are broken down into progressively less complex substances which are then absorbed.

The mouth is the point of food entry into the gastrointestinal tract. Mastication begins the mechanical breakdown of food and the digestion of starches is begun. Saliva, with which the food is mixed, is largely water but also contains the enzyme, salivary amylase, and several proteins, for example mucin, IgA and a growth factor. The latter is also found in the saliva of many animals and may aid the healing of licked wounds. Saliva is secreted continuously in small amounts which increase enormously when food enters the mouth. Irritation of the lower gastrointestinal tract, particularly when accompanied by feelings of nausea, also increases salivation.

The stomach furthers the chemical and mechanical breakdown of food and then delivers the resulting chyme to the small intestine. The stomach usually empties completely within four hours after a meal, but the rate of emptying is highly variable. Stress and anxiety delay gastric emptying – traffic accident victims may still have food in the stomach up to ten hours after eating. Fat also delays gastric empty-ing, as the presence of fat in the stomach brings about the release of the hormone enterogastrone which inhibits gastric motility. It is for this reason that patients with peptic ulcers used to be prescribed a bland low fat diet. Such measures have been superceded by the new generation of drugs, for example cimetidine. For an individual who has little appetite a pre-prandial glass of sherry may be the answer. The sherry promotes the release of the hormone gastrin which brings about the release of hydrochloric acid and enzymes which aid digestion. Most of the chemical digestion occurs in the small in-testine; enzymes from the pancreas and bile from the liver aid the process. Some ten litres of gastrointestinal secretions are produced every day, but only 5–10 per cent reaches the large intestine. For an individual with a small bowel obstruction, much of the fluid will be lost by vomiting as it cannot be absorbed. Such fluid and electrolyte loss would cause severe dehydration if not treated.

Most nutrients are absorbed through the intestinal villi into capilla-ries and are then transported to the liver via the portal system. In new born infants intact proteins may be 'absorbed' by a process, similar to phagocytosis, known as endocytosis. The baby's immune system 'recognises' the protein as antigenic and mounts an 'attack'. This accounts for the food allergy of babies weaned too early.

The large intestine is primarily concerned with propulsion, absorp-tion of water and salts, and defaecation. Colon peristalsis is very sluggish. Roughage, or fibre, in the diet increases the strength of colon contractions and physically holds water molecules, thus soften-ing the faeces. One of the best ways of avoiding constipation is to eat a diet high in fibre, i.e. plant products. If the volume of residue is small, the colon narrows and its contractions become more powerful, increasing the pressure on the colon wall. This increase in pressure may force the lining of the colon (mucosa) between the muscle fibres creating little pouches of mucosa, i.e. diverticuli. If the diverticuli become inflamed, a conditon known as diverticulitis, the patient will experience pain on the left side of the abdomen. Abscess formation may lead to perforation of the colon and peritonitis, all of which can be avoided with a high fibre diet. During old age gastrointestinal activity declines, fewer digestive juices are produced, absorption is less efficient and peristalsis slows. No wonder that most patients with diverticular disease are elderly. Additionally, taste and smell are less acute and thus eating may become less appealing. For the elderly patients in hospital, in the absence of other diversions, mealtimes become the highlight of their day. Providing both tasty and nutritious meals that are high in fibre may tax the ingenuity of the nurse.

Low income groups may have difficulty in providing themselves with a balanced diet. Lack of time and/or education may also give rise to problems. Nurses need to be able to recognise when professional dietetic help may be required.

Some nutrients are used to build cell structures or replace worn ones but many are used as metabolic fuel. To provide fuel nutrients are metabolised and adenosine triphosphate (ATP) is produced, the substance used by cells to power their many and varied activities. However, without vitamins, all the carbohydrates, fat and protein we eat would be useless. Most vitamins function as co-enzymes. Co-enzymes act in concert with an enzyme to catalyse a particular reaction. For example, the B vitamins are all co-enzymes and most are involved in the oxidation of glucose for energy, although vitamin B_6 (pyridoxine) is also required for the formation of antibodies. Although an adequate intake of vitamins is essential for normal function, it can be dangerous if the intake is excessive; for example the fat soluble vitamins A, D, E and K are all stored in the liver. A high dose of vitamin supplements, not actually required by the body, could have detrimental effects on liver function, and is not to be recommended. Water soluble vitamins, B and C, are excreted in the urine and thus rapidly lost from the body. Most Western governments have published recommended daily requirements and these figures should be consulted before going to the expense of purchasing costly vitamin supplements which may be unnecessary or even harmful.

Once inside body cells, nutrients are involved in a variety of biochemical reactions known collectively as metabolism. Glucose is the major fuel molecule of ATP production. It can enter body cells by facilitated diffusion, a process that is enhanced by insulin. In the absence of insulin glucose accumulates in the blood, a condition known as hyperglycaemia. Neurones are freely permeable to glucose and are thus particularly vulnerable to changes in blood glucose levels. Hence the neurological changes, i.e. coma, that occur with hyper- or hypoglycaemia. In the condition known as diabetes mellitus there is either a deficiency of or an inability to utilise insulin. Glucose accumulates in the blood, fat oxidation is disrupted and metabolites known as ketones are produced. Ketones are organic acids and when present in the blood in large quantities cause metabolic acidosis. The body cannot excrete ketones quickly, hence the build up continues. One of the ketones, acetone, is vapourised from the lungs and such patients may have a smell of 'pear-drops' on their breath. The acid nature of the blood depresses nervous system activity even further and patients with hyperglycaemia and ketoacidosis require urgent treatment.

Individuals with insulin dependent diabetes mellitus have to balance calorie intake and energy output against their insulin injections. Failure to do so may result in a sudden severe reduction of blood sugar (hypoglycaemia) which could prove fatal. Insufficient insulin or an excessive calorie intake will lead to hyperglycaemia and ketoacidosis, which takes longer to develop but may also prove fatal. In addition to learning about diet and how to inject insulin, patients must learn how to test their urine, how to recognise the onset of hypoglycaemia and to manage their lives in order to maintain a reasonably stable blood-sugar level. Nurses can play a crucial role in both teaching and supporting patients.

- What are the long term effects of diabetes?
- What is the role of the nurse in detecting such complications?

Before amino acids are oxidised for energy their amine (NH_2) group is removed. In the liver the amine groups are combined with carbon dioxide to form urea which is then execreted by the kidneys.

When energy intake and output are in balance, body weight remains stable. If energy intake exceeds output, obesity will result. Current theories of eating behaviour relate to four factors; namely total energy stores, hormones, body temperature and psychological factors (Marieb, 1989). As yet there is no magical solution to obesity other than to reduce the calorific intake and/or increase the energy output, or, more simply, eat less and exercise more. Considerable interpersonal skills, as well as dietary expertise, are required if people are to be persuaded to adopt healthy eating habits.

Renal system

The kidneys play a major role in eliminating nitrogenous waste, toxins and drugs from the body. In addition to these excretory functions, it is the kidneys which maintain the pH and salt and water balance of the body. As mentioned earlier (p. 129) the kidneys produce erythropoietin. The kidneys also produce renin, which is involved in the regulation of blood pressure, and 1,25 dihydroxycholecalciferol which is involved in calcium and phosphate regulation. As can be imagined, an individual with end-stage renal failure has many signs and symptoms, for example hypertension and anaemia, as a result.

The kidneys have a very rich blood supply and normally receive almost 25 per cent of the cardiac output every minute. Each kidney contains over one million nephrons. It is the nephrons, the functional units of the kidney, that produce urine (Fig. 5.6). Each nephron consists of a tuft of capillaries known as the glomerulus which is enclosed by a blind-ending, cup-shaped Bowman's capsule. The glomerulus is extremely permeable, as is the Bowman's capsule, and virtually all substances, except blood cells and plasma proteins, can pass into the lumen of the Bowman's capsule (Lote, 1982). The proximal convoluted tubule contains 'deproteinized' plasma which

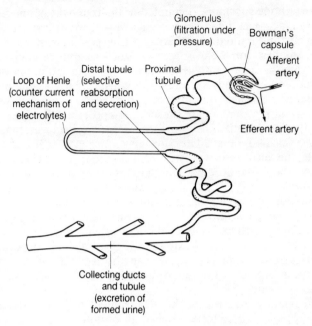

Fig. 5.6 Structure of a nephron (from Hinchliff *et al.*, 1989; p. 60).

has been filtered from the blood. The remainder of the nephron, i.e. loop of Henle and distal convoluted tubule, then reabsorbs much of the filtrate allowing unwanted substances to pass out in the urine.

Between them, the kidneys process about 180 litres of filtered fluid every day. Only 1 ½ litres leaves the body as urine. This is the equivalent of filtering the body's blood volume some sixty times a day, a prodigious task.

Urine formation, as already stated, begins with glomerular filtration. Insufficient pressure of blood in the glomerular capillaries leads to a cessation of filtration and no urine is produced. Hence a severe drop in blood pressure, such as occurs during haemorrhage, may lead to an inadequate filtration pressure and anuria. If the kidney tubules are deprived of blood, and hence oxygen, for a sufficient length of time necrosis occurs and kidney function is lost. The patient will suffer from acute renal failure. This is one of the reasons why post-operative patients and trauma victims have their blood pressure monitored carefully – i.e. to detect early signs of haemorrhage.

In the proximal convoluted tubule (PCT) active transport processes reclaim much of the filtered substances and the water in which they are dissolved. Substances that are actively reabsorbed include glucose, amino acids, vitamins and the ions of sodium and potassium as well as chloride and bicarbonate ions. Sometimes the active transport of one substance is coupled to the transport of another, for example glucose and sodium ions. However, the transport systems are specific and limited, i.e. there is a transport maximum (Tm). In general, the Tm for useful substances such as glucose is high but if excess glucose is present, as in diabetes mellitus, the Tm may be exceeded and glucose is excreted in the urine. Any plasma proteins that squeeze through the filter are removed by pinocytosis (cell drinking) but if too many are present then protein will appear in the urine. It is to identify the presence of such substances that urine testing is carried out. Some substances are not reabsorbed, for example the nitrogenous wastes such as urea, uric acid and creatinine. Although the entire length of the nephron is involved in reabsorption, the PCT cells are the most active.

In the loop of Henle more salt and water is absorbed as the result of a series of events which produce an osmotic gradient (Fig. 5.7). To illustrate the principle, consider the foot of an Arctic Tern. It walks on ice but does not get 'frostbite' (Bligh *et al.*, 1976) because of counter-current exchangers present in the legs. Blood moving towards the foot warms the blood returning to the heart, i.e. a heat gradient is created.

In the kidney, because of the arrangement of blood vessels, the loops of Henle and collecting ducts, an osmotic gradient is created and more salt and water can be reabsorbed. Reabsorption of the remainder of the filtrate takes place in the distal convoluted tubule (DCT) and collecting duct and is regulated by hormones. The hormones include aldosterone which controls the reabsorption of sodium and potassium; antidiuretic hormone which affects the permeability of the DCT to water thus altering the final concentration; and natriuretic hormone, released by atrial cardiac cells when blood

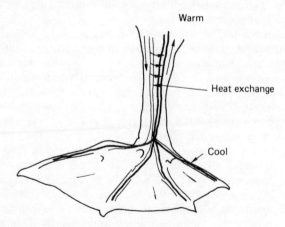

Fig. 5.7 Model of a counter current exchanger

pressure is high, which inhibits sodium reabsorption. Failure to produce the required amount of hormone may result in electrolyte imbalance, for example a tumour of the adrenal glands producing aldosterone results in excessive retention of sodium and thus water, leading to hypertension, and excessive loss of potassium giving rise to cardiac arrhythmias and/or muscle weakness. This collection of signs and symptoms is known as Conn's syndrome.

Diuretics are substances that increase urinary output. Alcohol increases diuresis by inhibiting the release of antidiuretic hormone from the posterior pituitary gland. Some of the symptoms of a 'hangover' are due to the dehydration that results from an excess of alcohol. It is for that reason that many people advocate drinking a pint of water after over indulgence! Spironolactone (Aldactone A) competes with aldosterone bringing about the loss of sodium ions and therefore water, but not potassium ions. Frusemide acts on the cells of the loop of Henle and DCT causing loss of sodium and potassium together with water. To avoid the dangers of low blood potassium (hypokalaemia), which can result in, for example, cardiac arrhythmias, potassium supplements are given to patients prescribed frusemide.

Consider Mary Black, aged 48. Mary is married and has 3 teenage children. Following repeated kidney infections she has developed chronic pyelonephritis. So far her illness has been managed by careful diet but her condition is steadily deteriorating. Renal failure occurs when the number of functioning nephrons is insufficient to maintain normal kidney function. Nitrogenous wastes accumulate in the blood, and electrolyte, water and pH imbalance occurs. Signs and symptoms include diarrhoea and vomiting, thought to be due to the build-up of waste products; oedema due to salt and water retention; cardiac arrythmias due to potassium retention; and anaemia, due partly to lack of erythropoietin and partly to toxic depression of the bone marrow. Until now, reducing Mary's fluid intake to 600 ml plus the equivalent volume of her previous day's output and reducing her protein intake, to avoid the build-up of nitrogenous waste, has sufficed. However the condition of her kidneys continues to deteriorate and continuous ambulatory peritoneal dialysis (CAPD) is commenced. The principle upon which this is based is that blood, flowing through peritoneal vessels, is allowed to equilibrate with dialysis fluid, in the peritoneal cavity, over a period of time. The dialysis fluid is then removed together with its waste and fresh fluid is introduced, thus repeating the cycle. Given the equipment currently available, patients are able to carry on a reasonably normal life while dialysing. However, for a variety of reasons, for example peritonitis and development of adhesions, CAPD cannot be continued indefinitely. After a number of minor complications it was decided to start Mary on haemodialysis. During haemodialysis the patient's blood is passed through membranes which are semi-permeable. Dialysis fluid, similar in composition to plasma, flows past on the other side of the membrane. Waste and excess salts and water leave the blood by diffusion and pass into the dialysis fluid. The 'cleaned' blood is returned to the patient, and the waste has been lost from the body. Although the process of haemodialysis is efficient, it cannot ever be as effective as functioning kidneys and thus the hope of all renal failure patients is for a renal transplant. Mary is no exception. She is required to dialyse for eight hours three times a week and to accept considerable dietary restrictions. A kidney transplant would give her the freedom to go on holiday and not to have to rely on a machine three nights a week.

- Bearing in mind a fluid restriction of 800 mls a day and the need for a low protein, low salt diet, attempt to construct a menu for Mary for one day, in order to be able to discuss Mary's diet with her.
- What support would Mary and her family require at this stage of her illness?

Nervous system

Maintenance of homeostasis depends on the body's ability to respond to change in an organised and co-ordinated manner. There are two systems for communication in the body, i.e. the nervous and endocrine systems. Both perform the same general functions of communication, control and integration, but the nervous system produces rapid, short-lasting responses whereas hormones, generally, produce longer-lasting responses (Stein, 1982).

The nervous system can be divided into the central nervous system (CNS) and the peripheral nervous system (PNS). The CNS contains some ten thousand million neurones, i.e. the cells which generate and propagate electrical signals as well as neuroglia, the supporting cells, which assist neurones in a variety of ways.

Neurones are normally long-lived and can function optimally for a lifetime. However, they cannot undergo mitosis and thus are unable to reproduce themselves or to be replaced if destroyed. Additionally they have a high metabolic rate and require a continuous and plentiful supply of both oxygen and glucose. Indeed, unless cooled to below normal body temperature neurones cannot survive for more than a few minutes without oxygen. It is for this reason that resuscitation attempts should be started within 3 minutes of the patient's heart stopping.

Neurones are large, complex cells, with a cell body and one or more processes extending from it. The plasma membrane is the site of electrical signalling. When a neurone is in its resting state, i.e. not conducting, the outer surface of the membrane carries a different amount of electrical charge than its inner surface, known as the resting potential. The cause of the resting potential is an active transport process 'pumping' sodium ions out of and potassium ions into the cell, in a ratio of 3:2, thereby keeping the outside more positive than inside.

If an adequate stimulus is applied, at the point of stimulation the permeability of the membrane to sodium ions is increased. Sodium ions rush in, the membrane potential dwindles and the membrane is depolarised at that point. This change in current acts as a stimulus for the adjacent piece of membrane and the 'action potential' moves on. Meanwhile, the original piece of membrane is re-polarised. The process is repeated until the end of the axon is reached (see Fig. 5.8). Thus, a nerve impulse is a self-propagating wave of electrical negativity that travels along the surface of a neurone's plasma membrane. When the impulse (action potential) reaches the axon filaments, vesicles present in the terminal boutons release a chemical known as a neurotransmitter. The neurotransmitter diffuses across the synaptic cleft, i.e. the gap between one neurone and another, or between a neurone and a muscle, and makes contact with receptors present on the post-synaptic membrane. The effect of the chemical may be to decrease the post-synaptic membrane potential, i.e. the chemical is excitatory, or to increase the potential and thus make the membrane more difficult to depolarise, i.e. the chemical is inhibitory.

Most neurones receive both excitatory and inhibitory inputs from many other neurones. The outcome depends on the neurone 'performing algebra' on the incoming signals, a process known as synaptic integration.

Acetylcholine was the first neurotransmitter to be identified. Acetylcholine (ACh) is released by neurones that stimulate skeletal muscle, and, after binding to the post-synaptic receptors, is inactivated by the enzyme acetylcholinesterase. Any chemical that destroys ACh, inhibits its formation or prevents its action will stop synaptic transmission. For example, curare competes with ACh for receptor sites and blocks them; botulinus toxin prevents the release of ACh.

Extremely small amounts of neurotransmitters underlie all our moods and the balance is delicate. Noradrenaline and adrenaline are the primary 'I feel great' neurotransmitters. When brain levels of noradrenaline are too low, depression results. Noradrenaline is inactivated by monoamine oxidase, thus monoamine oxidase inhibitors, for example phenelzine, raise levels of noradrenaline and lift depression. The tricyclic antidepressants prolong the activity of noradrenaline and thus enhance the mood-elevating effects of noradrenaline. Noradrenaline receptors are also present on arterioles and

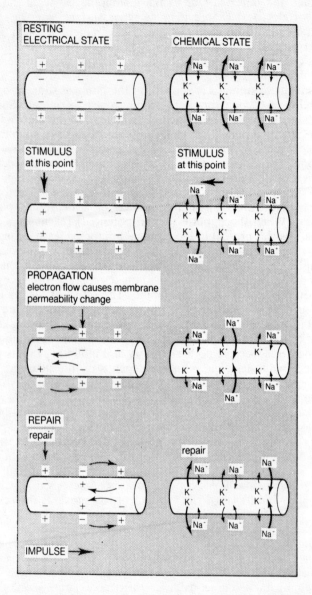

Fig. 5.8 Resting membrane potential and action potential (from Hinchliff *et al.*, 1989; p. 62).

hence monoamine oxidase inhibitors (MAOIs) can have serious side effects. They may potentiate the actions of many drugs and foods. Severe hypertensive episodes leading to stroke or heart failure may occur if these inhibitors are given with sympathomimetic amines, for example pethidine, levodopa or amphetamines. Foods such as cheese, Bovril, Oxo, Marmite, broad beans, pickled herrings, wines, beers and other alcohol all contain amines, for example tyramine, the precursor substance for catecholamines, i.e. adrenaline, noradrenaline and dopamine. High levels of tyramine may provoke severe hypertension. Not only must patients be informed of such possible reactions but patients taking MAOIs should have a 14-day drug free period prior to elective surgery to avoid possible complications.

Many nerve fibres are covered with a segmented phospholipid structure known as the myelin sheath. Myelin protects and electrically insulates the nerve fibres from each other and increases the speed of nerve transmission. Some fibres transmitting pain impulses are myelinated and some are not. Most other sensory nerves are myelinated. Given the differing speeds of impulse transmission it is possible to 'interfere' with the perception of pain by the central nervous system. For example the use of heat or rubbing the area of injury (pressure) stimulates sensory receptors and nerve impulses are passed rapidly to the brain. Some of the pain messages are travelling in slower conducting fibres (unmyelinated routes) and in some way the other sensory messages (heat and pressure) interfere with the perception of pain. Melzack and Wall (1965) described a 'gate control' system modulating sensory input before it evokes pain reception and response – the 'gate control' theory.

The catecholamine neurotransmitters, for example adrenaline, are excitatory, i.e. make it easier for a nerve to depolarise. Anxious patients have high levels of adrenaline and therefore nerve pathways are facilitated. This may result in a reduced pain threshold, and the patient's pain is perceived as 'worse than before'. Hayward's (1975) research showed that a fully informed patient was less anxious and experienced less pain. An appreciation by nurses of the nature of pain responses may mean they can find ways of alleviating pain other than the use of analgesics alone.

Individuals who develop multiple sclerosis lose myelin sheathing and thus nerve transmission is impaired or absent. Optic nerves may be affected as may be the muscles of limbs or bladder.

Regions of the brain and spinal cord containing many myelinated fibres appear white and are referred to as white matter. Grey matter consists of nerve cell bodies and unmyelinated fibres. The outer layer or cortex of the cereral hemispheres and cerebellum are grey matter. The cerebral cortex enables us to perceive, communicate, remember, understand, appreciate and to initiate movement (Marieb, 1989). Each hemisphere is largely concerned with the motor and sensory functions of the opposite (contra lateral) side of the body. The hemispheres appear similar in structure but, as there is specialisation of the cortex, the functions are not similar. For example the motor speech area (Broca's area) develops in one hemisphere only, usually the left. Damage in this area causes an expressive dysphasia. An individual who suffers a stroke affecting Broca's area can understand what is said to them but may not be able to respond in the way they intend, for example they may say 'yes' when they mean 'no'. In most people it is the left hemisphere which controls language abilities and the ability to reason logically and analytically. The right hemisphere is usually more involved with visual-spatial skills, intuition, emotion and appreciation of music. It is poetic, creative and far better at recognising faces (Marieb, 1989). Individuals with space occupying lesions, or those who suffer a stroke, will reflect the specialisation of the cortex in their specific signs and symptoms. As the left hemisphere is concerned with the motor and sensory functions of the right side of the body, an individual who suffers a left middle cerebral artery thrombosis will have a right hemiplegia and have problems with speech.

- Identify the actual and potential problems of a patient with a left hemisphere lesion.
- How may the nurse help this patient optimise his or her independence?

The brainstem contains the vital centres and also provides transmission pathways beween the higher centres and other neural centres. The vital centres include the cardiac, vasomotor and respiratory centres, but centres for vomiting and coughing are also present. Deep within the cerebral hemispheres is a small area known as the hypothalamus. Although only small, it is of importance to homeostasis. The hypothalamus regulates the autonomic nervous system and thus can influence blood pressure, cardiac output, respiratory rate and many other activities. Nuclei involved in the perception of pain, pleasure, fear and rage as well as biological rhythms are also located in the hypothalamus. In addition, the regulation of body temperature, water balance and sleep-wakefulness cycles is the responsibility of this crucial structure. By producing releasing factors it controls the release of hormones from the anterior pituitary gland. Antidiuretic hormone and oxytocin are produced in the hypothalamus and then stored in the posterior pituitary gland. This small area of brain is an integrating centre for both neural and endocrine function (Greenspan and Forsham, 1983).

Circadian (circa = about, die = day) rhythms are the daily rhythms that all humans display, for example sleep-wakefulness cycles. Levels of adrenocorticotrophic hormone (ACTH), which stimulate the adrenal glands to produce cortisol and other corticosteroids, are secreted with a circadian rhythm. The peak of secretion is between 6.00 a.m. and 10.00 a.m. and low levels between 2.00 a.m. and 5.00 a.m. – one of the reasons for feeling 'at low ebb' at 4.00 a.m. This has implications for shift workers and for people moving between time zones, for example translantic passengers. Slight variations in the morning peak are thought to account for the description of individuals as being 'larks' or 'owls'. Circadian rhythms are related to day length and to daylight. Hence some of the difficulties for nurses working internal rotation of shifts. Also, for some individuals, lack of daylight during the winter produces a type of depression known as seasonal affective disorder (SAD), which can be treated with phototherapy.

● What are the possible problems faced by nurses during night duty with regard to the circadian rhythm of ACTH secretion?

The endocrine system

The endocrine and nervous systems interact to coordinate and integrate body cell activity. The endocrine system produces its response by releasing chemicals (hormones) directly into the bloodstream. Tissue responses, once initiated, tend to be more prolonged than those produced by the nervous system. Although a large variety of hormones are produced they can be classified chemically into two main groups, steroids and amino acid based. Steroids are synthesised from cholesterol and include oestrogen, testosterone, aldosterone and cortisol. Although hormones circulate freely in the blood to all body cells, they only influence the activity of specific target cells. The ability of a target cell to respond to a hormone depends on the presence of specific receptors present on the cell membrane, or inside the cell, to which the hormone can bind. For example, thyroxine is involved in the regulation of basal metabolic rate and therefore most body cells have receptors for thyroxine.

Hormones may
   (*i*) bring about changes in the permeability of plasma membranes, e.g. insulin and glucose;
   (*ii*) initiate the synthesis of proteins, e.g. erythropoietin, on the production of red cells;
   (*iii*) activate enzymes, e.g. hormones of alimentary tract; or
   (*iv*) induce secretory activity, e.g. adrenocorticotrophic hormone (ACTH) on the adrenal gland

(Greenspan and Forsham, 1983)

Hormones are strong chemicals and exert their effect at low concentration. However, the duration of action is limited, as they are removed from the blood by the liver and kidneys. The 'half-life' or persistence of a hormone in the blood stream varies from seconds to some 30 minutes. Thus hormone levels have to be precisely controlled to meet the body's changing needs. Hormone secretion is generally triggered by some event and the rising hormone levels not only produce the desired effect on the target cells but also inhibit further hormone release – a mechanism known as negative feedback.

Failure of this mechanism will result in hormonal imbalances which may result in illness. For example overactivity of the adrenal cortex produces a condition known as Cushing's syndrome. The administration of large doses of steroid drugs such as prednisone, prednisolone or hydrocortisone will produce similar effects. Hydrocortisone has an effect on glucose metabolism and, as a result, blood glucose levels are raised. The level may overwhelm the glucose transport mechanisms of the proximal convoluted tubule and glycosuria results. Thus patients on steroid therapy have their urine tested for glycosuria. Additionally glucocorticoids, such as hydrocortisone, depress the activity of fibroblasts and the mobility of white blood cells and hence delay wound healing. Collagen fibres are weakened and the skin is thinned and easily bruised. Fat metabolism and protein synthesis are altered, giving rise to the pathognomic features of Cushing's syndrome, i.e. stick-like arms and legs, obesity of the trunk, and moonshaped face. The body's ability to produce its own glucocorticoids is depressed and at times of 'stress' the prescribed dosage may have to be adjusted, for example for surgical operations. Patients receiving steroid therapy must carry a card so that, in an emergency, the relevant information would be available.

- How would you explain to a patient having steroid therapy the need to carry a card at all times?

The male and female sex organs produce gonadal hormones. The paired ovaries not only produce eggs (ova) but the hormones oestrogen and progesterone. Oestrogen is responsible for the appearance of the female secondary sexual characteristics. It also influences the level of cholesterol in the blood and may be the reason for the comparatively small number of females developing a coronary thrombosis before the age of forty. Oestrogen also affects the activity of bone cells and hence the amount of calcium present in bones. Following the menopause some 10 per cent of females develop osteoporosis. It is for its protective effects that hormone replacement therapy (HRT) may be prescribed for menopausal females. Progesterone works with oestrogen to establish and then regulate the menstrual cycle. Oestrogen alone causes the lining of the uterus (endometrium) to proliferate. HRT of oestrogen alone increases the risk of endometrial carcinoma. HRT with oestrogen for 28 days, supplemented by progesterone for the last 15 days, produces the equivalent of a normal uterine cycle and endometrium is shed. Thus the benefits have to be offset against continuing to have 'periods'.

● Do the benefits of HRT outweigh its risks?

Testosterone is not only involved in spermatogenesis, but various anabolic (building) processes throughout the body. When the hormone is deficient or absent the accessory reproductive organs, for example the penis, and various ducts and glands, atrophy. Additionally, the volume of semen decreases and erection and ejaculation are impaired. Thus, a man lacking testosterone becomes sterile and impotent. Testosterone enhances muscle mass and boosts basal metabolic rate as well as increasing red cell production. Hence the notoriety of one particular athlete in the 1988 Olympic games.

Reproductive system

Genetic sex is determined when the genes of a sperm combine with the genes of an ovum. If gametogenesis (meiosis) fails to distribute sex chromosomes properly, then a fertilised egg may contain abnormal combinations of sex chromosomes leading to abnormalities of sexual development. For example, females with a single X chromosome, a condition known as Turner's syndrome, fail to develop ovaries, whereas females with three or more X chromosomes are sub-fertile and may be mentally retarded. Any interference with the normal production of sex hormones in the embryo results in some peculiar abnormalities. For example if the embryonic testes fail to produce testosterone, a genetic male will grow up with female external genitalia and accessory structures. Thus gonadal hormones can and do have major effects on the body. Indeed, the growth and development of an individual depends on the translation of the DNA code of the gene-bearing chromosomes. These are obtained from one's parents via sperm and egg, and we are back where we started – with a cell.

Cells, like amoeba, perform all the activities necessary for life. In the multicellular human body, cells cannot and do not work in isolation. Instead they form cooperatives that are coordinated by the highly specialised nervous and endocrine systems. Each system is interdependent; for example, when resuscitating a patient it is not much good performing external cardiac massage and thus creating a blood flow without ventilating the lungs to provide the oxygen necessary for tissue respiration.

Summary

The life sciences embrace biology, physiology, microbiology, pharmacology and biochemistry. A knowledge of all of these will prove crucial when trying to explain to patients the nature of their illness or their treatment. Signs and symptoms are the outward manifestation of disordered physiology. A great deal of knowledge, anticipation and planning is required for the relief of signs and symptoms. Even more knowledge of the life sciences is required to help patients come to terms with disability, to promote their independence, explain their drug therapy and discuss the need for changes in life-style. Knowledge of the biological sciences is not enough; nurses also need to be able to communicate that knowledge effectively. Keeping up-to-date with advances in technology, new drugs and therapies against a background of rapid patient turnover is not easy. However, it is vitally important if patients' needs are to be met. Miller (1985) showed greater morbidity and mortality occurred in individuals with task-oriented rather than individualised patient care.

Individualised patient care is about identifying problems, planning, implementing and evaluating care to manage the problems. This requires a good knowledge base. The inference which can be drawn from Miller's (1985) findings is that unthinking, routinised care may not diminish ill-health and may lead to even greater ill-health. If this inference is true, then patients have the right to expect informed nursing care. The life sciences can provide much of the rationale for such informed nursing care.

References

Akinsanya, J. (1985). Learning about life. *Senior Nurse*, **2(5)**, 24–5.
Atkinson, R. L., Atkinson, R. C., Smith, E. E. and Hilgard, E. R. (1987). *Introduction to Psychology*, 9th edition. Harcourt Brace Jovanovich, San Diego.
Bligh, J., Cloudsley-Thompson, J. L. and Macdonald, A. G. (Eds) (1976). *Environmental Physiology of Animals*. Blackwell Scientific Publications, Oxford.
(COMA) Department of Health and Social Security Committee on Medical Aspects of Food Policy (1984). *Diet and Cardiovascular Disease. Report*. H.M.S.O., London. (Report on Health and Social Science No. 28.)
Gould, D. (1989). Homeostasis: the key to normal function. In *Nursing Practice and Health Care*, S. M. Hinchliff, S. E. Norman, and J. E. Schober (Eds), pp. 45–69. Edward Arnold, London.
Greenspan F. S. and Forsham, P. H. (1983). *Basic and Clinical Endocrinology*. Lange, Los Altos.

Guyton, A. C. (1981). *Textbook of Medical Physiology*, 6th edition. Saunders, Philadelphia.

Hayward, J. (1975). *Information –a Prescription Against Pain*. Royal College of Nursing, London.

Lote, C. J. (1982). *Principles of Renal Physiology*. Croom Helm, London.

Marieb, E. N. (1989). *Human Anatomy and Physiology*. Benjamin/Cummings, Redwood City.

Martin, P. (1987). Psychology and the immune system. *New Scientist*, **114(1555)**, 46–50.

Melzach, R. and Wall, P. D. (1965). Pain mechanisms, a new theory. *Science*, **150**, 971–9.

Miller, A. (1985). Nurse/patient dependency – is it iatrogenic? *Journal of Advanced Nursing*, **10(1)**, 63–9.

Montague, S. E. (1981). The contribution of biological sciences to the art of nursing. In *Nursing Science in Nursing Practice*, J. P. Smith (Ed.), pp. 133–51. Butterworth, London.

Stein, J. F. (1982). *An Introduction to Neurophysiology*. Blackwell Scientific Publications, Oxford.

Williams, G. (1989). Concepts of Health. In *Nursing Practice and Health Care*, Hinchliff et al., Edward Arnold, London.

6 Sociology – its contributions and critiques

The Nursing Problem

How can sociology promote understanding of nurses and their practice? What insights into nursing problems does sociology offer that are not already available in nursing theories? The purpose of this chapter is to provide an overview of the ways in which nursing dilemmas become issues in mainstream sociological theory. The study of the changing nursing order requires reference to explanations concerning the organisation of the social order. The study of nursing theories requires investigation of social theories and professional ideologies. While nurses are aware of the limitations of the biomedical model in understanding the influence of personal, cultural and social factors in health, they have been reluctant to view their own roles in the wider social context. The social function of nursing and nursing knowledge has, until recently, remained in obscurity in nursing history (Davies, 1980; Maggs, 1987; Dingwall, et al., 1988).

Traditional debates in nursing concerning questions of 'Who should be allowed to nurse?' and 'How should they do it', in response to 'Whose needs and what definition of health?' have been discussed as progressive or retrograde steps in the move towards professionalism. These visions of how nursing 'ought to be' tell us little about the social reality of nursing; its location in the health hierarchy and the effects of competing ideologies, professional and bureaucratic, on nurses' positive and negative attitudes to their work.

General nursing has been taken to be the norm, and acute clinical specialism the ideal. Nursing models tend to be grounded in physical care and purposive action, that is self-help, even though the majority of hospital patients are suffering from psychiatric illnesses or extreme vulnerability in old age. While physical care may be 80 per cent of the nursing and social imagery, what is the reality? For instance, what is the reality for trained staff with their supervisory, management and educational responsibilities; for psychiatric and community nurses whose work involves understanding a combination of health and social problems; for those working with sophisticated machinery in intensive care and operating theatres or midwives whose historical purpose, deflected at times, has been women's health and not just symptom relief? Meanwhile, bedside or physical care is mainly carried out by student nurses along with auxiliary and domestic staff. Nursing practice is, therefore, a multilayered occupational structure: it is not a socially isolated cloister of women.

Despite the formal change to the 'whole person' approach in nursing, it can be seen that elitist hospital medicine continues to exert a strong influence on nursing practice. It contributes to status divisions between different areas of nursing such as general nurses and health visitors, and patients grouped according to clinical categories (Pearson and Vaughan, 1986).

In the absence of accessible knowledge based upon what nursing is when it is happening, nurses have used bureaucratic definitions to describe their reality, i.e. the accomplishment of tasks. In the absence of forums to develop understanding of their social roles on the wards or in the community, many problems arising out of service provision have been seen as personal inadequacy. In the absence of clear ideas about the situations in which people find themselves, they resort to moral codes to clarify confusions and make important decisions. In nursing, professional ideology has been the only acceptable explanatory theory. Nurses have to make conceptual leaps from the worst mess of reality 'on duty' to the humanitarian codes governing the disinterested practice of the real professions. These are the negative effects.

What nurse, at the end of an exhausting shift, has not appealed to the caring philosophy to help her or him decide whether to return the next day? Or, as a student watching over a dying person has suddenly become aware of the symbolic meaning, the human trust, involved in this aspect of the nurse's role. These sacred beliefs have an important place in nursing, ensuring a kind of loving care and integrity in the face of someone's life/death struggle. As theories which explain more mundane events or the reasons underlying 'the rules', they are not very efficient. For many nurses problems arising from objective conditions tend to be relegated to the complaints department, thus maintaining compliance at work (Turner, 1987).

At present nursing knowledge and nursing practice can be seen in a dualistic relationship, like parallel lines. The work ethic and bureaucratic objectives dominate actual practice, while professional ethics are mainly perpetuated through formal education in schools of nursing. English National Board (ENB) courses with their lists of behavioural objectives are supposed to help to bridge the theory/practice gap and ensure equality in nursing care. Nurses are in control of setting professional standards in their practice, at least on the educational front. This may be an improvement upon service imperatives and medical directives but these 'ethical responsibilities' are largely based upon normative assumptions of what nursing ought to be; that is, a unified profession. This could mean, as it does with family imagery, that only a tiny minority of nursing realities will continue to correspond to the ideal. Most importantly, one learns little about the critical evaluation of the role change from direct patient care to management; or the imposition of nursing models as naturally beneficial to the patient and not just the nurse management function.

The theory/practice gap is not just a nursing problem but prevalent throughout many, especially industrial, societies. Differences between social activities labelled as intellectual or manual work closely follow class, gender and wealth/hardship divisions. Middle class jobs are characterised by mental capabilities, educational qualifications and ethical responsibilities and manual work by skill divisions. Craft skills, where judgement is not totally separated from the creator and transferred to a machine or management function, come somewhere in-between. In the present occupational hierarchy, manual work, reduced to skill definitions, does not command high status and rewards in the market place, no matter how socially useful.

New technology gives rise to new ways of working and professions rise and fall for complex reasons; their status is neither simple nor assured. For instance, surgery was once a manual occupation providing a 'fee for services' to physicians who tended the wealthy. Barber-surgeons/apothecaries with their sharp instruments were called in to perform the 'dirty tasks' of blood letting, lancing boils or pulling out teeth. They also provided over-the-counter chemicals and drugs to the general public. Over a considerable period of time, members of this self-employed group became associated with the elite physicians whose status and prestige they have now overtaken (Parry and Parry, 1976).

The fundamental ambivalence in the nurse's role has been attributed mainly to its subordinate status to medical authority to initiate caring actions (Chapman, 1977). This is compounded by its location in the occupational and class hierarchy. It is an intermediary or manual occupation with aspirations of middle class gentility; in other words, a lower middle class job performed largely by women.

If nurses, along with the patients, do not want to be victims of the health service, they need to overcome the situation in which they are currently located. Nurses do not need to be professional social scientists, but they do need the tools of sociological analysis to understand the social foundations on which their practice is based. Nurses have been informal and largely unrecognised generalists of health: representatives of humanity in an increasingly impersonalised service. Sociology is one of the disciplines which can be used by nurses to reveal and assert these skills in social caring.

Introductory and advanced nursing courses in sociology and health vary according to the specific vocational and professional interests of the students. The material presented here will be necessarily selective, focusing on two main themes from which many nursing, health and social issues can be discussed. These are:

(i)   the significance of sociological analysis in drawing together numerous nursing debates concerning autonomy and compliance in nursing and patient care; and

(ii) the relevance of sociological theory to the understanding of organisational diversity and change in nursing.

Increasing recognition of sociology in nursing can be shown by the production of textbooks on the subject, notably Chapman (1982), Lopez (1982), Cox (1983) and, more recently, Bond and Bond (1986).

Issues in nursing and social care

Many nurses are concerned to maintain continuity with their traditional caring ethos and constancy in the physical care of patients. Nurses have based their claims for higher status on their central role as the patient's advocate; specialists and technical experts having an intermittent or casual relationship. Other 'welfare occupations' or 'feminine professions', such as teaching and social work, are also facing restructuring problems. Administrative, supervisory and management tasks replace time and energy allocated to face to face contact with students or clients. Though many nurses, teachers and social workers are keen to analyse these changes, it is difficult to obtain the necessary leave of absence and secondment to attend up-dating and specialist courses. While professional goals emphasise caring as a personal relationship rather than a fee-for-service, bureaucratic objectives encourage impersonality or standardised procedures in order to get the work done quickly. Clashes between the work ethic of service provision and the moral or professional values of service delivery are not, therefore, confined to nursing.

Is caring being further devalued? Current conflicts between social carers and their employers, government departments, would indicate that this is so.

'Professional services are being reduced, with a greater burden of responsibility for the sick shifted to kin and the private sector.'

(Locker, 1986; p. 135)

Further cutbacks in social provision therefore affect informal carers in families as well as professionals. Caring in nursing has been seen as largely adjunctive to medical prescription and cure. Its validity has been as the means or medium in which medical outcomes are assured. This problem is taken to be the fault of doctors rather than the establishment of technological values throughout western societies. The natural and biological sciences have a long history of accepted validity in their application to human problems of food production (agriculture) and human misery (medicine). Caring or learning theories can be demoted as 'unscientific' and amateurish by comparison. What are the consequences for nurses?

'. . . the traditional 'craft' skills of health care may be jeopardized if the training of health workers concentrates exclusively on the technological and bio-medical dimensions of health care'.

(Fitzpatrick *et al.*, 1984; p. 1)

Criticisms of the growth of technologically-intense health care are increasingly linked to a more widespread dissatisfaction with scientific development as the cure-all for unhappiness, including ill-health. Weberian and Marxist perspectives have been very influential in the evolution of this critique (Smart, 1983; Doyal, 1979a).

Attempts to act positively and analyse the present reorganisation of health provision are aspects of the huge task confronting nursing (Jolley and Allan, 1989). In some cases it may be more a question of survival tactics rather than the adoption of professional caring strategies. Debates in nursing concerning the direction of change tend to focus on professionalisation and underestimate the complementary industrial strategy of trade unionism. Most professional groups, including doctors, use a variety of tactics to protect and develop their professional interests and public service ethic within a market economy dominated by materialistic values. In nursing, increasing bureaucratic regulation and the throughput goals of management have led to a decline in intrinsic rewards or job satisfaction and have increased demands for better pay and working conditions. Nurses and other health workers actively protect their work in the changing health industry using different educational, industrial and managerial strategies.

Nurses are now being educated for more highly differentiated roles in specialist areas. This process is largely due to the creation of more administrative and management grades. There are increased divisions in status and rewards between the various levels. Nursing, like other occupations, is not a homogeneous group: it has been divided in various ways, rather than unified (Bellaby and Oribador, 1980). Changes in nursing are not solely attributable to a recognition by policy makers of population changes and patterns of ill-health.

The redefinition of nursing practice largely stems from a combination of economic, social and political factors. First, the growth of highly specialised health disciplines or para-professions from chiropodists, occupational and physiotherapists, to cytologists and haematologists. Second, a response to the inabilities of governments to finance full hospital care for the general population. Third, the limited power of traditional health professionals in the political arena and in the market place: the independence of doctors is undermined by subjection to state regulation and the interests of drug companies (Worsley, 1987; p. 236). Fourth, the class, race, and gender composition of nursing has contributed to the change in the social image of the nurse. The ideal of vocational calling has shifted to technically competent professionals and the reality to heterogeneous groups of increasingly part-time, hospital and community carers (Salvage, 1985; Freidson, 1970a).

The sociology of nursing: care and castigation

The historical and current situation of nurses in health care is related to many wider social issues analysed by sociologists. For instance it is difficult to discuss whether nursing is, or should be, a vocation, a craft-skill or a profession without reference to the position of women in society and the lower social status associated with their work relative to the male 'norm'. Divisions and potential conflicts between nurses and doctors, and doctors and patients, are linked to gender and class based inequalities in the wider society.

Nurses have been instrumental intermediaries between doctors and patients, and prescription and cure. Nurses meticulously follow medical directives; they do not have the formal authority to deal with a situation as it arises as social workers do. If a patient is not progressing as the doctor ordered, the vigilant nurse calls the doctor, she or he does not vary the treatment. The pharmacist, who is not a doctor, will say 'try this or that', but she or he is not responsible; she or he has authority but not responsibility. Thus the nature of health professions varies in terms of control over work content and practices. In the sociology of the professions this fundamental ambivalence in the professional's role is located in the determinancy/indeterminacy debate (Jamous and Peloille, 1970).

In the powerful professions indeterminancy is seen as virtuosity; in less prestigious groups, it is labelled as a problem due to, or requiring, external and internal regulation or discipline. All professional occupations are hierarchical in structure but some individual practitioners have greater autonomy than others (Johnson, 1972). The history of nursing is located in the care of the poor; the diseases of poverty and custodial care of the dispossessed and the insane. The history of medicine is associated with doctors' consultative role to the wealthy. Thus the status of occupations is also linked to the status of the 'objects of care'; that is the groups of people cared for, thereby ennobling or debasing those who do the caring.

Nurses have not been theoretically uninformed practitioners. Instead, assessment of the work they do and the required standards of performance have been imposed by higher status groups. Nurses have gained knowledge from their observations of the varied nature of illnesses and treatments from the viewpoint of the sufferers. This often leads to conflicts between doctors and nurses; doctors feel they are being summoned by nursing staff for 'trivial' reasons. However, the patient's peace of mind may not be 'trivial' to nursing staff. Generally speaking, health professionals have relied upon the continuous flow of information relayed to them by nursing staff. Medical learning relied on the practice of nursing, particularly within the teaching hospitals. The working conditions and mental horizons of nursing have been defined and overwhelmed by 'significant others'.

These external controls over nursing, particularly the imperative of service provision, a source of cheap labour, have been reflected in the maintenance of a rigid, internal hierarchy and ritualistic practices. The nursing ideology of personal dedication is tied to social definitions of women as nurturers. Nursing is widely accepted as socially useful work. Other professions do not have this type of prestige. Accountancy might be a profession on which the commercial world, with some suspicion, depends but it is not dominated, as is nursing, by intense humanitarian ethics. This powerful social imagery and tradition in nursing can be seen as a compensation for a lack of economic reward. Nurses viewed as altruistic carers are therefore publicly valued; as careerists with a price on their work they may face derision. Is this the historical purpose of the iron rule of obedience in nursing?

Notions of middle class respectability, linked to ideas of the general nurse as a 'lady benefactor', have been emphasised in nursing history to the detriment of mutually supportive networks and unified strategies for real change. These ideas of gentility arose at a time when philanthropy was a recognised social force in the expansion of fairly limited poor law provision. Therefore the attainment of middle class status had an important historical 'truth' in the attempt to establish nursing as a profession for respectable women. It has, however, masked class, gender and age differences between nurses and doctors (Turner, 1987) and between general and psychiatric nursing, with its history as proletarian work in custodial care institutions. Could these internal divisions be the source of numerous internal conflicts in nursing?

The prestige hierarchy of clinical specialism in medicine, and increasingly in nursing, reflects social attitudes to 'non-productive' groups of people such as the elderly, the mentally ill and the long-term chronically sick. Nurses and doctors may not be elitist by nature, but the system rewards or benefits some professionals and patients more than others.

'Geriatric and long-stay patients in mental hospitals are probably the lowest priority in the distribution of National Health Service resources . . . But it has among the highest levels of commitment in an already committed workforce, not only among nurses but auxiliaries and orderlies too.'

(Campbell, 1984; pp. 124–5)

At its inception in the 1940s the 'welfare state' was based upon professionalism and the 'less eligibility' principle whereby certain groups of people were regarded as less deserving of resources than others. This process of stereotyping is expressed in the health sector in confused attitudes to cases of self-inflicted injury such as parasuicide, drug abuse, alcoholism to a lesser extent and psychosomatic illness such as anorexia (slow suicide). Though the stigma of suicide has lessened, being no longer a criminal offence, the attitudes of individual nurses fluctuate widely. Nurses are assailed by feelings of shock, guilt and apprehension about their own actions and behaviour towards parasuicide patients and the relatives of those who succeeded in their attempt (Clark, 1985).

Individuals are seen to escape into illness because they are work shy, malingerers or unable to accept 'grown-up' responsibilities. In other words, illness is defined in terms of deviation from assumptions of normal social functioning. Maintaining one's expected responsibilities is taken as a sign of health; health, that is, as an individualistic responsibility. Talcott Parsons, an American sociologist, was the first to demonstrate that illness is always associated with a notion of purposive or self-motivated deviance (Parsons, 1964). Behaviour considered to be inappropriate or deviant is easily equated with anti-social activity. A patient not conforming to medical prescription in treatment, for whatever reason, can be seen as disruptive and unwilling to resume their prescribed social roles.

This is a serious problem for those who are sick. These views also affect 'well patients' such as pregnant women. In the medical model, obstetrics is directly linked to gynaecology or disease pathology rather than paediatrics or child health. The example below, from Oakley's research on the medical management of maternity, illustrates the medical equation of 'normal' with 'unusual'.

'Consultant: Interesting, very interesting, most unusual.
Registrar: You mean it was a normal delivery?
Consultant: Yes – pushed the baby out herself!'

(Oakley, 1980; p. 22)

Medical ideology equates health with medical intervention: thus justifying its role in *every* pregnancy and in many other aspects of human behaviour. Even though pregnancy can be seen as the statistical 'norm' for women in childbearing age-groups, medicine continues to define it in 'abnormal'terms. 'Isn't 35 a bit late, Mrs Jones, for having a *first* baby?' This social process or therapeutic strategy is known as 'medicalisation' (Illich, 1977). In the past the compliance of nurses to the doctors' orders ensured, to a great extent, the compliance of patients✗What is the present role of nurses in promoting positive self-image and self-esteem in patient-care✗Can nurses continue to carry out their contradictory tasks of organisational functionaries and patient advocacy?

Many nursing writers in the 'education versus training' debate have paid little attention to

(*i*) the social development of educational aspirations and opportunities, particularly among women, the working classes and ethnic groups, and

(*ii*) the growing importance of 'paper qualifications' throughout the world of work, i.e. credentialism regarding specialisation.

Since the health service has depended to a great extent on the labour of these minority groups, this is an important oversight in some discussions. Project 2000, however, does address the serious problem of providing pre-nursing courses and conversion training for enrolled nurses, particularly those from ethnic backgrounds (Pearson, 1987).

At the same time, there is little criticism of the present centralisation of caring expertise as a management and not a professional function. Caring expertise is being effectively separated from the direct control of professional groups (New Society, 1987). The pretensions of professional medicine may be criticised but that does not automatically lead to the wholesale closing down of the National Health Service. What are the implications for those seeking careers in professional nursing management? Does a career as a nurse leader necessarily imply a social distancing from practitioners and identification with management ideals? Nurses are overtly 'professionalising' at the same time as other caring professionals are facing a real decline in their expert status and control over the content of their work in the market place.

The key to a sociological interpretation of nursing and other professional or vocational groups lies in the occupational role and wider context in which practice takes place (Gomm,1982). This is not the whole story. It is the framework or setting in which the structure, ideology and social interaction of nurse/patient relationships can be examined critically. The sociology of nursing is not limited to a single contribution from any particular sub-field such as the sociology of health and illness or the family, relevant though these are. The impetus of many problems confronting nurses and patients is located in major processes in society. The study of nursing requires reference to, and understanding of, a selection of issues in sociological analysis.

Nurses and bureaucratic authority: an imposed order?

Nursing has been overshadowed by a traditional emphasis on medical and physical aspects of care. Nurses have had an intense responsibility for carrying out medicine's prescriptions to produce 'cured patients'. The nature of nursing and conceptions of health have been derived largely from the doctor-patient relationship and the hospital system of control over nurses' labour and work content. The occupational role of the nurse in society is largely dependent upon the structure of society and hospitalised medicine rather than a particular conception of health. Sociologists analysing changes in nursing refer to social stratification or status arrangements in the wider society to explain
 - the distribution of authority between medicine and nursing, nurses and other health professionals
 - the containment of health needs
 - the quality of existing provision, and
 - the passivity of patients within various institutional settings

(Stacey *et al.*, 1977)

It is sociologists who have put forward the shocking idea that authorities create deviance by defining 'normality' or what passes for conformity in their own terms (Burke, 1980; p. 59). Social control is the process whereby appropriate behaviour is rewarded and inappropriate behaviour disapproved of or punished. The problem is that these notions of normality are by no means consistently applied. Deviance is not a property inherent in certain forms of behaviour; it is a property conferred upon these forms by people who have the power to do it, and reasons for wanting to (Aggleton, 1987).

How can the subservience of nurses in health bureaucracies be understood without reference to the exercise of power by individuals or groups in authority positions? Some careerist individuals in organisations have a tendency to set up their own systems of patronage, i.e. sponsorship of those considered 'eligible', within large-scale institutions. This is an aspect of the hidden agenda in nursing and other large-scale bureaucracies. For example, a positive ward report may depend more on the personal preference of the authority figure, ward sister or charge nurse, than the competence of subordinate members of staff. The rewarding of certain individuals over others is not always based on overt organisational goals, i.e. the normative value-system or performance indicators of merit. This is creative use of the rules or inconsistency in valuing the performance of different individuals. Stated accomplishments are not rewarded but serving the interests of whoever the authority figure may be!

Marxists analyse power in terms of the dominance of middle class values in all capitalist institutions; respectability as ideology. Weber, the founder of interactionism, drew attention to the way individuals invested with authority may not always use it rationally. Institutions do not therefore only function at the level of appearances. Using Goffman's (1959) dramaturgical model, the way that some people devote their energy, and that of underlings, to promoting themselves symbolically as indispensable to the organisation while others use their energy to accomplish the necessary work tasks can be analysed. This is ambition based upon personal vanity, i.e. intense individualism and not public service. These people are the biggest time wasters in any organisation (Jacobs, 1969). They are often rewarded with more power by management, in the mistaken belief that the work only gets done because these people act as the 'coercive arm' of the organisation. As long as management goals appear to be served, the quality of the product and personal interaction between staff is not seriously questioned.

The promotion of these intense competitive values, expressed in authoritarian leadership styles and closed communication systems, may be particularly offensive and distressing to those who have chosen to work in caring occupations. This may be one of the reasons for the high turnover of staff in the semi-professional caring fields.

Michels' rule of power (Michels, 1949) states that those who rise to positions of authority tend to become corrupted. For power is not an abstract thing: it has to be constantly exercised to be real. While some individuals benefit from this, others do not. The distinguishing criteria between individuals are their personal credentials rather than their attachment and accomplishment at work. Living up to high standards of care may render an individual deviant within an organisation in which materialistic values hold sway in service delivery. If organisational theory is to be useful to nurses in the understanding of modern medical bureaucracies, then it needs to be interpreted critically. Otherwise one would have to accept that all those in positions of authority are the most talented and best suited for the posts (Davis and Moore, 1968). Also that individual complaints are personal grievances and not the result of problems in the organisation of work. Furthermore, it would need to be agreed that competitive ways of working naturally take precedence over democratic or more cooperative methods (Strong and Robinson, 1988).

·Sociological research on gender and race inequalities in employment have shown how informal and formal patronage in organisations operate as modes of discrimination in selection procedures (Jewson and Mason, 1986) and barriers to career opportunities (Crompton and Sanderson, 1986). Individuals are selected and judged on an unfair basis of personal characteristics or ascription, and not educational and work qualifications or achievement. This process is known as occupational segregation by gender, race and age (Blaxall and Reagan, 1976). Looking across the economy, it can be seen that women are concentrated in relatively few service industries.

Along with other minority groups they continue to occupy the lower status levels within all occupations.

The social practices of nursing and doctoring

The central issue which links sociological ideas with current nursing problems is expressed in the seemingly obvious question 'What is the relationship between nursing and the people's health?' Sociologists believe that concepts of health and the roles of health carers and patients are socially defined. Nursing is a process of social interaction; a complex carer-client relationship involving interpersonal skills, techniques of communication, collective responsibilities and the implementation of health and welfare policy. Nursing has personal, social and political concerns.

The structure and function of nursing, how it is organised and its internal workings, are important aspects of the way societies regard and allocate social support through political processes. In the USSR, for instance, medicine is an overwhelmingly female occupation: over 90 per cent of primary care physicians are women. Medicine, like nursing, is regarded as 'women's work': men take up better career options in industry, the armed forces or Party officialdom. The relatively low status of medicine is not because women do it; women do it because it is regarded socially as a lower status profession than, say, engineering (Navarro, 1977). In a society like the USSR the production of goods takes precedence over the health and welfare of individuals. In another industrial society, like Britain, profit-making enterprise takes precedence over individual need in health and social caring.

Modern nursing may be defined as a holistic response to actual and potential health problems in the population (Campbell *et al.*, 1985). Nursing practice, therefore, operates at different levels: that of individual patient needs as well as those defined by social institutions. The bureaucratic classification of patients'needs, for example definitions of disability defined by the Departments of Health and of Social Security, affect the labelling or assignment by the community nurse or health visitor of a client into a welfare category for receipt of benefits and services.

Nurses are not simply skilled domestic workers, hygienists or technicians whose work is amenable to management ideals of the timing and sequencing of appropriate acts. For instance, giving an injection could be broken down into detailed tasks, reduced to a skill only, rather than an action involving judgement, i.e. adjustment to the needs of particular patients. Apart from administrative and legal procedures informing drug use, nurses decide where is the best place to give the injection and the way to carry out the procedure carefully and gently. The nurse takes into account skin and muscle tone, age and condition and how to reassure and reduce the patient's apprehension or fear. Nurses learn how to approach patients as people, within a framework of intense caring, in accordance with nursing observations and the rules and values of a social-medical institution. The practice of nursing, like doctoring, does not take place in a vacuum but within various social relationships of mutual dependency and asymmetrical reciprocity between individuals and groups.

Nurses have an important social purpose ensuring that people are integrated into the patient role and the health organisation so that the doctor/patient relationship can be effective. At the same time their caring philosophy requires that they respond to the patient's personal needs. This causes many problems for nurses. If a surgeon cuts out a kidney instead of repairing a hiatus hernia, what does the nurse tell the patient? All studies of doctor/patient communication show how little meaningful information doctors give to patients (Gomm, 1979). Sociologists of medicine are therefore inclined towards a conflict view rather than a notion of security in shared goals. A high proportion of NHS patients feel guilty for taking up the doctor's time, confused by the medical advice given and at the same time frightened to find out the truth (Thompson, 1984).

Studying nursing in its social and occupational context helps to overcome the 'invisibility' of caring and carers in the hospital system and the wider society. It also provides insight into problems women face in having their work taken seriously, either in the home or in employment. While nursing was regarded as purely women's work it was not seen as a proper job but an interim occupation before women got down to the serious business of marriage and nurturing within their own families. Demographic change, especially the reduction in the number of school-leavers, means there will no longer be a ready supply of young recruits. Nursing, like many other occupations, is seeking new labour markets, i.e. mature entry and part-time work, and ways of retaining staff by means of mutual support and improved systems of communication. Nurses work in situations of high turnover, for staff and patients; they cannot rely upon a long term 'building up' of team or psychological harmony with colleagues and patients.

Curative science, anatomical pathology, pharmacology and other important disciplines have acted as a collective underpinning to a medical ethos which has perhaps marginalised people's experience of illness. It is social scientists who have begun to explore the importance of cultural and personal perceptions in the diagnosis, treatment and prescribed outcomes of illness behaviour. The overwhelming majority of ill people suffer from long-standing and obviously socially related conditions requiring support and care. Their needs cannot be totally defined by the purely biological approach of orthodox medical practice. Medical training is primarily based upon the distinction between urgent and non-urgent conditions and treatments. Doctors are not necessarily expert in the management of chronic conditions requiring long-term personal involvement with patients and their families.

The proposed change from hospital to community care implies that the careers of nurses and doctors are no longer solely based upon curative techniques. It also implies that all sick people should have decent homes and available relatives to look after them. Recent policy clearly states a diminishing role of the state and an increasing role for self-help and care by the family (Locker, 1986). Community care is seen as either supplementary to the resources available to individuals and families, or as a last resort. Sociologists question whether the modern family, limited to two generations, is capable of shouldering further social burdens, especially families with fragile resources. With the decline in family size, increased distances between ageing parents and their grown-up children and the large numbers of married women in employment, the resources of women as family carers are sorely stretched.

Historically nurses have been aligned with their patients in a subordinate relationship to hospital bureaucracy and the medical profession. As well as the negative effects of occupational control and discipline, there have been positive outcomes. Nurses have been highly successful in the management of the subjective aspects of illness as nurses and patients tend to agree. Nurses undertake complex social action. They attend to the patient's feelings; they provide emotional support and they make links between the patient's family, social identity and the medical institution. All this is invisible to the institution, unrecognised in terms of pay or a career, but embodied within notions of the personal qualities required, a priori, for the job. On the other hand these imaginative qualities of the nurse-patient relationship are absolutely visible to the patient. Who offers tea and sympathy to worried relatives waiting in the corridor while the doctor attends their dying loved ones? Patients expect, and appreciate with affection, this personal approach from nursing staff. However, within the biomedical framework with its emphasis on physical care, these expectations may not be always met.

Social theories and health ideology

Definitions of nursing and health have moved away from disease categories to consideration of the complex interplay of physical being with 'feeling states', cultural beliefs and living conditions. An obvious contribution of sociology in this field is the understanding of social factors in the aetiology of illness and disease. Sociologists and other theorists link the majority of illness conditions with poor housing and nutrition, industrial health hazards, family pressures, inherited social disadvantage and unhealthy lifestyles and beliefs.

British epidemiologists, Doll and Peto, estimated that over 75 per cent of cancer deaths in industrialised societies are avoidable, that is, preventable. They argue that the majority of cancers are caused by diet, i.e. food contaminated by additives, consumption of social drugs such as cigarettes, alcohol or betel nuts and industrial processes resulting in unhealthy working and living environments (Open University, 1985).

A less obvious contribution is sociology's understanding of the ways in which very abstract ideas, theories or explanations of human behaviour are real in their consequences. The expectations individuals have of themselves and others, the way behaviour is defined as normal or abnormal in terms of health or illness arise out of particular social conditions and the understandings or theories available through culture. An important aspect of the sociology of health is to investigate how these ideas arise and question their implication for health and health carers (Armstrong, 1983; Parrish, 1985).

People do not invent theories all by themselves; they find them ready-made in the culture in which they are brought up (Worsley, 1987). These theories lead to rule making and ways of enforcing them. In western or technological societies the natural sciences create the knowledge that modern states transform into power. Social progress is reduced to notions of the profits that modern economics brings, i.e. how many car-owners there are in the population. Similarly, a patient's recovery is measured in terms of responses to technologoical treatments such as surgery, radiation therapy or sophisticated chemotherapies and not his or her quality of life. Progress is thus equated with consumption patterns.

Patients are discharged back into the situations which gave rise to their health difficulties in the first place (Chapman, 1984). The patient's recovery, post-surgery, is confined to ensuring that they are still alive afterwards. Community nurses have to contend with post-operative problems such as infected suture lines which require stringent hygiene and take time to heal. Chemical treatments frequently have appalling consequences or side effects, such as long-term disability in the practolol syndrome and deformities in the case of thalidomide (Melville and Johnson, 1982). The widespread knowledge and use of the biomedical model in understanding illness and health means patients demand prescribed drugs and look to medicine and doctors for answers to many social as well as health problems.

Human societies are unequal societies. The ideas or theories available to explain 'how people should lead their lives' tend, therefore, to resemble closely the assumptions of those powerful enough to impose their views on others. These powerful meaning systems are called ideologies. According to sociologists these ideologies are the means whereby people interpret reality and professionals their professional practice. In order to understand professional nursing one needs to explore the connection between the ideas which inform its practice, the structures in which it takes place and the stated roles of nurses related to the patient's welfare. This dynamic or changing process is called social action or social interaction, terms preferred by sociologists to attitudes and behaviour which imply a mechanical or static relationship between the way individuals feel, reason and act.

The way one acts may be largely constrained by others: cultural expectations and social organisation. Many people struggle against these imposing forces in their lives. If sceptical sociologists have anything to import, it is that conventional or appropriate ways of doing things, i.e. institutional practices, may be harmful to spiritual and physical health. This perspective is shared by some health users who form themselves into pressure groups to effect more humane methods of treatment and care. Another example is medical fashion; it can be totally unrelated to better medical practice. This was the case with the dramatic decline in breastfeeding in the United States. Though this proved detrimental to health, it lasted until problems with bottled milk and pressure from women reversed the medical trend (Francome, 1986). Professionals may need to reflect upon the implications of their own truths or theories before advising clients.

The adoption of the holistic approach in nursing and its relevance in primary health care implies new ways of helping people through illness and its prevention. In this model health care is not an end-in-itself, but a process linked to relevant support systems in people's lives, and to the community in which they live. Health is not, therefore, purely the absence of disease. Increasingly theories of nursing care are located in the social and behavioural sciences rather than disease pathology. What type of sociology do nursing students need at the different levels? In order to develop a sociological understanding of nursing one needs to look at the contribution of specific ideas, methods and topic areas.

Sociology and health: health, illness and society

Sociologists believe that all significant human behaviour is learned. The less genetically programmed a species, the more highly complex the process of acquiring essential characteristics. In primary socialisation in the family children learn to become members of the human group. Subsequent socialisation in school, peer groups and work illustrates the sophisticated changes and conflicts encountered as individuals come into contact with new people and situations. In socialisation human beings not only learn to adapt to conventional ways of doing things. They also acquire the mental capabilities or the shared intellectual systems which means they can communicate with other human beings in meaningful ways. Whether this potential is expressed or repressed depends upon the nature of social constraints and opportunities for emotional warmth and security. These ideas are discussed in nursing models concerned with human growth and development. For example, the developmental model of King (1971) and the interactionist approach of Peplau (1952).

Occupational groups undergo intellectual or symbolic changes in preparation for their roles and professional status positions. For interactionists this process forces the professional to discard lay imagery, and to internalise the correct professional values. This personal identification is more than technical know-how. For novices it forms an introduction to the knowledge base relating to the claims of the occupational group (Gomm, 1982; Melia, 1984). In the case of medical students 'one might say that the learning of the medical role consists of a separation, almost an alienation, of the student from the lay medical world' (Hughes, 1958).

Another consequence of this esoteric learning is the use and justification of jargon which only the initiated understand. This perpetuates the alienation of patients from what is happening to them. They become objects of the caring process, clinic or disease categories, and not subjects or whole persons. According to most sociologists, what keeps caring professionals acting in basically human(e) ways is the moral or ethical systems which remind them of their connections with other people.

These values which govern and inform behaviour in roles and relationships have to be shared if societies and individuals are to function at a minimal level. It is important to grasp this point to understand why sociologists keep discussing values or the effects of other people's expectations on our behaviour. The source of these social imperatives and meanings is an important topic in sociology at basic level in the study of value-teaching institutions such as the family, education, religion and the mass media (Moore, 1987).

Human societies depend on the communication or knowledge business, from the family through the world of commerce to political parties. Sociologists attempt to answer why it is in consumer societies that loving care for the bodywork of a new car, a status symbol, takes precedence over caring for our own bodies. It is not true that lay interpretations of illness are totally distinct from the medical model.

'Most patients . . . have been conditioned to believe that the doctor alone knows what made them sick and that technological intervention is the only thing that will get them better.'

(Capra, 1982; p. 163)

Capra concludes that overcoming this medical dogma would require nothing short of a cultural revolution (Capra, *op.cit.*).

'Altered states': the experience of illness

Nursing education promotes an understanding of patients as complex human beings. The nursing process acknowledges the impact of the demands of the social world on an individual's physical and emotional resources for recovery and health. This holistic approach helps to overcome distinctions between physical, mental and psychosomatic illness. In psychoanalytic theory all illness is taken to be self-motivated though not in a self-conscious way. This means it is functional or necessary to a certain extent in the maintenance of a stable personality. In popular usage pyschosomatic has come to mean 'not really ill'. This assumption overlooks the nature of illness as a widespread and devastating experience and the significance of stress in producing vulnerability to a wide range of diseases from the common cold to myocardial infarction (Fitzpatrick, 1986).

It seems that some people react to stressors in their lives by having nervous breakdowns while others become physically ill. Whatever the trigger factor, these people are not suffering from imaginary illnesses. However, to understand the altered states brought about by illness – the solitude and heightened introspection – it is necessary to turn to literature rather than scientific texts (Green 1964, Solzhenitsyn, 1971). Little has been written from the viewpoint of medical learning. One learns about the experience of many illnesses, which have defied medical interpretation, from self-help groups organised around specific symptoms and conditions such as the Myalgic Encephalomyelitis (ME) Association.

Health and illness always involve psychological and physical causes and effects. Patients are thinking and reasoning individuals and not simply bedridden or ambulatory cases! This is in contrast to the biomedical model where the individual complaint is isolated from the physical presence and social identity of the patient.

According to Erving Goffman, doctors maintain their impersonality in treating patients by two main methods. First, they can anaesthetise the patient. By the time the powerful pain suppressing effects of the anaesthetic wears off, the patient has been turned over to the nursing staff. They are no longer medical problems but nursing problems. Secondly, they can treat the patient as a non-person by ignoring the fact that a person has to accompany their body to the medical workshop. Apart from greeting the patient 'with what passes for civility, and said farewell to in the same fashion, everything in between goes on as if the patient weren't there as a social person at all, but only as a possession someone has left behind' (Goffman, 1961, p. 298).

This non-person treatment is compounded by the use of a technical vocabulary which means the patient's fate can be discussed openly with colleagues without fear of the patient understanding. These practices enable physicians to evade communicating hasty diagnoses which they may feel uncertain about and to distance themselves from the anxiety which would result from identifying with a patient's suffering. In the medical model doctors, as leaders in the field, are impelled to intervene to effect cure (Morgan, 1986).

In western medicine doctors have an imperative to act. A first step is the legitimising of the illness by assigning it, in diagnosis, to a clinical category. The patient is rendered into a passive, subservient consumer of products of treatment over which she or he has little knowledge and even less control. Doctors receive job satisfaction by using their technical skills, applying their 'tinkering-services', according to Goffman (1961). Conversely, personal interaction with patients is essential to most nurses' stated satisfaction with their work (Chapman, 1976).

The impersonal approach of biomedicine can serve humane as well as bureaucratic functions. For example, it means that doctors accept the burden of the disease, as most healers do, and responsibility for the patient's recovery. In other cultures, healers are more concerned with the misfortunes of illness and not the causes: they do not automatically accept a responsibility to produce a cure. Working within this framework of impersonality, many health professionals, especially nursing staff, turn it into something positive. They use it to preserve the dignity of the patient. Nurses and auxiliary staff may present a matter-of-fact persona to the patient while dressing a foul-smelling gangrenous limb or removing bedpans from patients with typhus or dysentery.

Assuming the mantle of the professional means one has the authority to penetrate social norms in terms of physical and emotional privacy. Case histories, body treatments and procedures all involve a transgression of normal social rules and group expectations (Parsons, 1964).

To protect the patient's privacy and integrity, nurses may appear to lack the necessary professional curiosity in questioning the patient about their personal interpretation of the often strange and terrifying sensations which are part of the illness experience. Some health workers are aware, not usually in a self-conscious way, that there is nothing intrinsically noble about suffering: it does not necessarily make you a better person. To believe otherwise is a form of puritanism.

Medical authority may alleviate the aura of personal inadequacy from the sick person as all illness is associated with social deviance to some extent, ranging from carelessness, 'catching cold', to moral impurity or divine retribution as with sexually transmitted diseases

(Mangen, 1982; Brimacombe, 1985). To be ill means there has been a deviation from the norm of being healthy and this condition is judged by doctors not purely on biological grounds.

'Being ill is not a state, it is a status, to be granted or withheld by those who have the power to do so . . .'.

(Kennedy, 1983; p. 6)

Sociologists ask: Does society put a strain on sick people or are sick people a burden on society?

The sociological problem of defining health

Collectively the social sciences investigate the whole range of human behaviour from the point of view of history, society, economy or organised politics. Sociologists look at the regularities in people's behaviour that underlie the obvious originality of the lived experience at the level of the individual's biography. This applies to modes of treatment as well as patterns of health and illness. What is just routine to medical and nursing staff may be an unknown and frightening event from the patient's point of view.

Many nurses assume that taking the personal needs of individual patients into account means literally catering to their every need. This would be an impossible task and it would do little to encourage a healthy independence in the patient. In the sociological approach quality in nursing and health care is both an individual responsibility (behaviour) and a collective, social responsibility (public health and preventive measures). Unlike the nursing process ideal, healing is not only a fusion of patient and nurse goals; in other words, being healthy, is not totally dependent upon the isolated activity of professionals. It has wider implications.

Some people think that 'health' or 'human nature' are timeless truths. Sociologists would say these are social judgements located in culture, which vary between and within societies and social groups, over time. Health as a social or relative concept is a variable or a factor which changes according to different circumstances. Health and illness can be measured objectively in terms of frequency of conditions and changes observed over time, and subjectively by investigation of cultural attitudes and beliefs of different individuals and social groups. Health professionals are familiar with a variety of definitions ranging from health as medical treatment, a matter of personal opinion, to a perfect state as in the World Health Organisation's ideal (see Chapter 3).

Generally speaking, health is understood in functional terms as the absence of disease or disability and the ability to carry out one's social roles: the normal functioning of individuals. There are three main criteria to judge wellness:

(*i*)   the subjective feeling of well-being;
(*ii*)   the absence of symptoms; and
(*iii*) the ability to perform activities which those in good health can perform.

Criteria for judging illness is derivative, that is the degree to which it interferes with ordinary activities and the originality or novelty of the experience; when it has just happened and has not happened that way before (Pearson and Vaughan, 1986, p.43).

The medical profession has an important role in the formulation and maintenance of these concepts. Doctors regulate sickness behaviour in terms of social as well as physiological norms. This can result in a doctor's dilemma. In consultation, general practitioners frequently use a concept of social functioning (effects of work and family roles on the patient's condition) and then switch to purely clinical criteria (biological functioning) in diagnosis and prescribed treatment. This means that if the illness is not clinically ascertainable as 'abnormal' or 'debilitating', general practitioners are not supposed to regard it as serious, despite the excruciating difficulties this person may have trying to maintain an orderly existence. Doctors give instructions to patients regarding the social aspects, such as 'you need to rest' or 'change your job', and leave patients to sort this out themselves. Conversely, a disabled person may lead a well-adjusted and useful life and be regarded medically and socially as 'abnormal' because they are blind or confined to a wheelchair.

The holistic approach in medicine is similar to systems' analysis in social science (functionalism and behaviourism) and systems' theories and adaptation models in nursing (Orem, 1980; Roy, 1976; Neuman, 1980). All use a mechanistic model of 'integrated functioning' which presumes adjustments in the individual's behaviour to return to usual activities (Webb, 1986). According to these professional views, first life is worth living and, secondly, there is a given way of improving it, that is by professional prescriptions of fitness.

'Health workers ask the patients 'would you like to . . .' but they expect compliance'.

(Pearson and Vaughan, 1986; p. 39)

In the functionalist model of sickness, health is defined as 'the state of optimum capacity of an individual for the effective performance of roles and tasks for which he has been socialized' (Parsons, 1972). Healthy individuals are essential for the smooth running of the social system. Illness is an undesirable deviance from this social conformity.

Problems for functionalist theorists arise if health or illness are too highly valued. The sick role is therefore a conditional one and the acute interventionist approach of medicine perpetuates the view that all serious illness is of a temporary nature, even dying. If the patient role is not restricted and fairly unpleasant, people may find it more desirable than the continued struggle with their everyday lives. On the other hand, too low a level of health would represent a poor return on society's investment in its members. If health expectations continue to increase due to the rising standard of living, then the demand for medical services may exceed supply. This seems to imply that it is in society's interest, being cheaper and less disruptive, to keep certain groups of people excluded from the general prosperity. Functionalist theory is frequently criticised by other sociologists as a justification for the status quo; the acceptance of medical monopoly in health care and the dependence of people on the exclusive knowledge of the experts (Hart, 1985; Morgan *et al.*, 1985).

Sociologists question self-evident 'truths' about how normality is socially constructed, maintained and changed. It is by no means true in all societies that insane people came to be regarded as mentally ill and institutionalised, or that the cause of illness was to be sought in the individual examination and dissection of bodies: or that minor mental disturbances may automatically indicate a predisposition to outright lunacy or suicidal tendencies in certain groups of people. The relativity of these 'truths', as specific social and cultural judgements, usually only become obvious when viewed in retrospect, as historical interpretation.

The social order that exists may not exist because of *need* but because of the activity of men in controlling the behaviour of others. This is the basic assumption underlying Foucault's path-breaking analyses:

(*i*) 'Madness and Civilisation – A History of Insanity in the Age of Reason'

(*ii*) 'The Birth of the Clinic', and

(*iii*) 'Discipline and Punishment – the Birth of the Prison'
(Foucault, 1973a; Foucault, 1973b; Foucault, 1977).

Social class, ethnicity and social role as dimensions of health

Sociologists have shown that social class, ethnicity and social role have important consequences in the distribution of mental illness. In America it is almost fashionable among white middle class professionals to seek support from an analyst for neurotic symptoms such as anxiety and depression. For these middle class people illness, to a certain extent, is a necessary part of health. Similar symptoms among the black population are more likely to result in a diagnosis of psychosis (schizophrenia) and admission to psychiatric hospitals as involuntary patients.

'An example of this differing experience is to be found in the high rate of referrals of black people by police, under section 136 of the Mental Health Act.'

(Hameed, 1989)

Brown and Harris' (1978) study of 600 women in London found that a far higher proportion of working class mothers were more vulnerable to depression and an inability to cope with crises than middle class mothers or working class women without children. Isolation in the home with three or more young children and little emotional support from husbands led to a lower level of self-esteem in these working class mothers.

Sociological perspectives and concepts provide insight into patterns, values, rituals, routines and their underlying structures which make up everyday practices. The particular expertise of the sociologist is in being able to draw readily upon a body of knowledge about the ways people are likely to act and why, within a variety of situations, cultures and societies including those distinct from our own. The process which links the mass of human activity into an on-going structure or *system* is termed the social division of labour or the specialisation of activities and tasks. It is also the key to the economy. If nurses were all busy manufacturing dialysis machines, there would not be any nurses!

It is commonly assumed that divisions between individuals and groups of people are natural divisions. Sex-based inequalities at work are often interpreted as an extension of natural or biological functions, based upon the assumption that men and women are, in some sense, immutable opposites. Though one may not expect to find women in top positions in male-intensive occupations, it is surprising that women do not appear to have 'made it' even within occupations in which they have been predominant over time. Nursing as an overwhelmingly female occupation illustrates these trends. While nursing is made up of over 90 per cent of women, men are over-represented in managerial and supervisory posts. Despite the equality legislation of the 1970s, male accomplishments in a patriarchal society tend to be more rewarded in work than the same or similar accomplishments in women employees. This is an aspect of the social control of women. Male nurses are seen primarily as men and managers and secondly as nurses (Gaze, 1987). More men in nursing does not automatically lead to improved conditions but more intense competition for career posts. The situation of women nurses in the health service reflects their female status in the wider society.

Until the confirming evidence of the Black Report (Townsend and Davidson, 1982) illness and premature death were not widely accepted by health educators as the products of class-based inequalities, but as individual mismanagement. This report showed that the distribution of health chances closely followed the distribution of income and wealth. Morbidity and mortality rates remain connected, as they have always done, to hardship and poverty. The researchers observed marked class distinctions for most causes of death, particularly in respiratory, infective and parasitic diseases and accidents. All these conditions were related to hazards in the socio-economic environment. These and other findings revealed that, relative to need, the middle classes tended to benefit more from the Health Service, particularly the preventive services, than the working classes. It is true to say that as the need increases the number and quality of the services available diminishes. This phenomenon is known as the 'inverse-care' law (Tudor-Hart, 1975).

Sociologists reject natural and individualistic explanations of the distinction between people's social roles and their health status. All societies have systems of organising activities and assigning differential prestige, usually along the lines of gender and age stratification. In complex industrial societies there are additional dimensions of class power/powerlessness and ethnic status. The assumption that all societies have rules for regulating and rewarding the behaviour of individuals and social groups may not be acceptable to individuals who believe they are free to choose their rulers, their employers and their religion (Bilton *et al.*, 1981). Sociologists do not disregard the importance of individual experience. Instead they regard certain aspects of people's lives as worthy of independent study.

Sociologists study patterns of behaviour and patterns of meaning and the way some people benefit from this structure more than others. In the study of the 'closed' or elite professions, sociologists investigate the way some groups of people use knowledge to exclude others and maintain an advantage or monopoly over certain personal services (Freidson, 1970b). They draw attention to the social conventions and values perpetuated by institutions as expressed in professional pratices and the way people use these moral codes to judge the behaviour of themselves and others.

When nurses are empathising with a patient's problem, they may ask themselves, 'How would I feel if it happened to me?'. This is the world of individual feelings; of emotional needs binding us to different people and situations – the psychological life drama. When nurses begin to question their roles or the patient's behaviour in terms of their own expectations and that of others, they enter the framework of sociology. They may say 'that is not fair' or 'I do not think nurses/patients should act that way'. These statements begin to unravel sociological relationships between nurses, patients and the purposes of health care. What is defined as health, who is labelled as a patient and the way these groups of people are treated or cared for depend upon the structure of society.

Sociological perspectives on health

Methods of investigation
Sociologists of health question:

(*i*)   purely biological definitions of health and illness;

(*ii*)   the authority of professional medicine in the definition of sick-people and the moral regulation of illness behaviour;

(*iii*)   understandings of patterns in illness and health as random or natural events, e.g. 'Why are some groups of people less healthy than others?' and 'Why are some illnesses more socially acceptable than others?'; and

(*iv*)   health care systems, modes of treatment as necessarily beneficial to the health of the population just because these institutions exist and continue to function for this stated purpose.

In order to carry out their investigations sociologists use a variety of methods and techniques.

Despite the popularity of the laboratory experiment in the natural sciences and psychological studies on compliance, it is almost never used in sociology. The reasons are both practical and ethical. Sociologists often study large groups of people and how they are affected by a number of social factors. Sociologists go into the 'field' to study group activities and attitudes because in a clinical situation people would not act as they usually do (O'Donnell, 1981). For instance, Erving Goffman's participant observation sprang from his fieldwork in an American psychiatric hospital as a member of staff (Goffman, 1961).

The experimental method as used in other disciplines involves a control group and an experimental group. The experimental group is subjected to a particular stimulus while the other is not. The experimental group is then compared with the 'control' so that an estimate can be made of the effects of the stimulus or cause. In clinical trials this means that one group of patients will be given a new drug treatment while others will receive placebos or nothing at all. Patients receiving placebos cannot be informed of the true nature of the research, otherwise it would be redundant. This type of manipulation of people is considered to be morally dubious in sociology. However, there are a number of romantics in social science and nursing research who seem to think that the experimental method is the end product rather than the beginning or a stage in the research process. Sociology has other comparative methods it can offer nurses

in research such as surveys and content analysi:
in survey analysis.

The most popular way of obtaining informa\
illness beliefs and behaviour is the social sur\
probably familiar with the techniques of quesi
viewing associated with attitude testing of whole
tative samples of populations. Surveys provide a i
from the characteristics of populations such as the
income and occupations, to epidemiological studi   ..⌣au of
sickness and communicable disease. Survey anaiysis at its most
productive involves coding and identifying significant features and
tendencies which will answer or at least clarify the original research
questions (see Chapter 2). This is a recognised method for assessing:

   (*i*)   health and safety at work and in the home
   (*ii*)   people's health needs
   (*iii*) the quality of existing service provision
   (*iv*) the benefits of clinical treatments, and
   (*v*)   the use of technology in medical practice
(Cartwright, 1983).

Theories

There are three main theoretical approaches within sociology: functionalism, social interactionism and marxism. These traditions were
founded by Durkheim, Weber and Marx in the nineteenth century
when the study of explanations of human behaviour (social theories)
devolved from metaphysics (philosophy and theology) into social
science. In other words, social knowledge as cultural values became
associated with particular forms of secular society. These three
perspectives are represented, in varying degrees of relevance, within
the sociology of health and illness and other specialist areas.

Functionalists as consensus theorists view unequal relationships
between doctors and patients as benign. They accept the clearly
defined roles of doctors, nurses and patients within the biomedical
framework as an essentially cooperative enterprise which prevents
sick people from being isolated and regarded as social deviants.
Illness as potentially disruptive behaviour is integrated and controlled
via institutionalised medicine (Parsons, 1964).

Interactionists and marxists analyse the organisation of health care
and the roles of professionals and clients in terms of different interest
groups. In the interactionst framework the nurse's role is a contradictory one. These theorists ask: 'Is the primary obligation of the nurse
to the doctor, the organisation or the patient?' Symbolic interactionists have studied the socialisation of carers in personal service
occupations such as doctoring (Becker *et al.*, 1961) and nursing

75). This form of professional education perpetuates the and identities of professionals: understanding of the needs of clients is a secondary consideration. Furthermore, social institutions, particularly mental hospitals, adhere to bureaucratic goals and nurses have an important role in the coercion of patients into routinised procedures. This is not the whole story; individuals may resist the 'imposed order' of institutional reasoning (Stacey, 1988).

There are important contributions made in other sub-fields. For instance, in the sociology of the family feminists and psychotherapists have provided radical critiques of the role of the modern family in the production of healthy individuals. Using data on mental illness, such as rates of depressive neurosis and case studies on schizophrenia, they suggest that normal family life produces passive and neurotic rather than creative and emotionally stable individuals (Oakley, 1976; Morgan *et al.*, 1985).

Contributions of specific theorists: family, economy and society

Sociologists have been concerned with the influence of social isolation on health for some time. In 1897 Emile Durkheim published his famous study on 'Le Suicide': defined as the ultimate retreat from the performance of social roles. Durkheim argued that suicide, like crime and divorce, was a symptom of problems in society rather than a weakness in the individual's personality. He believed that an individual's health came from involvement in social roles and relationships. A lack of shared norms and values would lead to a sense of failure and suicide. In particular, Durkheim was concerned with the negative effects of rapid social change (industrialisation) and the break-up of traditional communities and their ways of life on social order and stability. This study concluded that suicide rates were the consequence of the degree of a person's integration within social groups. Changes in suicide, crime and divorce rates are analysed as the effects of changing social values and norms, i.e. breakdowns in roles, family, communities and society generally.

The patterns he identified are still prevalent today. The suicide rate, and general mortality rate, is higher among single and divorced people than married couples. More men commit suicide than women, though the rate of depression is higher in women than men, and the rate increases with advancing age due to increasing social isolation and poverty. This approach provides insight into those 'at risk', the parasuicide rate being much higher, and has relevance for all those in health care. Personal and caring relationships are shown to have a great influence on the maintenance of emotional and physical well-being (Ashton, 1986).

In the 1950s American sociologists developed the study of illness and the institutions of medicine in the wider context of deviance and social control. According to this perspective, illness is largely a response or reaction to pressures and tensions building up in people's disrupted lives. Functionalists have concentrated on the role of temporary illness in maintaining a healthy social system. Talcott Parsons, above all others, is known for the development of 'sick role' theory and his analysis of the function of medicine in the social distribution of illness behaviour (Parsons, 1964; Gerhardt, 1987).

The work of Parsons, like Durkheim before him, signifies the move away from viewing illness and disease as inadequacy on the part of the individual. Parsons sees overcoming of the sick role in the patient's acceptance of medical prescriptions for cure. Doctors control entry to the sick or patient role and the length of stay permissible, given the patient's biological condition. A doctor will give a patient two weeks off work and be surprised, even irritated, when the patient reports back still feeling unwell. If the signs, detected via the stethoscope, appear to have abated, the patient's reporting of persistent symptoms can be overlooked. Patients are relegated to a very subserviant role and Parsons regards this as essential to avoid the sick forming themselves into a legitimate group of 'non-productive' people. This 'social sickness' model closely resembles the anatomical pathology focus of biomedicine: both have difficulty accommodating health disorders which are not of a short term nature.

Symbolic interactionists have contributed to an understanding of the problems arising out of the impersonal values which characterise modern, large-scale bureaucracies. Using a concept of the 'total institution', Goffman viewed the process of becoming an 'inmate', a mental patient, as a humiliating and de-personalising experience; literally 'mortification' of the self or 'soul murder'. In large mental hospitals patients have to act deferentially to staff. They have to ask humbly for a glass of water or for permission to use the telephone; they have to take medications whether desired or not; and to eat when not hungry. Through a complicated system of punishments and rewards, the inmate is induced to conform to the 'house rules'. It is hardly surprising that release becomes the ultimate goal rather than rehabilitation. This is institutional rationality taken to its logical extreme. Care is organised along lines of bureaucratic efficiency, which, over time, become rituals or taken-for-granted practices. This does not, says Goffman, render all patients and staff totally func-tional to the 'machine', i.e. the production of mentally ill people. He provides examples of individual resistance to the imposition of the system's values on personal identity. This critical theory of negotiated order within organisations has implications for those working throu-ghout the monolithic health industry (Goffman, 1961).

Further developments in the critique of health, illness and health professionals have come from marxists, feminists and medicalisation theorists such as Freidson (1970b) and Illich (1977). Marxist and feminist writers have discussed the role of women as the main producers and consumers of health care in capitalist and patriarchal societies (Doyal, 1979b; Doyal, 1985; Ehrenreich and English, 1976). They see women's position in the family and employment as the effects of a repressive society; not purely a matter of individual choice. Women have the prime responsibility in the family for maintaining emotional stability and mental health, a hygienic environment, and support of the sick and dependent. The study of the family therefore requires an understanding of its relationship to concepts and patterns of health and illness; to existing 'welfare state' and voluntary provision, and to the essential role of women as formal and informal health carers (Graham, 1984). Instead of the family being a place of stability and respite from competitions in the world of work and politics, feminists have revealed the numerous conflicts and abuses of power in relationships between husbands and wives, parents and children, young and old (Pizzey, 1974; Dingwall, 1987; O'Byrne, 1988).

Sociologists define the modern family mainly in terms of its caring functions such as parenting and provision of a secure home life. They are concerned that many families do not have the resources to cope with social pressures arising from increasing divorce, unemployment, poverty and long-term sickness as well as class and race inequalities and the decline in social and health care provision. Illness in the family can be devastating, as providers cannot work and carers cannot look after children or relatives.

Sociologists use statistics from various government publications in the analysis of families, households and health. They take into account a host of demographic variables such as the distribution of age, gender, mortality, fertility, occupations, immigration, income and poverty. This mass of material, especially illnesses and causes of death, is obtained notably from the General Household Survey, Social Trends and the Office of Population Censuses and Surveys (OPCS).

Why do nurses need to know about the family? One of the principles of nursing education is absolute equality of care for all patients. Nurses are involved with patients or clients from many walks of life. When they encounter unusual or unexpected relationships in their patient's lives, they may have to battle against their own stereotyped images and prejudices. Nurses need to be sensitive to the wide variety of needs of individuals if nursing care is to be effective.

Recognition among nurses that Britain is a multicultural society has led to the belief that all immigrants from the Indian subcontinent tend to live in groups of nuclear families where support is assured. In her study of Asian women in Britain, Wilson (1978) showed that this was not necessarily the case; many lived in almost total isolation suffering from the effects of loneliness in an alien culture. Although there is a recognition that many immigrants are poor and live in depressed inner city areas, there is little discussion of the links between social class and ethnicity in the onset of illness (Fitzpatrick and Scambler, 1984; Pearson, 1986). A critical perspective on 'normal' family life would help to avoid embarrassing presumptions about who is the patient's closest relative, who would be responsible for the home care and whether there is anyone to care for them at all.

It would be a great leap forward if nursing staff disseminated the use of the term 'partner' to describe a patient's cohabitee rather than 'live-in-lover'. The use of the term 'households' is another example. Households are defined in industrial societies as families. Previously they were work groups among the poor and the means of consolidating and passing on social advantages, including the inheritance of political power and wealth, in the aristocracy. Many children are raised in nuclear families but a considerable number are cared for by foster parents or in institutions. Many adults live in single households or in institutions such as residential care, prisons or hostels for homeless people.

Divorce has replaced death as the main terminator of the marriage contract. There has been recognition that high rates of remarriage carry particular stresses in the combining of children and relationships from the previous marriage with those of the new. To accommodate the prevalence and problems of establishing new family relationships, sociologists and other social commentators have brought into currency the terms, the reconstituted or blended family (Burgoyne and Clark, 1982).

Single parent families and illegitimacy have increased. These groups of individuals are still viewed as deviants but the label of stigma has been considerably reduced. There is a growing awareness that babies born out of wedlock may be born into a stable relationship between parents. The Women's Movement and other pressure groups, such as the Child Poverty Action Group, have been influential in presenting alternative views on stable household arrangements, apart from the nuclear or conjugal family. Furthermore, homosexual men and women live in households or relationships as stable as any contemporary marriage. The difference and discrimination, of course, is that one is legalised, the other is not. Recently New York courts have set up a series of legal guidelines stating that 'a family should not be rigidly restricted to those people who have formalised their relationship by . . . marriage' (Botsford, 1989). In other words gay people, as partners or family of the deceased, may legally inherit the property.

What about non-sexual households such as groups of single people who share a mortgage? Until very recently single individuals not sharing a sexual relationship had great difficulty obtaining finance to purchase property. One begins to see why people who live together resort to marriage to clarify their relationship socially and legally. Marriage is the licensing of adult heterosexuality but, more importantly, the legitimising of relationships for purposes of inheritance (O'Donnell, 1985).

The Black Report's emphasis on prevention rather than medical intervention in health focused on increased benefits to families and communities. The Working Party recommended a major increase in community services for the elderly and disabled, as well as child allowances and welfare benefits, to bring the UK in line with the more generous payments in other EEC countries. Contrary to popular opinion, 87 per cent of the disabled aged over 65 years are cared for in private households and not institutions, representing approximately one and a half million people. These include some of the most severely disabled (Locker, 1986).

Feminist sociologists and historians have also addressed the question of professionalism in nursing (Gamarnikow, 1978; Davies, 1976). They see the position of women in the domestic and public health domains as the product of social divisions. Consequently they reject the view of the early nurse reformers, such as Ms Nightingale, that women are naturally suited to make a specific contribution to health care. Women are basically cheaper workers; historically their paid work has been undervalued by employers. Occupations successful in their claim to elite status have been male intensive with upper class connections and those not succeeding have been predominantly female semi-professions with open recruitment coming largely from the skilled manual, and lower middle, classes and immigrant labour (Stacey, 1988; White, 1986).

Marxists as political economists have drawn attention to a fundamental tension in health care. This is the problem of trying to operate as a public service and at the same time as an industry, subject like any other to free market forces. This makes democratic management, particularly at middle management level, almost an impossibility. Interestingly, nursing management and administrative posts are concentrated below this level. On the one hand, the public service philosophy attempts to induce or coerce members of its labour force to be spread equitably between branches of the service so that all the work, even the less desirable, is accomplished. On the other hand, as an industry, free market forces result in high labour shortages in low wage, low prestige sectors of the service. In a capitalist economy, the health industry with its market-driven strategy has to realise profit; that is, all health institutions are committed to the consumption of health goods and services. The market controls the demand for products of the industry rather than political decisions to allocate resources for humanitarian or social reasons (Widgery, 1988; Le Grand, 1982).

Sociologists of health have a strong, if critical, belief in preventive care. This represents a departure from the biomedical model, in which resources are concentrated towards coping with the disease after it has occurred. People swallow pills in an effort to relieve the symptoms because the causes remain a mystery. This means an increase in the demand for more expensive technology in medicine which, in turn, means high profits for medical equipment corporations. For example, foetal monitors used routinely in obstetrics cost thousands of pounds. Huge profits are made by the Pharmaceutical Industry which relies for its existence on the continued emphasis on symptom relief rather than holistic health care with its emphasis on prevention. It appears that health care has become increasingly limited to drug taking through prescription and self-medication (Inglis, 1983).

Ivan Illich sees this 'clinical iatrogenesis' as an inevitable consequence of medical care in western industrial societies. Students of sociology and health studies will be familiar with Illich's devastating critique of modern medicine as 'a major threat to health' (Illich, 1977). This major contribution to the critique of western ideals of technological progress uses the concept of iatrogenesis; i.e. disease caused by medicine. Illich explores the damaging effects of chemical and technological solutions to the health problems of whole populations and societies. He presents carefully constructed arguments and a mass of epidemiological data to support his view that all human problems have become subordinated to medical definitions of illness and the technical solutions of health experts. Contrary to the view of the medical establishment, Illich argues that the environment, in particular diet, working conditions, housing and hygiene, rather than medical chemotherapy, are the main determinants of health. The dynamic of human behaviour, including health, is less biological than social (Haralambos, 1980).

Changing patterns of health

With the development of industrialism in British society all manner of relationships between people changed. To some sociologists the most relevant were:

(*i*)   the separation of the family from the working environment, resulting in specific problems of combining childcare and work for working class families; and

(*ii*) the coming together of different classes of people in the industrial towns, giving rise to public health and social problems associated with widespread poverty (Young and Willmott, 1975).

The establishment of sociology as an academic discipline arises out of an analysis of these 19th century conditions relating to the effects of technological change and social upheaval in people's work and family lives. These humanitarian concerns are reflected in classic texts such as *Capital* (first published 1867: Marx, 1974), *The Division of Labour in Society* (first published 1886: Durkheim, 1933), and *The Protestant Ethic and the Spirit of Capitalism* (first published 1904: Weber, 1958).

'In 1917 it was safer to be a soldier on the Western Front than to be born in England. For every nine soldiers killed in France, twelve babies died within their first year of life, in Britain. The infant casualty rate was 1,000 per week'.

(Iliffe, 1983; p. 11)

The Registrar General's social class scale was introduced in 1911 to help analyse variations in demographic statistics in general, and infant mortality statistics in particular. The greatest gaps between the death rates of the upper classes and the rest of the population occurred predominantly in infancy and childhood (Leete and Fox, 1977). Western disease patterns have changed dramatically, from infectious epidemics to degenerative conditions associated with increasing age. According to Illich, those who die young are more often than not victims of accidents, violence or suicide (Illich, 1977; New Society, 1986).

Control of the infectious epidemics in the late 19th and early 20th centuries is often attributed to developments in medical science and technology. Instances cited have included the safer techniques of modern surgery and the use of anaesthetics; the discovery of antibiotics; the widespread implementation of immunisation programmes, and improved diagnostic testing. However, the many doubts which exist concerning medicine's effectiveness make it difficult to accept this view uncritically. After all, one of the major effects of the increasing scale of medical organisation has been the increase in the numbers of people diagnosed as sick (Gomm, 1979). Sociologists and some medical historians believe that social change has had a greater impact on patterns of health than developments in medical science. Improved diet and working and living conditions have enabled people to build up resistances to infectious diseases. Furthermore, the decline in malnutrition, combined with a reduction in family size, have had a significant effect on rates of maternal and infant mortality. Medical intervention is but one aspect of social health promotion (Hart, 1985; Perry, 1987).

Sociologists of health are interested in the patterns of inequality between different classes and groups which persist over generations. The Health Education Council itself, following the Black Report, confirmed that:

'. . . most of the major and minor killer diseases . . . affect the poorest occupational classes more than the rich. This applies equally well to coronary heart disease, stroke and peptic ulcers, which are still sometimes misleadingly referred to as 'diseases of affluence' or 'executive diseases' when in fact they are more common in the manual classes.'

(Whitehead, 1988; p. 231)

While there has been a rise in general standards of health since the establishment of the National Health Service, marked class differences are evident at every stage of life (Stacey, 1988).

Health: a nursing or medical science?

Health care is not an isolated scientific endeavour between individual patients and professionals, whether doctors or nurses. It is largely a social responsibility requiring a system of integrated caring. Nursing theories do not account for the wider social context in which the majority of changes in nursing practice are located. In the adoption of a professional strategy, nursing has recognised scientific and humanitarian concerns. For the particular expertise of the professional is located in an exclusive and verifiable knowledge base for practice. In order to do this nursing theorists, mainly American, have drawn upon ideas from social and learning theories as well as the logic and methods of the life sciences. Nursing theory, models and research literature demonstrate the application of established methods of scientific reasoning to practical problem-solving in nursing. The fundamental idea is to extend the nurse's understanding from particular to generalised knowledge or empathy, which all nurses can use. This is the ideal, but what is the reality?

The point of nursing theory is the imposition of an intentional link between professional practice and the health outcomes of individual patients. Are these models just attempts to foster a pre-conceived harmony between scholarship and the purpose of nursing practice? This is an area where there is a certain amount of published criticism and even more informal discussion (Webb, 1984; Hardy, 1982).

There are obvious dilemmas in implementing personalised caring in a climate of financial constraints and chronic understaffing. Unfortunately, a considerable amount of criticism can be too easily labelled as either resistance to change from direct practitioners, or the careerist notions of nurse educationalists. Debates on current trends in nurse education and practice continue to be discussed in terms of historical differences between the caring ideals encouraged in schools of nursing and the real context of service provision. Nurses are part of the changing institutions of health care, policy decisions governing provision, technological change and increasing credentialism in vocational and technical occupations. In order to retain one's place in the hierarchy, 'paper qualifications' are necessary to justify a status position alongside other competitors. The dynamic of theoretical and practical change is based in the changing technical division of labour with its emphasis on supervisory and managerial tasks. Yet nursing theorists continue to present nursing as a unified profession. In other words, if nursing does not follow the separatist path, like medical science, to elite status and therefore therapeutic control of caring, it will lose its place in the current restructuring of the health industry. Sociologists ask: 'What price professionalism?' (Oakley, 1984).

Despite the technical and chemical component of hospital medicine, some nurses have struggled to retain their almost domestic involvement in caring interaction. Professionalism and managerialism in nursing imply a distancing from the traditional 'hands on' physical care of patients. Many nurses are concerned about this aspect of the proposed changes.

This is a dilemma of the professional/client relationship. How do professionals resolve clashes between their stated humanitarian values, such as integrity to the client's needs and scientific concerns relating to the development of nursing theories? One solution is for certain generalists or lower status members within professional groups to deal with the welfare problems while others are engaged in more prestigious areas of research and technological specialism. A considerable amount of the work of 'high street' lawyers is of a welfare nature, intervening and providing legal solutions to family and neighbourhood disputes. Their reality is fairly distant from the corporation lawyers who supervise the million dollar deals between huge multinational corporations.

The same generalist/specialist divisions in status, prestige and rewards applies to general practitioners compared with hospital based technical specialists such as surgeons. A basic problem in medicine has been the mixture of medical solutions to health problems with the elite status of the profession. Medicine has been accused of pursuing its speciality, not the patient's welfare. Is nursing science to follow suit?

Nursing models demonstrate an uncritical acceptance of the value of scientific knowledge and clinical or technical 'know how'. Social and psychological factors tend to be mere supplements to models overwhelmingly based in physical care, clinical practice and individual functioning. The main disadvantage of these conceptions is that they largely overlook the implications of the social context; the production of healthy individuals is not a purely individual responsibility of the professional or the patient. Medical science is rejected on these grounds, but nursing science, which concentrates on care rather than cure, is presumed to be acceptable.

Many nurse researchers are concerned with standardising *all* nursing procedures in the interests of safe practices. Other professional groups try to prevent this because the mystery of their skills in judging or diagnosing problems is revealed; therefore other people know how to do it. This could result in deskilling and the imposition of standardised procedures which do not allow for a wide range of possible responses to different problems. We are back to square one where the patient has to fit the procedure, not the other way round. Arguing for the uniqueness of nursing is the antithesis of the holistic approach. Healing is not a concept exclusive to nursing; it is a recognition of the multiple causes of health and illness, and of the involvement of other health disciplines, including nursing. This implies the development of interprofessional learning and a shared basic education or a core curriculum between all health carers, including doctors, prior to specialism.

The self-care concept prevalent in models is, first, a great improvement on the 'helpless' patient confined to bed, and second, where social provision should have started over a hundred years ago; instead of hospital development to the exclusion of everything else. Third, it is a real attempt to link health care with the personal interests of the patients, as in the 'activities of living' model and not just the interests of medicine (Roper *et al.*, 1980).

Critics of the self-help approach see it as a way of pushing the responsibility back to individuals in an attempt to justify the reduction in social provision (Pearson and Vaughan, 1986). It may be applicable to patients suffering from short-term illness or well people wanting to lead healthier lifestyles, but what about those with mental and physical handicaps? How do such people sustain the required positive self-image and self-esteem over long periods of time? It is one thing to mend a broken leg and another to mend broken minds and broken lives.

The modular health care industry: specialism or fragmentation?

Hospitals are no longer socially isolated places to contain the infectious poor or the insane. In a privatised system they become expensive hotels for the wealthy or the comprehensively insured. Health insurers become confronted with the 'demographic puzzle'. The proportion of the over-65s in British society is increasing steadily. Technological medicine calls for high premiums but the majority of patients suffer from the long term, chronic conditions associated with this stage of life. Furthermore, due to the dominance of throughput methods, more people require post-operative care outside the acute sector, as present policies impose community care as opposed to ward care upon them. Thus the cost of the health industry rises: a high proportion of its budgets consist of wages and salaries. This rise in costs inflates health insurance premiums, while:

'the cover is for acute surgical illness in otherwise well people
with the odd 'multi-phasic' health checks of dubious utility'.

(Widgery, 1988)

With the move to community care, the majority of nurses who work
there will become social carers; one of a wide range of therapists from
social workers to drama and art teachers, who support individuals
and families with long-term health and social problems. This could be
an imaginative and comprehensive caring system for those most in
need. Unfortunately, community care, caught up in a technological
and commercial system, will continue to be a poor relation. Furthermore, closing the asylum doors does not mean mental illness will go
away.

Nurses may witness the rise of the 'massified' community worker
similar to the deskilling of manufacturing crafts in the 1920s and
1930s with the advent of factory production (Fordism) and scientific
management (Taylorism). This fragmentation of caring into discrete
units or modules may produce conflicts rather than cohesion in the
divisions between different community workers. Where does one
specialist's job end and another's begin? This has been the main bone
of contention between groups of hospital workers for the past forty
years. For the patient, increasing specialism implies greater confusion
regarding who is responsible for what part of their treatment and
care. Will an army of care coordinators or managers overcome many
of these difficulties?

While some nurses may benefit, as they have in the past, from
medical or technical specialisation and increasing managerial functions, others will not. However, nurses as 'handmaidens to medicine'
do not have an assured place. Laser beam surgery for cancers
requires not caring nurses but laboratory technicians.

Sociological perspectives are essential to the understanding of
current changes and future developments in nursing and health care.
Many nurses may want to keep the theory and the politics out of
nursing, but the contemporary health industry may have overtaken
them.

Learning activities

Social science disciplines require students to be imaginative: to 'put
themselves in another person's shoes'. Students learn ways of transforming themselves, through ideas, into the world of others, without
losing the immediacy of the lived experience for those involved. In
psychology we enter the world of individual 'feelings' which underlie
cultural traits; in sociology we enter the systems of meanings which

people use to interpret their everyday reality. The discussions outlined below will help students to develop the 'sociological imagination'; to have empathy towards social activities which may differ from their own experiences.

Topic area 1: the sociological problem of defining health

Working in pairs consider the questions below from a sociological perspective.

1. What is health/mental health?
2. Who are the sick/mentally ill?
3. Why are some people healthier/sicker than others?
4. What are the main killers today?
5. What were the main killers in the past?
6. What are society's attitudes to mental illness, disability, the elderly, death and dying, drug use and HIV/AIDS?
7. What does it feel like to be a professional?
8. How do you think people's health could be improved?

Further discussion
1. Interview your partner to identify his or her health needs regarding medical, psychological and social aspects.
2. What does it feel like to be a patient?
3. How do you think your own health could be improved?

Topic area 2: health and social stratification

Small group discussion. Each group should select a note-taker and a speaker to present the group's findings to others in a forum discussion.

Within the social model of health, how would you account for the variations in health status between men and women *or* middle and working class groups *or* young and old, *or* different ethnic/cultural groups, in relation to the following.

1. Infant mortality rates.
2. Rates of mental illness.
3. Violence in the family.
4. Health and safety at work.
5. The distribution of circulatory and/or respiratory diseases.
6. Greater life expectancy.

References

Aggleton, P. (1987). *Deviance*. Tavistock, London.

Armstrong, D. (1983). *An Outline of Sociology as Applied to Medicine*, 2nd edition. Wright, Bristol.

Ashton, J. (1986). Preventing suicide in hospital. *Nursing Times and Nursing Mirror*, **82(52)**, 36–7.

Becker, H. S., Geer, B., Hughes, E.C. and Strauss, A. L. (1961). *Boys in White: Student Culture in Medical School*. University of Chicago Press, Chicago.

Bellaby, P. and Oribador, P. (1980). 'The history of the present' – contradiction and struggle in nursing. In *Rewriting Nursing History*, C. Davies (Ed.), pp. 147–74. Croom Helm, London.

Bilton, T., Bonnett, K., Jones, P., Stanworth, M., Sheard, K. and Webster, A. (1981). *Introductory Sociology*. Macmillan, London.

Blaxall, M. and Reagan, B. (Eds) (1976). *Women and the Workplace*. University of Chicago Press, Chicago.

Bond, J. and Bond, S. (1986). *Sociology and Health Care*. Churchill Livingstone, Edinburgh.

Botsford, K. (1989). Gays go to court to seek salvation. *The Independent*, 22 July, 19.

Brimacombe, M. (1985). The stigma of epilepsy. *New Society*, **72(1167)**, 202–3.

Brown, G. and Harris, T. (1978). *The Social Origins of Depression*. Tavistock, London.

Burgoyne, J. and Clark, D. (1982). Reconstituted families. In *Families in Britain*, R.N. Rapoport, M. P. Fogarty and R. Rapoport (Eds), pp. 286–302. Routledge & Kegan Paul, London.

Burke,P. (1980). *Sociology and History*. Allen & Unwin, London.

Campbell, B. (1984). *Wigan Pier Revisited: Poverty and Politics in the 80s*. Virago, London.

Campbell, J., Allport, C., Erickson, H. C. and Swain, M. A. P. (1985). A theoretical approach to nursing assessment. *Journal of Advanced Nursing*, **10(2)**, 111–15.

Capra, F. (1982). *The Turning Point: Society and the Rising Culture*. Fontana, London.

Cartwright, A. (1983). *Health Surveys in Practice and Potential*. King Edward's Hospital Fund, London.

Chapman, C. (1976). The use of sociological theories and models in nursing. *Journal of Advanced Nursing*, **1(2)**, 111–27.

Chapman, C. (1977). Concepts of professionalism. *Journal of Advanced Nursing*. **2(1)**, 51–5.

Chapman, C. (1982). *Sociology for Nurses*. 2nd edition. Baillière Tindall, London.

Chapman, P. (1984). Specifics and generalities: a critical examination of two nursing models. *Nurse Education Today*, **4(6)**, 141–3.

Clark, J. (1985). The sociology of suicide. *Australian Nurses Journal*, **14(9)**, 43–4.

Cox, C. and Mead, A. (Eds) (1975). *A Sociology of Medical Practice.* Collier-Macmillan, London.

Cox, C. (1983). *Sociology: An Introduction for Nurses, Midwives and Health Visitors.* Butterworths, London.

Crompton, R. and Sanderson, K. (1986). Credentials and careers: some implications of the increase in professional qualifications among women. *Sociology*, **20(1)**, 25–42.

Davies, C. (1976). Experience of dependency and control in work: the case of nurses. *Journal of Advanced Nursing*, **1(4)**, 273–82.

Davies, C. (Ed.) (1980). *Rewriting Nursing History.* Croom Helm, London.

Davis, F. (1975). Professional socialization as subjective experience: the process of doctrinal conversion among student nurses. In *A Sociology of Medical Practice*, C. Cox and A. Mead (Eds), pp. 116–31. Collier-Macmillan, London.

Davis, K. and Moore, W. E. (1968). Some principles of stratification. In *Class, Status and Power*, R. Bendix and S. M. Lipset (Eds), pp. 47–53. Routledge & Kegan Paul, London.

Dingwall, R. (1987). No need to panic. *Nursing Times and Nursing Mirror*, **83(5)**, 28–30.

Dingwall, R., Rafferty, A. and Webster, C. (1988). *An Introduction to the Social History of Nursing.* Routledge, London.

Doyal, L. (1979a). A matter of life and death: medicine, health and statistics. In *Demystifying Social Statistics*, J. Irvine, I. Miles and J. Evans (Eds), pp. 237–54. Pluto, London.

Doyal, L. (1979b). *The Political Economy of Health.* Pluto, London.

Doyal, L. (1985). Women and the NHS. In *Women, Health and Healing*, E. Lewin and V. Olesen (Eds), pp. 236–69. Tavistock, New York.

Durkheim, E. (1933). *The Division of Labour in Society.* Free Press, New York.

Durkheim, E. (1952). *Suicide.* Routledge & Kegan Paul, London.

Ehrenreich B. and English, D. (1976). *Witches, Midwives and Nurses: A History of Women Healers.* Writers & Readers Publishing Cooperative, London.

Fitzpatrick, R., Hinton, J., Newman, S., Scambler, G. and Thompson J. (1984). *The Experience of Illness.* Tavistock, London.

Fitzpatrick, R. and Scambler, G. (1984). Social class, ethnicity, and illness. In *The Experience of Illness*, R. Fitzpatrick, J. Hinton, S. Newman, G. Scambler and J. Thompson (Eds), pp. 54–84. Tavistock, London.

Fitzpatrick, R. (1986). Social causes of disease. In *Sociology as Applied to Medicine*, D. L. Patrick and G. Scambler (Eds), pp. 30–40. Baillière Tindall, London.

Foucault, M.(1973a). *Madness and Civilization: a History of Insanity in the Age of Reason.*Vintage Books, New York.

Foucault, M. (1973b). *The Birth of the Clinic: an Archaeology of Medical Perception.* Tavistock, London.

Foucault, M. (1977). *Discipline and Punishment: the Birth of the Prison.* Penguin, Harmondsworth.

Fox, R. (1975). Training for uncertainty. In *A Sociology of Medical Practice*, C. Cox, and A. Mead (Eds), pp. 87–115. Collier-Macmillan, London.

Francome, C. (1986). The fashion for caesareans. *New Society*, **75(1203)**, 100–1.

Freidson, E. (1970a). *Professional Dominance.* Aldine Atherton, New York.

Freidson, E. (1970b). *Profession of Medicine: a study in the Sociology of Applied Knowledge.* Dodd Mead, New York.

Gamarnikow, E. (1978). Sexual division of labour: the case of nursing. In *Feminism and Materialism: Women and Modes of Production*, A. Kuhn and A. Wolpe (Eds), pp. 96–123. Routledge & Kegan Paul, London.

Gaze, H. (1987). Man appeal. *Nursing Times and Nursing Mirror*, **83(20)**, 24–7.

Gerhardt, U. (1987). Parsons, role theory and health interaction. In *Sociological Theory and Medical Sociology*, G. Scambler (Ed.), pp. 110–33. Tavistock, London.

Goffman, E. (1959). *The Presentation of Self in Everyday Life.* Anchor Books, New York.

Goffman, E. (1961). *Asylums: Essays on the Social Situation of Mental Patients and other Inmates.* Penguin, Harmondsworth. Also Pelican edition (1968).

Gomm, R. (1979). Social science and medicine. In *Perspectives on Society*, R. Meighan, I. Shelton and T. Marks (Eds), pp.240–60. Nelson, Sunbury on Thames.

Gomm R. (1982). Teaching sociology on vocational courses. In *Handbook for Sociology Teachers*, R. Gomm and P. McNeill (Eds), pp. 272–3. Heinemann, London.

Graham, H. (1984). *Women, Health and the Family.* Wheatsheaf, Brighton.

Green, H. (1964). *I Never Promised You a Rose Garden.* Pan, London.

Hameed, A. (1989). Black and blue: where does rage at racism and schizophrenia begin? *New Statesman and Society*, **2(46)**,24–5.

Haralambos, M. (1980). *Sociology: Themes and Perspectives.* University Tutorial Press, Slough.

Hardy, L. K. (1982). Nursing models and research – a restricting view? *Journal of Advanced Nursing*, **7(5)**, 447–51.

Hart, N. (1985). *The Sociology of Health and Medicine.* Causeway,

Ormskirk.

Hughes, E. (1958). *Men and Their Work*. Free Press, Illinois.

Iliffe, S. (1983). *The NHS: a Picture of Health?* Lawrence & Wishart, London.

Illich, I. (1977). *Limits to Medicine. Medical Nemesis: the Expropriation of Health*. Penguin, Harmondsworth.

Inglis, B. (1983). *The Diseases of Civilization*. Granada, London.

Jacobs, J. (1969). Symbolic bureaucracy: a case of a social welfare agency. *Social Forces*, **47**, 413–22.

Jamous, H. and Peloille, B. (1970). Professions or self-perpetuating systems? Changes in the French university hospital system. In *Professions and Professionalization*, J. A. Jackson (Ed.), pp. 111–52. Cambridge University Press, Cambridge.

Jewson, R. and Mason, D. (1986). Modes of discrimination in the recruitment process: formalisation, fairness and efficiency. *Sociology*, **20(1)**, 43–63.

Johnson, T. (1972). *Professions and Power*. Macmillan, London.

Jolley, M. and Allan, P. (Eds) (1989). *Current Issues in Nursing*. Chapman & Hall, London.

Kennedy, I. (1983). *The Unmasking of Medicine*. Granada, London.

King, I. M. (1971). *Towards a Theory for Nursing*. Wiley, New York.

Leete, R. and Fox, J.(1977). Registrar General's social classes: origins and uses. *Population Trends*, **8**, Summer 1–7.

Le Grand, J. (1982). *The Strategy for Equality*. Allen & Unwin, London.

Locker, D. (1986). The family, social support and illness. In *Sociology as Applied to Medicine*, 2nd edition, D. Patrick and G. Scambler (Eds), pp. 135–47. Baillière Tindall, London.

Lopez, F. (1982). *Sociology and the Nurse*, 2nd edition. Saunders, Sydney.

McGilchrist, I. (1985). Review of J. Meyers' 'Disease and the novel 1880–1960'. *Times Literary Supplement*, 13 December, 1415.

Maggs, C.(Ed.) (1987). *Nursing History: the State of the Art*. Croom Helm, London.

Mangen, S. (1982). *Sociology and Mental Health*. Churchill Livingstone, Edinburgh.

Marx, K. (1974). *Capital: a Critical Analysis of Capitalist Production*. Volume 1. Lawrence & Wishart, London.

Melia, K. M. (1984). Student nurses' construction of occupational socialisation. *Sociology of Health and Illness*, **6(2)**, 132–51.

Melville, A. and Johnson, C. (1982). *Cured to Death: the Effects of Prescription Drugs*. Secker & Warburg, London.

Michels, R. (1949). *Political Parties*. Glencoe, Illinois.

Moore, S. (1987). *Sociology Alive*. Stanley Thornes, London.

Morgan, M., Calnan, M. and Manning, N. (1985). *Sociological Approaches to Health and Medicine*. Croom Helm, London.

Morgan, M. (1986). The doctor-patient relationship. In *Sociology as Applied to Medicine*, 2nd edition. D. Patrick and G. Scambler (Eds), pp. 55–68. Baillière Tindall, London.

Navarro, V. (1977). *Social Security and Medicine in the USSR*. Heath, Lexington.

Neuman, B. (1980). The Betty Neuman health-care systems model: a total person approach to patient problems. In *Conceptual Models for Nursing Practice*, 2nd edition. J. Riehl and C. Roy (Eds), pp. 119–34. Appleton-Century-Crofts, New York.

New Society (1986). New Society database: the grim reaper. *New Society*, **76(1220)**, back cover.

New Society (1987). Fall of the expert. *New Society*, **82(1293)**, 3.

Oakley, A. (1976). The family, marriage, and its relationship to illness. In *Introduction to Medical Sociology*. D. Tuckett (Ed.), pp. 74–109. Tavistock, London.

Oakley, A. (1980). *Women Confined: Towards a Sociology of Childbirth*. Martin Robertson, Oxford.

Oakley, A. (1984). What price professionalism? The importance of being a nurse. *Nursing Times*, **80(50)**, 24–7.

O'Byrne, J. (1988). High abuse figure indicates low status of old people. *Geriatric Nursing and Home Care*, **8(9)**, 6.

O'Donnell, G. (1985). *Mastering Sociology*. Macmillan, London.

O'Donnell, M. (1981). *A New Introduction to Sociology*. Harrap, London.

Open University (1985). *Experiencing and Explaining Disease*. Open University Press, Milton Keynes. (Course U205, Health and Disease, book VI.)

Orem, D. E.(1980). *Nursing: Concepts of Practice*, 2nd edition. McGraw-Hill, New York.

Parrish, D. (1985). Sociology and the community psychiatric nurse. *Community Psychiatric Nursing Journal*, **5(5)**, 9–12.

Parry, N. and Parry, J. (1976). *The Rise of the Medical Profession*. Croom Helm, London.

Parsons, T. (1964). *The Social System*. Free Press, New York.

Parsons, T. (1972). Definitions of health and illness in the light of American values and social structure. In *Patients, Physicians and Illness*, 2nd edition. E. G. Jaco (Ed.), pp. 107–27. Free Press, New York.

Pearson, A. and Vaughan, B. (1986). *Nursing Models for Practice*. Heinemann, London.

Pearson, M. (1986). The politics of ethnic minority health studies. In *Health, Race and Ethnicity*. T. Rathwell and D. Phillips (Eds), pp. 100–16. Croom Helm, London.

Pearson, M. (1987). Racism: the great divide. *Nursing Times and Nursing Mirror*, **83(24)**, 24–6.

Peplau, H. E. (1952). *Interpersonal Relations in Nursing*. Putnam, New York.

Perry, A. (1987). Sociology in the curriculum. In *The Curriculum in Nursing Education*. P. Allan and M. Jolley (Eds), pp. 126–48. Croom Helm, London.

Pizzey, E. (1974). *Scream Quietly or the Neighbours Might Hear*. Penguin, Harmondsworth.

Roper, N., Logan, W. and Tierney, A. (1980). *The Elements of Nursing*. Churchill Livingstone, Edinburgh.

Roy, C. (1976). *Introduction to Nursing: an Adaptation Model*. Prentice-Hall, New Jersey.

Salvage, J. (1985). *The Politics of Nursing*. Heinemann, London.

Scambler, G. (Ed.) 1987. *Sociological Theory and Medical Sociology*. Tavistock, London.

Smart, B. (1983). *Foucault, Marxism and Critique*. Routledge & Kegan Paul, London.

Solzhenitsyn, A. (1971). *Cancer Ward*. Penguin, Harmondsworth.

Stacey, M., Reid, M., Heath, C. and Dingwall, R. (1977). *Health and the Division of Labour*. Croom Helm, London.

Stacey, M. (1988). *The Sociology of Health and Healing*. Unwin Hyman, London.

Strong, P. and Robinson, J. (1988). *New Model Management: Griffiths and the NHS*. University of Warwick, Nursing Policy Studies Centre, Coventry.

Thompson, J. (1984). Compliance. In *The Experience of Illness*. R. Fitzpatrick, J. Hinton, S. Newman, G. Scambler and J. Thompson (Eds), pp. 54–84. Tavistock, London.

Townsend, P. and Davidson, N. (1982). *Inequalities in Health: the Black Report*. Penguin, Harmondsworth.

Tudor Hart, J. (1975). The inverse care law. In *A Sociology of Medical Practice*. C. Cox and A. Mead (Eds), pp. 189–206. Collier-Macmillan, London.

Turner, B. S. (1987). *Medical Power and Social Knowledge*. Sage, London.

Webb, C. (1984). On the eighth day God created the nursing process and nobody rested! *Senior Nurse*, **1(33)**, 23–5.

Webb, C. (1986). Introduction: towards a critical analysis of nursing models. In *Women's Health: Midwifery and Gynaecological Nursing*. C. Webb (Ed.), pp. 1–12. Hodder & Stoughton, London.

Weber, M. (1958). *The Protestant Ethic and the Spirit of Capitalism*. Scribner, New York. (Translated by T. Parsons.)

White, R. (1986). *The Effects of the NHS on the Nursing Profession 1948–1961*. Oxford University Press for King Edward's Hospital Fund, London.

Whitehead, M. (1988). The health divide. In *Inequalities in Health*. P. Townsend, N. Davidson, and M. Whitehead (Eds), pp. 221–356. Penguin, Harmondsworth.

Widgery, D. (1988). *The National Health: a Radical Perspective*. Hogarth Press, London.

Wilson, A. (1978). *Finding a Voice: Asian Women in Britain*. Virago, London.

Worsley, P. (Ed.) (1987). *The New Introducing Sociology*, 3rd edition. Penguin, Harmondsworth.

Young, M. and Willmott, P. (1975). *The Symmetrical Family: a Study of Work and Leisure in the London Region*. Penguin, Harmondsworth.

7 Psychology – themes in nursing

The main aim of this chapter is to identify the relevance of psychology for enhancing nursing practice, and to familiarise the reader with a number of specific areas of psychology which are likely to have significance for all nurses whatever their specialist field of activity.

In an attempt to meet this broad aim, three forms of knowledge with specific relevance for nursing practice are identified: these are implicit, experiential, and empirical knowledge. A psychological perspective is used to integrate and elaborate on these.

The focus of this text is nursing. Nursing is an activity which is influenced by the three forms of knowledge outlined above. This chapter will therefore start by focusing on specific nursing activities and then introduce psychological themes in relation to these.

Research by Watts (1988) on shared learning in nursing, focused in part on nursing activities identified by student psychiatric nurses as significant to their nursing role. Ongoing research is focusing on nursing activities identified by student nurses at different stages of training, and also those identified by teaching staff as significant to a student nurse's role. Although large numbers of specific activities have emerged these can be grouped according to certain themes, these being broadly consistent for all groups. The overarching theme is of nursing as an activity involving communication and relationships between people, in particular the patient or client, relatives and colleagues. One of the primary purposes of the research is to identify students' attitudes to and perceptions of various nursing activities.

Nursing activities identified by psychiatric nursing students (Watts, 1988) included 'therapeutic' activities, talking to patients, assessing a patient, giving or receiving the ward handover report, physical care-giving and activities involving relatives. Activities from current research with first level students and tutors include educating patients about their health and health problems, helping patients cope with their worries, and carrying out and assisting patients with a number of physical activities, for example helping a patient maintain personal hygiene and comfort. The activities identified by students have psychological as well as physical dimensions and require nurses to have knowledge and skills which go way beyond the purely physical. They are also activities which are likely to be influenced by nurses' own attitudes to and perceptions of their nursing role, and health and illness related issues. Sundberg and Tyler (1963) suggested that the first task of the clinician should be to discover the conceptual framework under which he or she is operating. They, like Caine and Smail in 1969, recognised the link between impersonal theory and personal practice. Caine and Smail (1969) argued, in relation to the treatment of mental illness, that the basic assumptions of those who give and of those who receive treatment, significantly influence the course of treatment. However it is not only in relation to mental illness that basic assumptions play a part. For instance, if a nurse believes that patients should passively receive without question, whatever nursing care is provided for them, this is likely to be incompatible with the notion of a patient being actively involved in maintaining or promoting his own health. This in turn may have implications for health promotion activities.

Nursing is an interpersonal activity. The types of activities that nurses engage in and the specific ways in which they engage in them are influenced by nurses' self awareness, including an awareness of the effect of self on others. Experience, knowledge and attitudes (often implicit) together combine to have a bearing on the interpersonal activity of nursing. This chapter will firstly focus on implicit psychology and the notion of the individual being a lay psychologist. It will then move on to integrating experience into this perspective, and finally focus in some detail on specific aspects of psychological knowledge of relevance to our understanding of health and illness.

Implicit Psychology

'Implicit psychology is the process of constructing theories about people and using the theories to predict people' (Wegner and Vallacher, 1977). Here the word 'people' refers to ourselves as well as others. We all act as lay psychologists when we try to make sense of our own, or others, behaviour. Often the sense we make of people and events is influenced by our implicit assumptions or theories. These are likely to have an effect on our own and others behaviour and it is for this reason that Sundberg and Tyler (1963) and Caine and Smail (1969) suggest that implicit assumptions should be made explicit. Implicit psychology is particularly relevant in relation to beliefs, attitudes and our perceptions of people and events, and these three all have a bearing on the interpersonal activity of nursing. Moss (1988) suggests that although the nursing process provides, in theory at least, an effective framework for practice, nursing attitudes are very significant determinants of patient care.

Attitudes

Definitions of attitudes vary considerably although there is general agreement that a person's attitude to a specific object or situation represents a predisposition to respond to that object or situation in a particular way. Attitudes can be represented in terms of thoughts, feelings and behaviour. An attitude is more than just a belief or an opinion. A belief may not entail an emotional component. However in practice the distinction between beliefs and attitudes becomes fuzzy as feelings and emotions can accompany beliefs to a greater or lesser degree and are not always clearly identifiable.

Further, there is no precise relationship between the thought and feeling components of an attitude and behaviour. Behaviour can be influenced by external factors such as positive or negative consequences of behaving in a particular way; by anticipation of these consequences, and also by an individual's perceptions of whether they feel capable of success if they behave in a particular way. This last point relates to Bandura's theory of self efficacy and is elaborated within the context of his social learning theory (Bandura, 1977). Social learning theory (SLT) attempts to provide a unified theoretical framework for analysing human thought and behaviour. It is based on the notion of a continuous reciprocal interaction between the individual and the environment. Central to this interaction are an individual's observations of events and behaviour and their awareness of the relationship between behaviour and its consequences. Thus nurses may have a positive attitude towards talking to patients and listening to their worries, believe that this aids recovery, but may modify their behaviour to make it compatible with the dominant ethos of the ward or clinical environment in which they are working so as to avoid criticism from peers or seniors. Nurses may also modify their behaviour if they believe they do not have the knowledge or skills necessary to be successful in what they do. This may reflect a valid assessment of themselves or a lack of confidence in their effectiveness.

Behaviour, and thus nursing practice is influenced by beliefs, attitudes, assumptions and perceptions of ourselves and others, and the nature of the relationship between these two and environmental factors. Studies by Copp (1971) and Larson (1977) suggest that nurses believe that people categorised as patients are dependent. Patients are vulnerable to the attitudes and role expectations of professional staff, and nurses form a very large and influential core of health care staff. Viney (1985) suggested that, even if communication is good between patients and staff, some patient constructs will receive more validation than others from staff, for example helplessness constructs receive more validation than competence constructs. (The notion of constructs will be addressed more fully later in the chapter in relation to Personal Construct Theory.) Research also indicates that patients' descriptions of themselves contain many references to helplessness and few to competence (Raps *et al.*, 1982; Westbrook and Viney, 1982).

Do nurses' perceptions and attitudes matter? Evidence would suggest that they do. A number of research studies supporting this position are cited by Moss (1988) who, following a review of these studies, states that:

'While nurses today claim to be concerned with the whole patient, developing nurse-patient relationships, and individualised patient care, there is considerable evidence to suggest that nurses deal with types of people, types of behaviour and types of illness, rather than individual patients. That is, nurses' perceptions of, and the labels they or others apply to the patient, influence their behaviour towards that patient'.

Moss quotes studies by Wallston *et al.* (1976; 1983), De Vellis *et al.* (1984) and Woods and Cullen (1983) to support this statement.

Learned helplessness and attribution theory

Several references have been made to 'helplessness', i.e. professional staff perceiving patients as helpless and patients perceiving themselves as helpless. Again the question can be asked 'Do perceptions of helplessness matter?' Does it matter if a patient perceives himself to be helpless, or if a nurse perceives either a patient or herself to be helpless? The basic question of interest is 'What happens to people when they are not in control of their environment?' A study by Seligman (1975) demonstrated that cognitive deficit can occur when people experience helplessness. He found that individuals exposed to a controllable unpleasant event – a loud noise which could be turned off by pressing a button – were more successful at solving anagrams whilst exposed to the noise than individuals who were exposed to an uncontrollable unpleasant event – a loud noise which could not be turned off at will but which stopped of its own accord. Hyland and Donaldson (1989) described four different psychological phenomena that can occur under conditions of helplessness.

These are:

'1.Cognitive deficit: Problem-solving ability is reduced; people are less able to find solutions to new problems and less able to adapt to new situations. The cognitive deficit is a 'thinking' deficit.
2. Motivational deficit: Activity and the desire for action is reduced. The motivational deficit is a 'wanting' deficit.

3. Sad effect: People feel and appear depressed.
4. Low self-esteem: People feel worthless, of little value.'

(Hyland and Donaldson, 1989)

Maier *et al.* (1969) described learned helplessness as the perception of independence between one's responses and the onset or termination of an aversive event. What is significant is an individual's perception of the controllability of an event rather than its actual controllability. Hence attribution theory is crucial to an understanding of the learned helplessness situation.

Attribution theory focuses on how an ordinary person understands the causes of an event or behaviour. It stems from the work of Heider (1958) who was interested in what he called the 'naive psychology' of the 'man in the street'. Attribution research attempts to determine the rules an average person follows when analysing the causes of events and behaviour. Clearly the average person does not analyse all behaviour looking for its causes. The tendency is usually noted when an event is either important or unexpected. Nurses often observe that patients try to make sense of their illness asking questions such as 'Why has this happened to me?' or 'What is the cause of my illness?'. According to attribution theorists, the lay person acts as a scientist in trying to make sense of events and uses a number of dimensions to explain them. Of particular significance are the dimensions concerning internality/externality, stability, controllability and globality. In relation to the experience of being ill, the sick person may make internal attributions – blaming self; or external attributions – blaming someone or something else. The identified cause may be perceived as (i) stable and unchangeable, or (ii) unstable and thus changeable. An individual might perceive their illness as being caused by external factors which they have the power to change – they are thus controllable and unstable. This person is unlikely to feel helpless or suffer from the psychological deficits outlined by Hyland and Donaldson (1989).

Another sick individual may make internal attributions: they may blame themselves for their situation and believe they cannot change it since it is uncontrollable, yet stable. They experience 'helplessness'. If, in addition, helplessness is perceived as global ('I am a helpless person'), a lowered self esteem is likely to follow. Abramson (1977) demonstrated that lowered self esteem occurs only in personal helplessness. The longer the helplessness is experienced, the greater the psychological deficits that are likely to occur.

It is now possible to return to the question posed earlier: 'Do perceptions of helplessness matter?'. If helplessness is perceived by a patient to be short term then the psychological phenomena outlined by Hyland might not occur. However, even if helplessness is likely to be short term, for example as with a short hospital admission, many people go through an initial stage of reactance when they try and regain control by fighting back. These people will probably present as hostile, angry and 'difficult', and they may fall into the unpopular patient category described by Stockwell (1972). Giving control back to these patients is likely to be a more effective way of helping them than being authoritarian and taking it away.

If helplessness is perceived to be long term then reactance is likely to be followed by cognitive and motivational deficits, sadness and lowered self esteem. This is a common phenomena in institutionalised patients and is well described by Goffman (1961).

Under conditions of uncontrollability internal attributions are more likely to lead to psychological deficits than are external attributions. On the other hand external attributions can be associated with behavioural deficits. Research by Eiser and Gossop (1979) demonstrated this in relation to drug dependency. They found that the addicts in their study had no confidence that they could control their own behaviour and get better through their own efforts, and they tended to see their addiction as an illness requiring medical intervention to bring about a cure. These addicts were making external attributions for continuing their addictive behaviour, which had an ego enhancement effect, but this is likely to have reduced attempts at self control. Responsibility had been shifted to the professional. If this dependency is reinforced by professional staff, effective behaviour change is unlikely to occur.

Returning to the question 'Do nurses' perceptions and attitudes matter?', the evidence is that they do and that Caine and Smail (1969) and Sundberg and Tyler (1963) were correct in advocating that clinicians discover the conceptual framework under which they are operating. For this to occur, implicit assumptions and theories must become explicit. One psychologist who developed a theory and a methodology consistent with this goal was George Kelly.

Personal construct theory and repertory grid technique

Kelly was responsible for Personal Construct Theory (PCT), a carefully built or developed and, in many ways complex, psychological theory (Kelly, 1955). Repertory grid technique represents a method – or in reality a number of methods which have evolved from the theory – for investigating an individual or group of individuals' personal constructs. Put more simply, the method represents a way of exploring an individual's implicit or explicit view of the world, i.e. their personal psychology. Exploration of this kind is considered valid in PCT terms, since Kelly suggests in his theory that each person holds a representational model of the world which enables him to chart a course of behaviour in relation to that model. Kelly's theory focuses on the experience of the individual and the way in which these experiences are construed. He describes his theory as being 'a theory of man's personal inquiry – a psychology of the human quest. It does not say what has or will be found, but proposes rather how we might go about looking for it'. (Kelly, 1970.)

A person's experience is central to Kelly's theory. Kelly believed that we all make sense of experiences by considering them in relation to our very personal system of construing, i.e. by applying personal constructs to them. Personal constructs are mental constructions, or ideas of a bi-polar kind, which represent a perception or thought relating to a specific object, event, person or behaviour.

Kelly's view of man was of 'man the scientist' and central to this notion were his assumptions concerning constructive alternativism.

'Constructive alternativism holds that man understands himself, his surroundings and his potentialities by devising constructions to place upon them and then testing the tentative utility of these constructions against such ad interim criteria as the successful prediction and control of events.'

(Kelly, 1970)

Constructions of reality are constantly tested out and modified to allow better predictions in the future. A reciprocal and dynamic relationship exists between an individual and his experience which results in an individual's representational model of the world being subject to change. However experience, even experience which does not support an individual's system of construing, does not always result in modified constructions of reality.

Kelly believed that if we never alter our constructions, all that occurs during our life is a sequence of parallel events which have no psychological impact. In other words the experience is not used to allow us to become more effective 'scientists' or to increase our personal knowledge and self awareness.

Kelly construed the unit of experience as a cycle having five phases: anticipation, investment, encounter, confirmation or disconfirmation, and constructive revision (Kelly, 1970; p. 18). This can be reproduced in diagrammatic form as in Fig. 7.1. Within this theory experience is not represented by the number of events in which an individual engages 'but by the investments he has made in his anticipations and the revision of his constructions that have followed upon his facing up to consequences.' (Kelly, 1970).

Therefore the theory of constructive alternativism states that we make sense of our world in an individual and personal way, that there are always alternative constructions which can be explored, but that we do not always allow ourselves to do this even if our experience disconfirms already held constructions. When this occurs we expe-

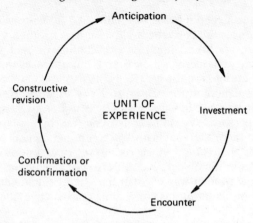

Fig. 7.1 Diagrammatic representation of the five phases of the unit of experience (Watts, 1988; adapted from Kelly, 1970).

rience a sequence of parallel events with no psychological impact. Learning is restricted by occurring within a closed system of personal constructions.

Personal construct theory is reflexive. In other words, it applies equally to exploring and understanding ourselves as it does to understanding others. Returning to an earlier part of this chapter, it was suggested that a dominant feature of the nursing activities outlined by students was their interpersonal nature. This implies communication and relationships between people, for example between the nurse and the patient, between different professionals and so on. Kelly believed that for interpersonal relationships to occur one person construes the construction processes of another and is thereby able to play a role in a social process involving the other person. To form a relationship with another we need to try and understand their perspective or outlook. Understanding does not have to be complete, nor reciprocal, but the degree of understanding and reciprocity will influence the nature of the relationship.

Therapeutic relationships require the 'stepping inside of somebody's shoes'. If a nurse construes a patient solely in terms of her own construct system she is in danger of creating a reality to which the patient is expected to conform and in many instances will conform. Patients who do not conform are in danger of being perceived as 'problem patients' and coming within the unpopular patient category identified by Stockwell (1972).

Following a review of the popular/unpopular patient research, Kelly and May (1982) conclude that: 'The good patient is one who confirms the role of the nurse; the bad patient denies that legitimation.' Unfortunately, confirming the role of the nurse is often synonymous with letting the nurse take charge and the patient becoming dependent.

It was suggested earlier (Viney, 1985) that helplessness constructs receive more validation than others from staff. Helplessness is not compatible with self-determination, yet health maintenance and health promotion ultimately depend on individuals taking responsibility for themselves.

Kelly's theory provides a useful conceptual framework which can be applied to understanding ourselves and others. Repertory grid techniques – which have evolved from the application of Kelly's theory – are a useful tool for learning about the system of constructs held by an individual or a group of people and can enable individuals to gain greater insight into their personal construing of situations and events. These techniques allow for exploration of the conceptual links between a person's ideas by demonstrating the statistical association between them. PCT does not depend on the techniques to support it, but the techniques can provide a useful way of exploring the 'implicit psychology' of an individual, monitoring change in this, and allowing the individual to learn more about themselves, including their reactions to situations and events and their anticipations concerning the future. Good reviews of the techniques and their applications can be found in Fransella and Bannister (1977), Beail (1985), Button (1985) and Dunnett (1988). A detailed review of an application within nurse education is provided by Watts (1988).

At the start of this chapter it was suggested that nursing practice is influenced by implicit, experiential and empirical knowledge. An attempt has been made to identify some ways in which implicit knowledge can influence the experience of being nursed and of nursing. The way an individual reacts to an experience, and the effect an experience has on future experiences is closely bound up with their attributions, beliefs and attitudes. Personal construct theory provides a theoretical framework for uniting implicit knowledge, experience and the individual. The third dimension to this is empirical knowledge. This does not mean knowledge which has been empirically tested by each individual, but knowledge which is presented as being grounded in some concrete and testable evidence. An example of this would be knowledge about the links between smoking and ill-health, and between Type A personality and coronary heart disease. Nursing behaviour, and patient behaviour are influenced by a combination of all three types of knowledge and these three also, inevitably, have a bearing on one another. They do not exist in the individual in isolation as they are influenced by others with whom the individual is in contact. For example the nurse influences or has a bearing on the patient and vice versa. The relationship between these variables is demonstrated in Fig. 7.2.

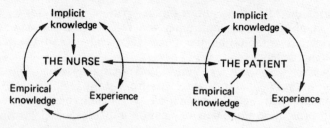

Fig. 7.2 The relationship between implicit, experiential and empirical knowledge on nurse and patient behaviour.

Clearly the nurse and the patient are not only influenced by each other, as other people such as relatives and colleagues will feed into the system and the relative weight or power of any influence will, in part, be situationally determined.

Behaviour is not only influenced by what people think or believe they know, but also by environmental factors. Not all behaviour is actually thought about. Numerous examples can be found of learned behaviour which is carried out routinely or habitually. Traditional learning therories of operant and classical conditioning can help us understand these. Social learning theory as outlined by Bandura (1977) provides a more personal dimension and draws attention to the reciprocal relationship which exists between the person and the environment.

This relationship will inevitably be influenced by specific factors which relate to the environment (e.g. does the ward environment lend itself to patients being actively involved in self care?) and also by factors which relate to the individual (e.g. are the knowledge base and skills of the nurse(s) compatible with a particular approach to care?).

Empirically supported knowledge is playing an increasingly significant part in determining nursing care and also patient behaviour. There is today a large field of knowledge linking psychology, health and illness, of which both health professionals and the general public are becoming increasingly aware. The following section of this chapter will outline a number of these areas.

Psychology and health

The twentieth century has seen a number of major health related changes. One of these is the shift from the prevalence of infectious diseases to chronic diseases with multiple causes. Pneumonia, tuberculosis and enteritis, once major killers, have been replaced by, amongst other diseases, heart disease, cancer, injuries, respiratory disease and diabetes mellitus. Increasingly it is becoming recognised that the major diseases of today have a number of determinants associated with individual, environmental and life style factors. That there is a relationship between behaviour and health is becoming increasingly clear. Factors such as diet, smoking and drug abuse, excessive drinking, unsafe driving, lack of exercise, working conditions and pollution, all have a bearing on the health status of the individual and whole communities. Recognition of the behaviourally linked nature of many illnesses makes health promotion and illness prevention more possible. Unfortunately, not all illness is prevented and the very nature of current health problems demands an approach to care which takes account of the multiple causation of ill health, the chronic nature of many disorders, and the stress and anxiety associated with many of the medical interventions available.

Health and illness can be conceptualised and defined in a variety of ways. They can be identified as constructs and thus by implication have an opposite pole. Individuals will have their own view of what constitutes the opposite end of the pole to healthy, and also what can be defined as either healthy or not healthy. The opposite poles, for example healthy/unhealthy, can represent end points on a continuum and an individual's health state at any time will fall somewhere on the continuum. Where it falls will reflect many factors including personal, social and medical definitions of health and illness, and the perception of the person or people making the judgement. It is possible for discrepancies to occur between an individual's own judgement about their health status, and the judgement of others, for example health professionals, friends, colleagues, and so on.

Age and sex factors are known to influence definitions of health. 'Children define health as feeling good and being able to participate in desired activities . . . in contrast, adults typically define health as a state enabling them to perform at least minimal daily activities and including physical, mental, spiritual and social components. The adult's perception, as well as life situation, influences the definition of health.' (Murray and Zentner, 1989).

Health and illness are defined differently by men and women. Women visit the doctor and are hospitalised more frequently than men, including cases of emotional illness (Briscoe, 1970). Murray and Zentner (1989) summarise a number of definitions of health, the most marked contrast occurring between that provided by the World Health Organisation, and Dunn (1961).

The United Nations World Health Organisation define health as a 'state of complete physical, mental and social wellbeing and not merely the absence of disease'. This definition makes no allowance for degrees of illness and health.

By contrast, Dunn (1961) defines health and illness in terms of a continuum, representing a relative and ever changing state of being.

'Health-wellbeing and disease-illness are now thought of as complex, dynamic processes on a continuum that includes physical, psychological (emotional, cognitive, and developmental), spiritual and social components and adaptive behavioural responses to internal and external stimuli . . .' (Murray and Zentner, 1989; p.5).

Final agreement on what constitutes health is never likely to be reached. Despite this, it is possible to identify factors which have a bearing on an individual's health status, and the ways in which these interact to produce health change. A person's health status is in a constant state of flux. What is important is the direction of change and the processes involved in that change. The more we can understand the influential factors in the process the better able we are to control it. This understanding has relevance for everyone, not just health care professionals. If it is confined to the professionals then the general public and patients immediately become reliant on others for their health. To prevent this happening, sharing knowledge becomes an important feature of health care.

Understanding the factors associated with the process of health change is of dual relevance for the nurse. On the one hand it has significance in relation to his or her professional role, but it also has personal significance. Health and ill health are something that we all experience and we can all play a role in promoting and maintaining our own health. It is all too easy as a health professional to focus exclusively on 'the patient' at the expense of caring for the self. What follows in this chapter has equal significance for the nurse and his or her health as it does for those in his or her care.

Before moving on to a number of specific psychological features associated with health a model will be outlined – a model which makes it possible to conceptualise health change in behavioural terms, and to demonstrate the relationship between environmental, social, psychological and biological influences on health (Fig. 7.3). Clearly this model represents only one approach to conceptualising

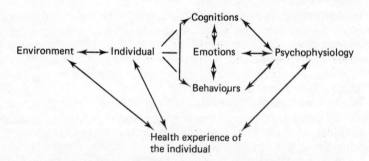

Fig. 7.3 The reciprocal relationship between the environment, the individual, psychophysiology and health.

health change but it provides a useful framework within which to place relevant aspects of psychological knowledge, and also to identify gaps in this knowledge.

As already stated, an individual's state of health is influenced by a multiplicity of factors which interrelate. Social learning theory centres on the reciprocal relationship which exists between the environment and the individual. When applying psychology to enhance our understanding of health and health behaviours, the relationship between the environment and the individual needs extending to include the relationship between psychology and physiology.

The term 'environment' refers to both the people and the physical objects in one's life.

'The concept of environment encompasses the total surroundings of an individual's life and its relationship to the person's behaviour. We all live surrounded by air, which can be clean, smoggy or full of sulphur and carbon monoxide. We all drink water, which can be pure or contaminated. We are all affected by radiation. We all live in neighbourhoods that are safe or too dangerous to walk in. All these factors are a consequence of some human behaviour.'

(Goldstein and Krasner, 1987)

But not only are they a consequence of some human behaviour, they also have an effect on it. This effect may or may not be compatible with health promotion and the avoidance of negative health changes.

Stress

Central to our understanding of the environment/individual/health equation is the concept of stress. The notion that stress correlates with ill-health is not new but it is only in recent years that the interrelationships between environment, the individual and their appraisal of environmental stressors and psychophysiology have been empirically investigated. Stress has been implicated in relation to the development of a number of conditions, including coronary heart disease, hypertension, cancer, asthma, backache and neuroses (Dobson, 1983; Cooper *et al.*, 1988).

Singer and Baum (1980) focused on three Cs of environmental stress – crowding, commuting, and cacophony (discordant sound or noise pollution). They emphasised that psychological and physiological responses to environmental threat were mediated by the cognitive appraisal of environmental stress factors made by the individual.

This is consistent with the interactional approach to stress adopted by Lazarus (1976), by Roskies and Lazarus (1980) and Cox and McKay (1978).

Interactional models go beyond considering stress as a stimulus, e.g. overcrowded, noisy working conditions, or as a response, e.g. Selye's (1956) General Adaptation Syndrome (GAS), but propose that stress occurs through a particular relationship between the person and the environment. It is suggested that self regulation of cognitive, emotional and behavioural coping strategies influence the impact of a stressor on the individual. The degree to which an event or situation is considered as a stressor by an individual will be influenced by whether that individual perceives they have the ability to cope with or control that situation.

Lazarus (1976) identifies two categories of coping. The first involves actual behaviour which is problem-focused and attempts to change the problematic aspects of the individual's relationship with his environment. The second Lazarus describes as 'palliative' or 'emotion focused' and is concerned with softening the impact of a stressor. An individual is thus allowed to detach himself emotionally from a situation. A resultant problem may be that the potentially threatening aspects of a situation may remain, and effective coping behaviour is not learned.

The way in which an individual perceives and copes with stress is significant both in relation to the development of ill health, and the way in which an individual copes with ill health. The experience of ill health in itself becomes a potential stressor, to which an individual has to respond and adapt and which, in turn, has a further cumulative effect on that individual's health state. We are all constantly having to adapt to external and internal stressors and there are considerable individual differences in the way we do this. Most people are probably unaware of their habitual ways of doing this, or the positive and negative consequences of these ways. However an individual's stress response is intricately linked with their health experience and the process of health change.

Returning to Fig. 7.3, each of the components can be viewed as a potential stressor or as a positive or negative response to a stressor, as indicated in Fig. 7.4.

Change can be either a threat or a challenge to an individual. Environmental change can result in an individual experiencing stress if they believe the demands made on them tax or exceed their adjustive resources (Lazarus, 1976). Change thus becomes a threat leading to feelings of uncertainty, loss of control, and mental, physical and behavioural manifestations of stress. The linkage between stress and illness is not new; however in recent years a greater understanding of the physiological and neuro-chemical dimensions of stress has resulted in interest in mechanisms which could explain the links between stress and illness. Empirical data is now available which suggests that there is a relationship between the functioning of the immune system and stress (Jemmott and Locke, 1984; Baker, 1987).

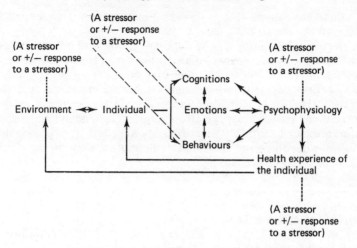

Fig. 7.4 The inter-relational model linking stress, the environment, the individual, psychophysiology and health.

In a study by Kiecolt-Glaser *et al.* (1986) a group of 35 volunteer medical students were assessed both before and during academic examinations. A number of measures of immunological function were taken including the percentage of various T-lymphocytes (some of the cells necessary to fight antigens) and the activity of natural killer (NK) cells. A reduction in T-lymphocytes or NK activity would reflect a reduction in the ability of the body's defences to fight off invasive agents.

The results showed that during the examination both T-lymphocyte percentage and NK activity were reduced. However, this reduction was modified in half of the subjects who had been instructed in a variety of relaxation procedures.

This finding is consistent with those of Arnetz *et al.* (1987) who, in an assessment of unemployed Swedish women, found that after nine months of unemployment they showed reduced lymphocyte reactivity to an antigen. However this effect was not found if the women were given a psychosocial support programme.

Anderson and Masur (1983) and Mathews and Ridgeway (1984) reviewed studies on the stress associated with hospitalisation. A number of these looked at procedures which teach and enhance coping strategies. They identified that a variety of techniques, including information giving, cognitive-behavioural coping strategies, and relaxation, can influence a patient's experience of hospitalisation and, to some extent, the results of that event. These, and other studies, are reviewed in Harvey (1989) who concludes that '. . . it is reasonable to argue that stress (however defined) has measurable and serious effects on the body and on people's health . . . . However

. . . there are enough data to show that intervention can alleviate the effects of the stressors.' (Harvey, 1989).

Effective intervention can be relatively simple and economical and can be taught by nurses in a number of settings. However it is worth remembering that a threat to one may be a challenge to another. Many people cope well with situations that others would find very stressful. There are individual differences in the ways that people perceive change and manage stress, and an understanding of these differences can add to our understanding of the personality/behaviour/health relationship and be helpful in assisting the person who is not well or not coping.

Individual differences

Type A behaviour and heart disease

During the last quarter of 1986 half of all deaths in England and Wales – over 60 000 men and women – were due to diseases of the heart and its associated blood vessels. The death rate from heart diseases is twice that from cancer, and, in the USA, it is calculated that it accounts for 1 620 219 years of potential lost life before the age of 65 (CDC, 1986). This represents enormous costs in human suffering and loss in economic terms.

In 1978 the Pooling Project Research Group was set up in the USA to coordinate and systematise data from eight prospective studies designed to identify factors which make it likely that some people will develop Coronary Heart Disease (CHD) rather than others. A summary of the data of five of these studies confirmed that hypertension, cigarette smoking and the amount of cholesterol in the blood are independent risk factors associated with the occurrence of CHD.

Psychological factors are associated with these risk factors. Diet (which influences cholesterol intake) and smoking are influenced by cognitive and emotional variables which in turn are likely to be associated with environmental factors. The idea of a direct link between behaviour and heart disease is also the subject of considerable interest. As early as 1910 Osler described the sort of person likely to have angina as not being, 'delicate or neurotic . . .' but '. . . robust, the vigorous in mind and body, the keen and ambitious man, the indicator of whose engines is always at "full speed ahead".' (Quoted from Harvey, 1989).

It was not until the 1950s, when Friedman and Rosenman noticed that many of their patients with heart disease had similar behavioural patterns, that systematic studies linking feelings, actions and cardiovascular disease, were started. Friedman and Rosenman (1974) identified the Type A behaviour pattern (TABP) and found that it constituted an independent risk factor in the development of CHD. This finding has significant implications for the management and prevention of CHD, and also for the development of testable models which link physical and psychological factors in health and illness.

TABP refers to specific patterns of behaviour which occur in some individuals under specific circumstances. It is referred to by some authors as a personality construct (Taylor and Cooper, 1988) and by others as a behaviour pattern (Harvey, 1989). The notion that there are Type A people with a specific personality trait carries the risk of implication that certain characteristics are fundamental to the individual's psychological make-up and thus fixed. However if certain individuals exhibit TABP this implies possibilities of change.

Type A behaviour is 'characterised by extremes of competitiveness, striving for achievement, aggressiveness (sometimes strongly repressed), haste, impatience, restlessness, hyperalertness, explosiveness of speech, tenseness of facial musculature and feelings of being under pressure of time and under the challenge of responsibility.' (Jenkins, 1971.) Individuals exhibiting this behaviour often have an extreme commitment to their work to the exclusion of other aspects of their life. The individual exhibiting Type B behaviour has been described by Friedman and Rosenman (1959) as 'having drive which acts as a steadying confidence-building influence, is more relaxed, unhurried, satisfied and easy going.'

Salient to the Type A construct is the consistent way in which individuals with TABP perceive demands, threats and challenges, and strive for control over people and events. The quest for control continues even when events are uncontrollable and it is likely that this response is stress inducing, maladaptive and detrimental to health. Strobe and Werner (1985) suggest that through striving to remain in control, Type A create their own stressful environment. We should note that Chesney and Rosenman (1980) identified that challenge and control are important factors for the well being of Type A Managers. These studies indicate both a positive and negative aspect to TABP.

Further conflicting results emerge from results of the Western Collaborative Group study reported by Ragland and Brand (1988). It was found that following an initial heart attack Type A and Type B deaths were approximately equal, but over a longer period of time Type A survivors outnumbered Type B. Taylor and Cooper (1988) suggest that a possible explanation for these findings might be within the framework of the control concept: There is some evidence to suggest that individuals who are 'internally' oriented, i.e. believe that they are controllers of their own destiny, engage in more generally adaptive health responses, both at preventative and remedial levels (Strickland,1978). Certain Type A individuals would possibly fall within this category. Therefore Type A behaviour might not always imply coronary-prone behaviour.

Studies identifying a positive dimension to Type A behaviour suggest that TABP cannot be considered globally and that global attempts to modify Type A behaviour could have negative consequences for some individuals.

Friedman *et al.* (1985) proposed two categories of both Type A and Type B individuals. They distinguished between charismatic and hostile Type A individuals, and relaxed and tense Type B. A charismatic Type A individual would be 'healthy, expressive, dominant, fast moving, in control, coping well and sociable.' They suggest that such individuals would remain healthy under stress. In contrast a hostile Type A individual would be competitive, expressive and dominant in a threatened and negative sense, and be coronary prone.

A relaxed Type B person, who Friedman *et al.* (1985) suggest could be less illness-prone, would demonstrate quiet, unexpressive and submissive behaviour, whereas a tense Type B person would be over controlled, unexpressive and inhibited but liable 'to explode under sufficient challenge', and could also be illness prone.

Three of the negative components which exist within the Type A behaviour construct are anger, hostility and aggression and have been termed the AHA syndrome by Spielberger *et al.* (1985). It appears that some Type A individuals exhibit more of these behaviours than others (Check and Dyck, 1986) and that such behaviours ultimately undermine health.

Measuring TABP

One of the problems associated with research has been the different methods of assessing the Type A/B construct. Measurement can be by structured interview (SI) designed to elicit TABP responses, with both the content and manner of responses to questions being assessed. The SI is dependent on being carried out by skilled personnel and is thus time consuming and costly as a measurement tool for large scale research. A number of self report questionnaires (Jenkins *et al.*, 1971; Haynes *et al.*, 1980) have been developed which can be more easily administered but which carry the risk of inaccurate reporting. The most commonly used self report questionnaire is the Jenkins Activity Survey (JAS) (Jenkins *et al.*, 1967) containing about 50 questions which ask the subject how she or he behaves in certain situations. Jenkins *et al.* (1971) showed that the overall agreement in classification using the SI and the JAS was 73 per cent and thus acceptable. Other studies have found a much smaller margin of overlap (Chesney *et al.*, 1981; Matthews *et al.*, 1982). This indicates that caution must be taken when comparing studies which use different measures.

Intervention

The identification of a behaviour pattern found to link directly with CHD raises a number of important questions.

- Can the TABP be changed?
- If it is changed does it lead to a reduction in CHD?
- What are the most effective change procedures?
- What are the ethics of change?

A number of studies (Roskies *et al.*, 1978; Levenkron *et al.*, 1983) have shown that it is possible to change aspects of TABP and that these changes may parallel measures of physiological change. Some studies have used patients who already have CHD. Friedman *et al.* (1982) used a group behaviour modification/cognitive behavioural approach to help people who had already suffered a myocardial infarct to develop self management techniques for reducing TABP. Their approach effectively reduced TABP and the reinfarction rate was only half what it was in a control group. Similar subjects were used in a study by Frasure-Smith and Prince (1985). The subjects were taught to self monitor stress and given the opportunity to talk about this to a specially trained nurse. The death rate due to cardiac disease was found to be significantly lower in the experimental group as compared to the control group.

The evidence so far is that TABP can be changed and that this can lead to a reduction in CHD. There is indication that there are positive as well as negative consequences of some aspects of TABP (see p. 215) Global attempts to change TABP may be less effective than programmes directed towards specific aspects of the behavioural pattern. A careful assessment of the potential costs and benefits of change must also be made, with the patient/client making their own decisions about what they believe is best for them, taking into account the many social, occupational and life-style factors likely to have a bearing on the decision.

Locus of control

A salient feature of research linking TABP to coronary heart disease is the role of control. Individuals with TABP strive for control over people and events. Locus of control is a personality variable which has its origins in Social Learning Theory (Rotter, 1954).

'It defines a generalised expectancy concerning the extent to which an individual believes that reinforcements, rewards or success are either internally or externally controlled. An *internal* locus of control implies a belief in personal power, control and influence over the outcome of events. An *external* locus of control implies a belief that personal power has a minimal effect on the outcome of events, these being influenced by fate, chance and powerful others.'

(Taylor and Cooper, 1988)

Extremes in either direction can be maladaptive (Rotter, 1966) and there is no such thing as 'internality' without 'externality'. To believe only in internality would be to deny the existence of any sources of external control (Reid, 1984). Externality comprises two components: 'fate/chance' and 'powerful others'. Jenner (1986) found that a belief in the influence of powerful others correlated with a greater perception of organisational stress. This study also found a positive association between organisational stress and relationship stress. Oliver (1983) found that employees in professional and managerial positions tended to be more 'internally' oriented. Lefcourt (1981) proposed that whereas most individuals react to stress, 'externals', unlike 'internals', continue to carry and add to this stress over a prolonged period of time, this ultimately having negative health consequences. In contrast to this 'internals' seek to change situations as a means to increasing personal control and reducing stress. However, in situations where personal control is not possible, if continued attempts to assert control are made – as in the case of the extreme Type A individual – this is likely to be detrimental to health. An assessment of locus of control can be made using Rotter's Internality-Externality scale (Rotter, 1966).

The notion of locus of control can be applied to the issue of who is responsible for an individual's health. Does the responsibility for one's health lie with the individual or the professional, or is it dependent on luck or fate, with nobody ultimately responsible for it? Since the development of Rotter's internal/external scale, health-specific measures of the construct have been developed and adopted by investigators in the health fields (Wallston and Wallston, 1981).

A measure of an individual's health locus of control (HLC) is a measure of their belief pattern at a particular point in time. It does not imply a fixed personality type. This distinction has significant therapeutic implications as it allows for individual change.

Wallston and Wallston (1982) provide a detailed review of HLC research literature. They conclude that 'most of the findings reported . . . attest to the construct validity of the HLC scales. The most consistent relationship is between depressive affect and the belief that one's health is unpredictable (i.e. Chance Health Locus of Control (CHLC).' (Wallston and Wallston, 1982; p. 74).

Strickland (1978) summarised the research, relating measures of locus of control to health knowledge and precautionary measures by saying:

'With some exceptions, the bulk of the reported research on I-E and precautionary health practices lends credence to the expected theoretical assumptions that individuals who hold internal as opposed to external expectancies are more likely to assume responsibility for their health. Internals appear to maintain their physical well-being and guard against accidents and disease to a greater extent than individuals who hold external expectancies.'

Wallston and Wallston (1982) suggest that the ideal partnership between health care provider and consumer is one in which each believes that the other has something to bring to the relationship and that they must work together to optimise outcomes. They suggest that a consumer belief pattern which is high Internal Health Locus of Control (IHLC), high Powerful Others Health Locus of Control (PHLC) and low Chance Health Locus of Control (CHLC) is the most conducive to a positive therapeutic relationship. Research is still needed to inform us of the health locus of control beliefs of health care professionals, their expectations of their clients' HLC beliefs, and the significance of these for the client/carer relationship and therapeutic outcomes.

Unfortunately there are numerous examples within the health care system indicative of an orientation towards removing control from patients and giving it to the professional. This is incompatible with the degree of responsibility for their health that many individuals find themselves expected to take once the acute phase of ill-health has passed. In turn, this indicates the need for a partnership between the client and the professional rather than a hierarchical relationship, and a role for health professionals in preparing their clients for responsibility and independence. Research findings bear this out, identifying a relationship between personal control and health.

However, both therapeutic interventions and future research on control and health care delivery

'must take into account actual situational potential for control, patients' perceptions and expectancies regarding control, and the expectancies of health care providers. Only by studying the complex interaction of these factors will we be able to predict health behaviour and thus intervene effectively to enhance health.'

(Wallston and Wallston, 1982)

Hardy personality

The correlation between stressful events and illness is typically only .30 and Kobasa (1979) demonstrated that many people are not becoming ill despite quite stressful lives. There has been a shift in the emphasis in 'stress and illness' research towards the study of 'resistance resources' that can neutralise the negative effects of stressful life events. Such resources include constitutional strengths (e.g. little family history of illness), social supports (e.g. social contacts and status centrality), health practices (e.g. jogging), and personality dispositions (Kobasa *et al.*, 1982). A major question is how these apparently different and diverse resistance resources operate in keeping the person healthy during their encounter with stress. An integrating theme was suggested by Kobasa (1979) when she proposed the hardiness concept – a personality variable combining several components and continuing the theme of control:

'. . . hardiness is a constellation of personality characteristics that function as a resistance resource in the encounter with stressful life events. The personality dispositions of hardiness are commitment, control, and challenge.'

(Kobasa *et al.*,1982)

Commitment reflects a disposition to become involved in rather than feel alienated from whatever one is doing. Committed people have a sense of purpose and find meaning in their activities and experiences, and they do not give up easily under pressure. They demonstrate 'active approach' rather than 'passive avoidance' behaviours.

The control disposition reflects a tendency to feel and act as if one is influential rather than helpless in regard to life's events. This does not mean that such people believe they can determine all events and exercise total control, but that by exercising imagination, knowledge, skill and choice they will have a definite influence on outcomes and events. This increases 'the likelihood that events will be experienced as a natural outgrowth of one's actions and, therefore, not as foreign, unexpected, and overwhelming experiences. In terms of coping, a sense of control leads to actions aimed at transforming events into something consistent with an ongoing life plan and is, thus, less jarring.' (Kobasa *et al.*, 1982). A feature of the challenge disposition is that change rather than stability is normal in life and change represents a challenge rather than a threat to security. Events are perceived as stimulating rather than threatening and lead to attempts to change oneself and 'grow' rather than cling to a former way of being. Challenge fosters openness and flexibility thus allowing for the effective appraisal of diverse and incongruent events.

Kobasa (1979) revealed that executives high in stressful events but low in illness showed greater commitment, control and challenge than executives experiencing similar life events but exhibiting much illness. This lends support to the hypothesis that commitment, control and challenge, i.e. 'a hardy personality', keeps people healthy despite encounters with events generally regarded as stressful. Retrospective studies such as this leave open the possibility that personality data could be the result of illness and stress. A five-year longitudinal study reported by Kobasa *et al.* (1982 op cit) suggests that the tendency towards commitment, control and challenge functions prospectively as a resistance resource, and that hardiness has its greatest health preserving effect when stressful life events mount.

Since hardiness has been identified as a significant resistance resource in buffering the effects of stressful life events, it is useful to consider (i) how hardiness develops, and (ii) what is its role with regard to other resistance resources? In regard to the second point, Kobasa *et al.* (1982) make a number of suggestions which relate to possible interactions among the resistance resources. They suggest that hardiness is especially effective in preserving health when constitutional strengths are low and that the likely mediating mechanism could be health practices. Positive health practices such as adequate rest, exercise, moderation in food and substance intake, may offset constitutional predispositions to some extent. By virtue of their approach to life, hardy people might engage conscientiously and effectively in positive health practices, as compared to people low in hardiness who might engage in more negative health practices and thereby exaggerate constitutional predispositions.

Another possible interaction they suggest is that social supports are more effective in preserving health when hardiness is high. When confronted with stressful events hardy people may actively seek out the kinds of social contacts that could decrease the stressfulness of the events, and attempt to learn from and possibly alter what is happening. In contrast, people low in hardiness might seek less support or concentrate on blanket reassurances and distraction from the events.

If future research continues to indicate the importance of hardiness as a resistance resource it will be important to learn more of how and why such a personality develops, and how people can be helped to acquire hardy personality characteristics. It is likely that existential personality theory and social learning theory can both offer something here.

Implications of research

Research on the individual differences/stress/health relationship has significant implications for individuals – including nurses and patients, and organisations. The significance of control has been highlighted in much of the research. It is important at an individual and at an organisational level to identify ways of managing and coping with change so that it becomes a challenge rather than a threat. Change leading to feelings of loss of control, threat and helplessness is associated with the experience of stress and negative health effects. This effect can occur in the health professional, the lay population and in the patient population. It can occur as a result of changes brought about by ill health and slow down recovery, and it can occur in apparently healthy individuals and precipitate ill health.

Nurses can play a role in implementing programmes to ameliorate these negative effects at a number of levels; at the organisational and managerial level, and at the individual level with staff and patients. Taylor and Cooper (1988)proposed that three processes – communication, control and counselling – are of particular importance. They suggest that organisations need effective two-way communication systems, that good communications help to reduce high stress and to lower job dissatisfaction, and that, in return, the organisation is more readily able to pinpoint areas of potential pressure and dissatisfaction.

Good communication means that employees have a greater understanding of policies and reasons for change, experience less uncertainty and have a greater perception of personal control.

The provision of counselling services and the open acknowledgement that organisational structures and change can lead to stress could help to offset the stigmatisation associated with stress. Marshall and Cooper (1981) found that this, combined with 'wellness' programmes including information on smoking, alcohol and drug abuse, and advice on diet and exercise had beneficial effects for the individual and the organisation.

Nursing management and organisation can be such that it generates stress and anxiety in both nurses and patients. Much of this could be prevented if its deleterious health effects were recognised and programmes focusing on communication, control and counselling implemented.

At the individual level, good communication reduces uncertainty and allows for the open discussion of problems and more realistic identification of problem areas. This allows for greater individual autonomy and control. It has already been identified that the perception of lack of control is associated with stress and ill health.

Individual counselling can increase self awareness and understanding of how personality variables interact to affect the stress/health relationship. This awareness is equally valuable to the patient population, nurses and the general population for promoting health.

If programmes to promote communication, control and counselling were implemented proactively to facilitate coping with the demands of life, rather than reactively, much ill-health could be avoided.

Summary and conclusion

This chapter started by focusing on nursing activities which had emerged during research with student nurses, identifying that they all potentially involved psychological as well as physical dimensions, and that the overarching theme was of nursing as an interpersonal activity involving communication and relationships between people. It moved on to identify ways in which implicit knowledge and experience could influence the nature of communications, relationships and therapeutic outcomes. Control emerged as a theme in the early part of the chapter and again in relation to empirical findings linking individual differences/stress/health.

Empirical evidence supports the position taken by Sundberg and Tyler (1963) that the first task of the clinician should be to discover the conceptual framework under which he or she is operating. A conceptual framework which ignores the importance of personal control and does not take account of the individual differences/stress/ health relationship may be capable of ameliorating physical ill health in the short term but will not effectively promote positive health in the long term.

Nursing is a complex activity requiring an immense range of knowledge and skills. The emphasis in this chapter has been on three forms of knowledge which can usefully integrate to be complementary – implicit, experiential, and empirical – and a psychological perspective has been taken in respect of each of these. Clearly the psychological perspective taken reflects inclusion of only a small selection of potentially relevant psychological knowledge; but sufficient material has been included to demonstrate that the combination of these three forms of knowledge, and a psychological perspective, can usefully be applied to inform nursing skills and attitudes, and promote effective nursing practice.

Learning Activities and Appendix 7.1

The following is an exercise based on Personal Construct Theory (PCT). It can be carried out individually or in groups.

Its main purpose is to increase the participants' awareness of their own and others' attitudes to nursing activities.

1. Write down a list of about ten nursing activities in which you have recently engaged. (If the exercise is carried out with a group the group decide together on ten activities.)
    Examples of activities could be:

    Assisting patients with personal hygiene
    Talking to patients
    Educating patients
    Giving medication

These activities are called *elements* in PCT language.

2. Take three activities at random from the list and think of a way in which two are similar and one different.

    e.g. I enjoy this . . . I do not enjoy this

This continuum is called a construct.

When this activity is carried out with a group, participants will identify a range of constructs relating to the same three elements (activities). There are no right or wrong constructs and these differences in construing can lead to interesting and useful discussion.

3. Another three elements (nursing activities) are selected from the list and the same procedure followed to produce further constructs.

    e.g. I felt well prepared for this . . . I did not feel well prepared for this
    Patient centred . . . not patient centred

4. This procedure is continued until no new constructs can be produced.
    The final list of constructs is that which the participant(s) commonly use to judge nursing activities.

The discussion generated by this activity will have increased participants' awareness of their own and others implicit assumptions and attitudes about nursing. Implications (which is not the same as correctness) of construing elements in particular ways can be usefully discussed.

It is important that this is done within a non-judgmental and supportive environment.

References

Abramson, L. (1977). *Universal Versus Personal Helplessness: an Experimental Test of the Reformulated Theory of Learned Helplessness and Depression.* PhD thesis, University of Pennsylvania.

Anderson, K. O. and Masur, F. T. (1983). Psychological preparation for invasive medical and dental procedures. *Journal of Behavioral Medicine*, **6(1)**, 1–40.

Arnetz, B. B., Wasserman, J., Petrini, B., Brenner, S. O., Levi, L., Eneroth, P., Salovaara, H., Hjelm, R., Salovaara, L., Theorell, T. and Petterson, I. L. (1987). Immune function in unemployed women. *Psychosomatic Medicine*, **49(1)**, 3–12.

Baker, G. H. B. (1987). Psychological factors and immunity. *Journal of Psychosomatic Research*, **31(1)**, 1–10.

Bandura, A. (1977). *Social Learning Theory*. Prentice-Hall, Englewood Cliffs.

Beail, N. (Ed.) (1985). *Repertory Grid Technique and Personal Constructs*. Croom Helm, London.

Briscoe, M. (1970). Sex differences in perception of illness and expressed life satisfaction. *Psychological Medicine*, **8(2)**, 339–45.

Button, E. (Ed.) (1985).*Personal Construct Theory and Mental Health*. Croom Helm, London.

Caine, J. M. and Smail, D. J. (1969). *The Treatment of Mental Illness: Science, Faith and the Therapeutic Personality*. University of London Press, London.

Check, J. V. P. and Dyck, D. G. (1986). Hostile aggression and type A behaviour. *Personality and Individual Differences*, **7(6)**,819–27.

Chesney, M. A. and Rosenman, R. H. (1980). Type A behaviour in the work setting. In *Current Concerns in Occupational Stress*, C. L. Cooper and R. Payne (Eds). Wiley, London.

Chesney, M. A., Eagleston, J. R., and Rosenman, R. H. (1981). Type A behavior: assessment and intervention. In *Medical Psychology*, C. K. Prokop and L. A. Bradley (Eds). Academic Press, New York.

Cooper, C. L., Cooper, R. D., Eaker, L. (1988). *Living with Stress*. Penguin, Harmondsworth.

Copp, L. (1971). A projective cartoon investigation of nurse-patient psychodramatic role perception and expectation. *Nursing Research*, **20(2)**, 100–12.

Cox, T. and McKay, C. (1978). Stress at work,. In *Stress*, T. Cox (Ed.). University Park Press, Baltimore MD.

De Vellis, B. M., Adams, J. L. and De Vellis, R. F. (1984). Effects of information on patient stereotyping. *Research in Nursing and Health*, **7(3)**, 237–44.

Dobson, C. B. (1983). *Stress: the Hidden Adversary*. Bogden, New Jersey.

Dunn, H. J. (1961). *High Level Wellness*. Mount Vernon Publishing Co., Washington.

Dunnett, G. (Ed.)(1988). *Working with People: Clinical Uses of Personal Construct Psychology*. Routledge, London.

Eiser, J. R. and Gossop, M. R. (1979). 'Hooked' or 'sick': addicts' perceptions of their addiction. *Addictive Behaviors*, **4(2)**, 185–91.

Fransella, F. and Bannister, D. (1977). *A Manual for Repertory Grid Technique*. Academic Press, London.

Frasure-Smith, N. and Prince, R. (1985). The Ischemic Heart Disease Life Stress Monitoring Program: impact on mortality. *Psychosomatic Medicine*, **47(5)**, 431–45.

Friedman, H. S., Hall, J. A. and Harris, M. J. (1985). Type 'A' behavior, non verbal expressive style and health. *Journal of*

Personality and Social Psychology, **48(5)**, 1299–315.

Friedman, M. and Rosenman, R. H. (1959). Association of specific overt behavior pattern with blood and cardiovascular findings: blood cholesterol level, blood clotting time, incidence of arcus senilis and clinical coronary artery disease. *Journal of the American Medical Association*, **169(12)**, 1286–96.

Friedman, M. and Rosenman, R. H. (1974). *Type A Behavior and Your Heart*. Fawcett, New York.

Friedman, M., Thoreson, C. E., Gill, J. J., Ulmer, D., Thompson, L., Powell, L., Price, V., Elek, S. R., Rabin, D. D., Breall, W. S., Piaget, G., Dixon, T., Bourg, E., Levy, R. A. and Tasto, D. L. (1982). Feasibility of altering type A behavior pattern after myocardial infarction. Recurrent Coronary Prevention Project Study: methods, baseline results and preliminary findings. *Circulation*, **66(1)**, 83–92.

Goffman, E. (1961). *Asylums: Essays on the Social Situation of Mental Patients and Other Inmates*. Penguin, Harmondsworth.

Goldstein, A. P. and Krasner, L. (1987). *Modern Applied Psychology*. Pergamon, Oxford.

Harvey, P. (1989). *Health Psychology*. Longman, Harlow.

Haynes, S. G., Feinleib, M. and Kannel, W. B. (1980). The relationship of psychosocial factors to coronary heart disease in the Framingham study 3: eight years incidence of coronary heart disease. *American Journal of Epidemiology*, **111(1)**, 37–58.

Heider, F. (1958). *The Psychology of Interpersonal Relations*. Wiley, New York.

Hyland, M. E. and Donaldson, M. L. (1989). *Psychological Care in Nursing Practice*. Scutari, Harrow.

Jemmott, J. B. and Locke, S. E. (1984). Psychosocial factors, immunologic mediation and human susceptibility to infectious diseases: how much do we know? *Psychosocial Bulletin*, **95**, 78–108.

Jenkins, C. D., Rosenman, R. H. and Friedman, M. (1967). Development of an objective psychological test for the determination of coronary-prone behavior pattern in employed men. *Journal of Chronic Diseases*, **20(6)**, 371–9.

Jenkins, C. D. (1971). Psychological and social precursors of coronary disease. *New England Journal of Medicine*, **284(5)**, 244–55; **284(6)**, 307–17.

Jenkins, C. D., Zyzanski, S. J. and Rosenman, R. H. (1971). Progress toward validation of a computer-scored test for Type A coronary prone behavior pattern. *Psychosomatic Medicine*, **33(3)**, 193–202.

Jenner, J. R. (1986). Powerful others, non-work factors and organizational stress. *Psychological Reports*, **58(1)**, 103–9.

Kelly, G. A. (1955). *The Psychology of Personal Constructs.* 2 volumes. Norton, New York.

Kelly, G. A. (1970). A brief introduction to personal construct theory. In *Perspectives in Personal Construct Theory*, D. Bannister (Ed.), pp. 1–30. Academic Press, London.

Kelly, M. P. and May, D. (1982). Good and bad patients: a review of the literature and a theoretical critique. *Journal of Advanced Nursing*, 7(2), 147–56.

Kiecolt-Glaser, J. K., Glaser, R., Strain, E. C., Stout, J. C., Tarr, K. L., Holliday, J. E. and Speicher, C. E. (1986). Modulation of cellular immunity in medical students. *Journal of Behavioral Medicine*, 9(1), 5–22.

Kobasa, S. C. (1979). Stressful life events, personality and health: an inquiry into hardiness. *Journal of Personality and Psychology*, 37(1), 1–11.

Kobasa, S. C., Maddi, S. R., and Kahn, S. (1982). Hardiness and health: a prospective study. *Journal of Personality and Social Psychology*, 42(1), 168–77.

Larson, P. (1977). Nurse perceptions of patient characteristics. *Nursing Research*, 26(6), 416–21.

Lazarus, R. S. (1976). *Patterns of Adjustment.* McGraw-Hill, New York.

Lefcourt, H. M. (Ed.) (1981). *Research with the Locus of Control Construct.* Volume one. Academic Press, New York.

Levenkron, J. C., Cohen, J. D., Mueller, H. S. and Fisher, E. B. (1983). Modifying the Type A coronary-prone behavior pattern. *Journal of Consulting and Clinical Psychology*, 51(2), 192–204.

Maier, S. F., Seligman, M. E. P. and Solomon, R. L. (1969). Pavlovian fear conditioning and learned helplessness: effects of escape and avoidance behavior of (a) the CS-US contingency, and (b) the independence of the US and voluntary responding. In *Punishment and Aversive Behavior*, B. A. Campbell and R. M. Church (Eds). Appleton-Century-Crofts, New York.

Marshall, J. and Cooper, C. L. (Eds) (1981). *Coping with Stress at Work: Case Studies from Industry.* Gower, Aldershot.

Mathews, A. and Ridgeway, V. (1984). Psychological preparation for surgery. In *Health Care and Human Behaviour*, A. Steptoe and A. Mathews (Eds), pp. 231–59. Academic Press, London.

Matthews, K. A., Krantz, D. S., Dembroski, T. M. and MacDougall, J. M. (1982). Unique and common variance in structured interview and Kenin's activity survey measures of type A behavior pattern. *Journal of Personality and Social Psychology*, 42, 303–13.

Moss, A. R. (1988). Determinants of patient care: nursing process or nursing attitudes? *Journal of Advanced Nursing*, 13(5), 615–20.

Murray, R. B. and Zentner, J P. (1989). *Nursing Concepts for Health*

Promotion, adapted for the UK by C. Howells. Prentice-Hall, New York.

Oliver, J. E. (1983). Job satisfaction and locus of control in control in two job types. *Psychological Reports*, **52(2)**, 425–6.

Osler, W. (1910). The Lumleian lectures on angina pectoris. *The Lancet*, **1**, 839–44.

Pooling Project Research Group. (1978). Relationship of blood pressure, serum cholesterol, smoking habit, relative weight and ECG abnormalities to incidence of major coronary events: final report of the pooling project. *Journal of Chronic Diseases*, **31(4)**, 201–306.

Ragland, D. R. and Brand, R. J. (1988). Type A behavior and mortality from coronary heart disease: a review. *Current Psychological Research and Reviews*, Winter, 63–84.

Raps, C. S., Peterson, C., Jonas, M. and Seligman, M. E. P. (1982). Patient behavior in hospitals: helplessness, reactance or both? *Journal of Personality and Social Psychology*, **42(6)**, 1036–41.

Reid, D. W. (1984). Participatory control and chronic illness adjustment process. In *Research with Locus of Control Construct*, volume three, H. M. Lefcourt (Ed.). Academic Press, New York.

Roskies, E., Spevak, M., Surkis, A., Cohen, C. and Gilman, S. (1978). Changing the coronary-prone (Type A) behavior pattern in a non-clinical population. *Journal of Behavioral Medicine*, **1(2)**, 201–16.

Roskies, R. and Lazarus, R. S. (1980). Coping theory and the teaching of coping skills. In *Behavioral Medicine: Changing Health Lifestyles*, P. O. Davidson and S. M. Davidson (Eds), pp. 38–69. Brunner/Mazel, New York.

Rotter, J. B. (1954). *Social Learning and Clinical Psychology*. Prentice-Hall, Englewood Cliffs, NJ.

Rotter, J. B. (1966). Generalized expectancies for internal versus external control of re-inforcement. *Psychological Monographs*, **80(1)**, 1–28.

Seligman, M. E. P. (1975). *Helplessness: On Depression, Development and Death*. Freeman, San Francisco.

Selye, H. (1956). *The Stress of Life*. McGraw-Hill, New York.

Singer, J. E. and Baum, A. (1980). Stress, environment and environmental stress. In *Environmental Psychology: Directions and Perspectives*, N. R. Feimer and E. S. Geller (Eds). Praeger, New York.

Speilberger, C. D., Johnson, E. H., Russell, S. F., Crane, R. S., Jacobs, G. A. and Worden, T. J. (1985). The experience and expression of anger: construction and validation of an anger expression scale. In *Anger and Hostility in Cardiovascular and Behavioral Disorders*, M. A. Chesney and R. H. Rosenman, (Eds), pp. 5–30. Hemisphere McGraw-Hill, New York.

Stockwell, F. (1972). *The Unpopular Patient*. Royal College of Nursing, London.

Strickland, B. R. (1978). Internal-external expectancies and health related behavior. *Journal of Consulting and Clinical Psychology*, **46(6)**, 1192–211.

Strobe, M. J. and Werner, C. (1985). Relinquishment of control and type A behavior pattern. *Journal of Personality and Social Psychology*, **48(3)**, 688–701.

Sundberg, N. D. and Tyler, L. E. (1963). *Clinical Psychology*. Methuen, London.

Taylor, H. and Cooper, C. L. (1988). Organizational change – threat or challenge? The role of individual differences in the management of stress. *Journal of Organization Change Management*, **1(1)**, 68–80.

Viney, L. L. (1985). Physical illness: a guidebook for the kingdom of the sick. In *Personal Construct Theory and Mental Health*, E. Button (Ed.), pp. 262–3. Croom Helm, London.

Wallston, B., De Vellis, B. and Wallston, K. (1983). Licensed practical nurses sex role stereotypes. *Psychology of Women Quarterly*, **7**, 199–208.

Wallston, K., Wallston, B. and De Vellis, B. (1976). Effect of negative stereotype on nurses' attitudes towards an alcoholic patient. *Journal of Studies on Alcohol*, **37(5)**, 659–65.

Wallston, K. and Wallston, B. (1981). Health locus of control scales. In *Research with the Locus of Control Construct*. Volume one. H. M. Lefcourt (Ed.). Academic Press, New York.

Wallston, K. A. and Wallston, B. S. (1982). Who is responsible for your health? The construct of health locus of control. In *Social Psychology of Health and Illness*, G. S. Sanders and J. M. Suls (Eds). Lawrence Erlbaum, Hove.

Watts, M. H.(1988). *Shared Learning*. Scutari, Harrow.

Wegner, D. M. and Vallacher, R. R. (1977). *Implicit Psychology: an Introduction to Cognition*. Oxford University Press, New York.

Westbrook, M. T. and Viney, L. L. (1982). Psychological reactions to the onset of chronic illness. *Social Science and Medicine*, **16(8)**, 899–905.

Woods, P. and Cullen, C. (1983). Determinants of staff behavior in long-term care. *Behavioral Psychotherapy*, **11(1)**, 4–17.

8 Caring: the nature of a therapeutic relationship

Introduction

The author, a practising nurse educator and psychotherapist examines his recent experience of hospitalisation and surgery for the purpose of analysing 'therapeutic' and 'non-therapeutic' influences in care. Events experienced as a patient provide the springboard to introduce those professional insights and interpersonal awarenesses necessary to the appreciation of a therapeutic relationship.

Much of this account is based on the author's observations of personal and social dynamics, skills and attitudes of direct care staff, the integrity of which has the power to maximise the therapeutic potential of the nurse-patient relationship.

Patient status, the clinical environment and the effects carers can have on the sick are first reported, then put under scrutiny and reflected upon, under heads of 'Insights for carers'.

Finally, the author draws together his insights to form a comprehensive reference of the social dynamics, skills and awareness that contribute to a relationship becoming therapeutic, and makes suggestions as to how clinical practice and professional education may be harnessed to supervision to maximise the therapeutic potential of the nurse-patient relationship.

It is hoped that the following experience, gained at a time of intense emotional and intellectual growth, shared within a personal action research frame will help to illuminate 'the client experience', provoke thoughtful reflection and enrich the reader's acceptance that 'therapeutic relationing' cannot afford to be under-credited.

On being well: the nature of health

In December 1987, accompanied by my wife, Anna, I travelled to my mother's home for a couple of days prior to Christmas. The Autumn Term, having being particularly busy for both of us in our respective teaching careers, caused us to view this as a well earned trip where we might combine family reunion with a little diversionary fun.

After a light tea we went out for a drink. This outing had the feel of 'a treat', the more so as we called along the way to collect David, a younger cousin we had not seen for many months.

Following a short drive we alighted at an old beamed inn adjoining an ancient village churchyard. The sharp night air made the warmth of the interior all the more inviting.

A couple of hours – and a few pints later – a troop of players resplendent in mediaeval costumes strolled in to offer entertainment, an impromptu mystery play of George and the Dragon. The main protagonists, a figure dressed as a jester, who gave a colloquial recitation, and two other fellows, dressed respectively as George and the dragon, frolicked around us. I joined with numerous other customers to become part of this fray, heckling and threatening George who, following each swipe of his sword, took a sup from the nearest pint to him, mine!

I had never felt so relaxed or had as much fun all year and was really starting to look forward to Christmas.

Over the course of the evening I drank three pints and, as Anna drove home, remembered feeling full and satisfied. It had been a good night with the family and Christmas had started well.

Insights for carers (1)

I am reminded in the above passage of just what the therapeutic relationship strives to achieve – 'health'. Health is substantially more than a sanitised or symptom free existence; it is rather 'for the sheer joy of it', a state of harmony between body, mind, spirit and our social community which permits us to live life adventurously. Health in this context relates to 'growth' and 'pleasure' and our ability to engage experientially with ourselves and to form intimate relations with others.

I am not alone in favouring an holistic definition. Other nurse theorists have observed health to be: an optimum level of energy when interpersonal and developmental activities are most productively performed (Peplau, 1952); the ability of an individual to meet his own needs (Henderson, 1969); one's position on a dynamic continuum of health-illness ever subject to change (Roy, 1979); a condition of personal integrity where all parts work to complement a whole (Orem, 1980); a value-laden word culturally denoting behaviours which are of high value (Rogers, 1970).

To be healthy is to have energy to play and self actualise, to be at home in dynamic movement, organismically whole and socially able. In sum, to live life creatively with the confidence to experiment with new ways of being. Nurses, within the bond of a therapeutic relationship must elicit and role model these qualities.

On becoming ill: regression and hospital symbolism

Back at my mother's home my sensation of fullness lingered on. At midnight, still feeling full I drank some water with Alka Seltzer. In bed the fullness persisted. About 3 o'clock I started to retch.

Anna brought a bowl to the bedside and suggested I saw a doctor – I refused. We were to drive back later that morning and I did not want to disturb my mother or make too much of a fuss. Lying in bed, occasionally retching but with nothing to show for it save an acidic taste in my mouth I passed the night. I guessed the beer I had drunk had been off. Five o'clock came – still retching I now knew something was really wrong. At 7 o'clock I took up the offer of a doctor. My body felt hot to the touch and I felt dizzy, tremulous.

My breathing was by now laboured and, with my heart rate and temperature up, I realised I could no longer go home without seeking aid. From this time on events speeded up and I lost appreciation of time. A general practitioner came, examined me and diagnosed an ulcer. I queried this – 'I'm not the personality type' I said. An ambulance was called and in due time arrived. Not until I tried to get out of bed did I realise how weak I was.

In the ambulance, on a narrow bed with the cot sides up, earlier memories were triggered of a similar ride when I was seven and had broken my leg. I had spent a discomforting night then also. I was surprised by how vivid these earlier memories were and how readily they had been restimulated by current events. It was difficult for a few moments to recollect if I was aged forty or seven. I made an effort to shake myself into present awareness, engaging the ambulance men in conversation to disengage from the past and a creeping sense of unreality.

I was by now feeling toxic; my mind swayed.

Insights for carers (2)

Distortions of time, memories of previous illness, unresolved fears relating to death and feelings of helplessness were all evoked in the acute onset described above. My being reminded of being seven again suggests that regressive influences were at work

Regression is defined as a return to earlier less sophisticated adaptive behaviour. This may take the form of a client demonstrating dependence; avoiding responsibility; losing their initiative; enacting 'child-like' behaviours such as sulks or projecting 'parent-like' roles on those who care for them.

Folklore relating to 'The Hospital' compounds this process.

It is cautionary to remember that to the public 'hospitals' represent much more than a workplace; imaginative perception causes them to be seen as taboo places where the mysteries of life and death unfold and where 'special others' – such as doctors and nurses – 'fight' with death and disease.

Few people have a value-free view of hospital life. Many individuals naturally associate hospitals with the 'rites of passage' of birth and death; especially the latter; 'places where people go to die'.

When frightened or caught in the midst of a life threatening event, it is all too easy to become haunted by fears of 'the worst possible outcome'. Dramatic interpretation and symbolic communication are the common currency of acute illness and hospital care.

My observations offer a good deal of support for 'symbolic interactionism', a view of the world which states:

- individuals respond to those unique meanings they carry with them rather than concrete situations or events;
- the meaning and/or definition of a situation is determined via an individual's social interaction with others; and
- the symbolic meanings an individual attaches to life events are modified through ongoing reinterpretation.

(Blumer, 1969)

This has considerable implications for the therapeutic relationship and the performance of 'individualised care', for it suggests that care professionals, if they are to perform in research-minded and process-aware ways, must appreciate:

- that each client views the world uniquely;
- that there are as many definitions of reality as there are clients;
- that all behaviour has meaning;
- that they need to be wary of invalidating a client's meanings in favour of their own 'professionalised values' and biases; and
- that through the medium of their therapeutic relationship they have a particular potential for helping clients to redefine their experience in health enhancing ways.

It is a tall order to ask the nurse to attend to the subconscious symbolism they portray to clients; far better they are exposed to professional preparation where their interactions are examined and to clinical supervision of a kind which feeds back to them 'how they are perceived'.

On entering hospital: establishing reality orientation and managing personal boundaries in the care relationship

On arrival at hospital events felt real enough but twice as fast. I was examined – wheeled down a whirl of corridors to the X- ray department – fed what I took to be barium – and eventually told I had an hiatus hernia. Knowing this brought a degree of relief; it was something I could start to make sense of events with.

Having a current diagnosis enabled me to speculate ahead; I envisaged bedrest, medical intervention and an early ride home. This was not to be. I was informed a nasogastric tube would be passed, after which I could expect to be conveyed to a hospital in Surrey, nearer my home. I swallowed the nasogastric tube – nothing came back. Several attempts later – with ever larger tubes – I began to cough up frothy blood. X-rays were taken. Eventually, it had to be admitted that my stomach was too distended and kinked to receive a gastric tube. All they could get were my lungs. Though the experience was uncomfortable I had not been anxious, but rather relieved and hopeful that a potential end might be in sight.

Insights for carers (3)

From a client's eyeview it was important to be told exactly what was happening to me and to be given a blow by blow account of investigations as they occurred. With my sensory world fragmented, fantasy started to predominate. Whenever a space of information was left amiss, I had a tendency to fill that space with anxiety. This suggests to me that:

- patients need as much information as possible to orientate to the crisis ridden world around them;
- factual information removes a lot of unncecessary drama and helps clients place their imagined fears on hold; and
- contact with a key worker – someone to provide consistency and to support the development of a relationship – is essential for psychological ease and reality orientation during admission.

Involvement and relationship with another is both necessary for the enactment of reality orientation (Glasser, 1965) and development of the therapeutic relationship (Peplau, 1952): Fig. 8.1 indicates that maintaining orientation while keeping a relationship therapeutic also necessitates that 'personal boundaries' be effectively managed.

To remain 'separate', as opposed to 'emotionally distant', is a key skill if carers are to balance 'empathy' and 'friendliness' with 'intellectual clarity'. Therapeutic distance is important, for a client needs to perceive the carer as sympathetic, yet undamaged by the distress they themselves are experiencing and able to emotionally contain them.

On awaiting surgery: defence mechanisms in times of crisis

Now I prepared myself for the worst – surgery.

The physician gave way to a surgeon. I was informed that, as my stomach was pushing up through my diaphragm to embarrass my lung, an operation would have to be performed. This information, delivered in a matter of fact way left little to discuss. Before this information had sunk in, or I was able to make enquiry, people had gone.

As evening fell I was wheeled into the surgical ward and my body was shaved and prepared for operation. The pre-medication stopped my retching and relieved most of my discomfort. I was alert and able to relay my medical history when asked.

A consultant anaesthetist now came to my bed. He was gentle, softly spoken, and for the first time I felt the busyness around me start to subside. His voice was slow and I felt supported and listened to.

I saw Anna and mother again at this time, and stayed light and jokey while they wished me the best. No need to 'make a drama out of a crisis' I felt. I was resigned to what had to be. As there was no

1 ORIENTATION:

Carer and client meet as strangers, orientate to each other and establish rapport while working together to clarify and define existing problem. Carer notes personal reactions to client and seeks to avoid stereotypic responses that limit therapeutic potential.

2 IDENTIFICATION:

Client and carer clarify each other's perceptions and expectations, examine past experiences that shade present meanings. Carer notes client's reaction to them, sources of trust and mistrust, dependence upon them or rejection of their interventions.

3 EXPLORATION:

Carer encourages client to take an active responsible role in their own therapy, to self explore and examine their feelings, thoughts and behaviour, and to trust to their own skills and resources. Carer seeks to convey acceptance, concern, and trust to facilitate this process. Wellness becomes a goal in itself, carer listens and employs interpretive skills to enable client's understanding of all those avenues open to them and agencies available to help their self adjustment.

4 RESOLUTION:

Termination of therapeutic relationship. Client encouraged to be less involved with helper. Carer also establishes independence from the client and works through issues of separation. Client's needs are met re original problem and new goals orientated to enriching wellness. Occupational and leisure interests encouraged.

(Adapted from Peplau 1952)

Fig. 8.1 Phases of the therapeutic relationship (adapted from Peplau, 1952).

real choice to make, I felt little anxiety. I felt detached, witnessing events, and determined not to give in to hopelessness.

In the pre-operation room I met the anaesthetist again. His voice remained soft and unhurried and I felt myself relax. I remember saying to myself that if these were to be my final moments I was going to live them with dignity.

As the anaesthetic flowed into me and I drifted from consciousness I caught snatches of a dream of a canal bridge I played under in childhood. I remembered I had dreamt this dream under dental gas at the age of four.

Insights for carers (4)

During the above period I drifted between internal sensations of discomfort within, to bewildering social relations without. If asked how I was, I said 'fine', as I could not, or rather chose not to attend to the gravity of my situation. I believe I was engaging in defence mechanisms of 'repression' and 'denial'.

Defence mechanisms, coping strategies which give respite from anxiety, protect the self via enabling an individual to deny or distort a stressful event so as to restrict their awareness and emotional involvement with it. They are unconscious and two or three may be combined together. When overused such defences narrow down an individual's perception of reality. At times like these a carer may need to educate a client to the other behavioural options open to them.

Resolving and working through defence mechanisms is a salient task of the therapeutic relationship; it is therefore necessary for carers to frequent themselves with the more common defensive behaviours.

Repression   This involves the exclusion of a painful or stress inducing thought, feeling, memory or impulse from awareness; it is the underlying basis of all mental defence mechanisms and moulds much socialised and professional behaviour. Repressed feelings, commonly sexual or aggressive, though generally out of awareness continue to exert pressure, and may be released in appropriate surroundings or expressed in times of extreme anxiety. Repression may also fail to function in febrile or toxic states.

Denial   Denial of reality shows itself when an individual discards or transforms an emotive event in such a way that it appears to be unrecognisable. Denial is typically present in the first minutes of an individual's adjustment to the death of a loved one. It may seduce the nurse into believing a client has less trauma or pain than is in fact experienced.

Rationalisation   Here reasoning is employed to deflect from the emotional significance of an event; i.e. the sudden death of a spouse may be rationalised as 'better than a long illness'; though the hurt is just as acute. If a carer takes what a rationalising client says at face value, they may well see only half the clinical picture.

Identification   The wish to be like and/or assume the personality characteristics of another, so much so that the individual concerned becomes estranged from their own personality. Simply, it represents unconscious imitation, an integral part of socialisation and sexual programming. In the hospital such passive receptivity, in contrast to relational reciprocity, can lead to the client confirming all we say and do. Such a client may validate all our biases, so causing us to be less exploratory than we might otherwise be.

Projection   An unconscious means of dealing with unacceptable parts of ourselves by splitting them off and attributing them to others; i.e. others are blamed for one's own shortcomings. A client may project his own distress and self absorption on to nursing staff and so view them as too busy or preoccupied to care for him.

Displacement The discharge of pent-up emotional energies on to objects or persons less threatening than the person or situation which caused them. I am reminded of the 'pecking-order' that may occur in families or work communities where anger is felt at the head but passed down amongst the ranks. The nurse a client feels safest with may receive the brunt of their emotional discharge. It is no accident that we show our tempers to those we trust or like the most.

Regression Reverting to an earlier, age inappropriate, level of behaviour to avoid responsibility and/or present environmental demands. This can be so easily compounded by patient status, bedrest and being placed at the mercy of a strange unfathomable clinical environment where people do things for you rather than with you.

Below, defences are related to their psychological roots and social use (modified from Kroeber, 1963). In this context they can be appreciated as exaggerated behavioural norms.

Psychological root	As a normal means of coping	As a defence
Impulse restraint	– Appropriate suppression	– Repression
Selective awareness	– Concentration	– Denial
Role modelling	– Socialisation	– Identification
Sensitivity	– Empathy	– Projection
Impulse diversion	– Sublimation	– Displacement
Time reversal	– Playfulness	– Regression

Note
Defence mechanisms are as common in the staff team as in the client population and form a basis for much professional behaviour; their presence and/or overuse presents a powerful argument for clinical team supervision.

On extraordinary experiences: altered states of consciousness and psycho-spiritual aspects of the care relationship

My next conscious moment was filled with darkness. I tried to open my eyes and speak, nothing moved or came out. 'Am I dead?' I wondered. Resigning myself to powerlessness, I reasoned I would just have to make the best of it.

I next heard a snatch of voices, seemingly far off, and felt myself being lifted and turned. I realised for the first time I was not dead. Many questions surfaced: 'Has the anaesthesia worn off?; Is this before or after the operation?; Will I feel the surgeons cutting into me?'. This was all very matter of fact – I was not allowing myself the luxury of an emotion.

Gradually I explored my bodily sensations. I became aware it was not me breathing; something was inside doing this for me. I remembered a film, 'The Alien', where a parasitic entity invades a human host; I smiled to myself but nothing moved. Strange to say, I also felt free to take stock: 'I have had a full life – do I really want to go back?'. I weighed things up for some time, remembering, reflecting on my life and relationships.

Anna and Marc, my son, were foremost in my mind. I had lived a fatherless childhood, I would not inflict this on my own son. Similarly I was determined not to leave the life I had with Anna in this way. In short, I contracted with myself to stay alive whatever it cost in terms of my personal resources. I never once during this time doubted it was in my power to live – or to die.

This state of suspended existence lasted for some hours. Eventually my consciousness became hazy, I thought I heard Anna's voice – but could not tell how much was real and how much imagined before floating into unconsciousness again.

My awakening to conventional reality was blurred, but recognisably on a ward with a cardiac monitor and tubes around me. I was aware of Anna and mother but could not focus upon them; like as a dream, the more I tried to focus the harder it was to see. I felt as if I was suspended in thick syrup – all my movements and senses were out of synchronisation and my thoughts formed in slow motion. Occasionally this slow other world of heavy haze would suddenly rip apart and pockets of alertness and clarity enter, to give way just as suddenly a little later to slow syrupy haze again. Even though my external world was fuzzy my internal one stayed clear. It was as if an internal 'other world' reality, one where I could witness myself – as in lucid dreaming – awoke, remained coherent and logical to its own laws and took over, to provide a venue where I could work things out in peace.

Insights for carers (5)

Lucid states, as the one described above, happen to clients more frequently than is imagined (Trevelyan, 1989; Oakes, 1981; Orne, 1986), but not enough time is given to attending to or processing them. Simply, there is often no heading for psycho-spiritual experiences in the nursing/medical records. Nevertheless, such experiences must be worked through for a return to full health; they are the meat of therapeutic relating in that they represent catalytic turning points. A little time spent in post-surgical counselling would do much to facilitate understanding and integration. Reintegration is the essential objective here. A counsellor attentive to spiritual aspects of care and the derivation of individualised meanings could do much in this area. If more clinical and managerial attention was directed towards balancing the view of 'client as an ailing body' with 'client as a spiritual being', I believe clinical environments would be much healthier places to live and work within.

As a nurse, I think I know what happened; while I was on the ventilator my anaesthesia wore off but my dose of muscle relaxant stayed effective, hence I could wake but not move.

On awaking from surgery: the case for individualised care

Gradually cohesion returned and I was able to glue my sensations back into a recognisable social world where I could start to relate to others. I checked my movement – I was stiff and full of heavy dull pain. Anna, mother, and my son Marc were present. 'So I'm not dead after all' I thought. For the next twenty four hours I slept, woke, passively received a blanket bath, drank 5 mls of water hourly and sucked lemon sticks. I looked forward to visiting when I could sample a little of the 'normal me', but everything else ran together.

On my second conscious day I was brighter; it was also dawning on me how limited my movement was. A sudden intake of breath or a cough and my generalised dull pain focused into a sharp one at the site of my chest drain.

A taped dressing spiralled from my right hip to my left shoulder blade. I joked I'd been mistaken for a potato. Joking, coping through displacement and denial, was the only means I had at my disposal to put things in perspective and relate in a more normal way.

During this period I tentatively explored the range of movement available to me. There were few comfortable positions and no painfree ones. Sleep was a series of intermittent catnaps, and whenever my breathing relaxed to a sleeping rhythm I would cough and awake in pain. Talking also presented a problem; anything above a whisper caused my diaphragm to jump into spasms. Nights were long, and days busy and tiring. I lived for those few lucid moments during visiting when I found the energy to feel really alive again

The day staff kept busy, superficial and distant. By contrast the night nurses drew close, chatted, took an interest in me and listened to the short whispered comments I could make. With them I felt a valued person first and a condition second. They answered my questions objectively, orientated me to what was going on and let a bond of friendship form. I felt I really needed friends at this time.

Insights for carers (6)

As a forty year old I was used to an independent life; as a male my assertion was linked with my sexual identity; as a teacher and psycho-therapist I was used to helping others from a position of strength. In the status of a patient these usual life roles were drastically reversed.

I felt myself becoming increasingly alienated from my previous sense of self worth by the transient relationships of carers who came in to perform intimate 'tasks on me' with little more than a superficial 'good morning' or 'how are we' and who left before I could answer.

I felt childlike and unimportant even though my body was being cared for. Being 'treated as an equal and valued in my own right' was an essential therapeutic need in this period. The day staff, in putting my condition first, failed to meet this need; the night staff, conversely, met it by attending to my person.

Rogers (1983) suggests person-centred care demands of practitioners that they:

– move away from facades, pretence and putting up a front;
– gain more self direction and value this in others;
– cultivate a reduced need to pretend and hide real feelings;
– value honest communicative relationships;
– be open regarding their own inner reactions and feelings; and
– be aware and sensitive to external events.

Carers, who give up their defences in favour of the above qualities are, I suggest, better able to:

– listen;
– demonstrate good contact with themselves and their own realities;
– stay open to and check out their perceptions;
– pay attention to those social processes that create fruitful interaction;
– share their own awareness and knowledge; and
– enable their clients to perform successfully without them (Barber, 1988).

Consequently, the therapeutic relationship they enact is more likely to:

– value the human condition;
– incorporate the client as a resource and cause them to feel valued;
– honour openness and honesty;
– volunteer information and invite questioning of the professional carer; and
– allow space for and encourage clients to express their fears.

A relationship founded upon such principles complements the nursing arts by creating a culture in which nurses may facilitate renewed energy via the medium of the nurse-patient relationship (Peplau, 1952); help patients meet components of basic care relating to breathing, eating and warmth (Henderson, 1969); analyse problems and potential problems while engaged in problem-directed activity (Roy, 1979); overcome the limitations of illness via supporting the patient's ability for self care (Orem, 1980); while re-establishing and promoting the interactive balance of an individual and their environment (Rogers, 1970).

Nursing, in this account, is seen to be an interpersonal process that works best when relating insights from the care sciences to clients in a humanistic and person valuing way, through the medium of an empathic relationship which incorporates the client as a care resource while facilitating them to ways of thinking, feeling and relating that maximise a potential for self-directed growth and health.

For care of this calibre to evolve, nurse educators must dovetail personal and professional development, and clinical managers need to make provision for peer support or supervision where the care practitioner may talk through those personal/professional distresses that emanate from the performance of care.

On the politics of experience: therapeutic and non-therapeutic intervention

On what I thought to be my third post operative day – but was in fact my fifth – I was approached just before visiting time by the Ward Sister who told me she was going to give me a pain-killing injection prior to getting me up and sitting me in a chair. As Anna was travelling up from Surrey to visit me, and as the injection cited made me sleepy, I enquired if this could be delayed so that I might remain alert during visiting time. This suggestion was not favourably received, and I was lectured on how important it was to get up. I agreed, but enquired whether two hours would make such a difference, and repeated my rationale. This did not go down well, and I was told that I must do as she asked.

The tempo now increased; we both had the bit between our teeth. I said, with respect, as a client I had a right to be heard; it was important to my own well-being for me to fully contact my kin; they were my lifeline. She objected. Surely, I argued, in these days of the nursing process and client-centred care my request was a reasonable enough one to make. She stormed off. My visitors came and went.

With their departure I had my injection, was helped out of bed and sat in a chair. While attending to me the Sister said nothing. I did not feel forgiven for querying her instructions. A few hours later I heard laughter; the junior nurses and Sister were playing, flicking water at one another. When she realised I was watching, the Sister stopped. I seemed to represent a problem for her, and suspected I had been 'hit by a projection' (see 'Insights for carers (4)'). A little after this a doctor was called and, following much flirtatious glancing, the Sister came out to tell me I was being transferred out from intensive care. I asked the Sister if this meant I was out of danger. She made no answer, but returned to the office where the doctor remained. More flirtatious glances ensued.

I checked myself, surely I was not becoming paranoid; I had earlier been told I would be here for at least a week more. A change of environment felt quite daunting, especially separation from that meaningful contact forged with the night staff. Within the hour porters came to collect me. When a nurse came over to carry the intravenous drips, I asked her to relay to the Sister and Doctor the message that I did not respect their professional cowardice; she looked embarrassed and I doubt if this message was relayed.

My move from Intensive Care felt ill prepared and emotive. On the positive side, I was aware that I had the resemblance of an emotion forming within me; a potential for anger; confirmation of my ability to experience emotions again.

Insights for carers (7)

A change of wards, a trivial thing for a healthy individual or nurse, can be a major event for a client emerging from a life crisis. Preparation is necessary. It felt like changing worlds, from a reality I knew to one I could not comprehend. The manner of this change put all my symbolic meanings in shift; those who pertained to care for me were now seemingly doing the most damage to my sense of orientation.

Attention to 'transitional periods', such as a change of ward, elevate care from a level of adequacy to one of excellence.

The need for carers to work through the 'resolution phase' of a therapeutic relationship, due to transfer or discharge, has been noted earlier (see Fig. 8.1).

Although it is important for a nurse to relay accurate information to a client, as information is what we construct our reality from, this is but half the story. Consideration must also be given to the 'intervention style' employed. When nurses act as guardians of the ward and its formalised medical systems, there is a tendency for them to behave in a manner reminiscent of a critical or/and controlling parent. This occurred with the Sister above, who made use of degenerative forms of authoritative intervention to:

'prescribe' what should happen;

'inform' me of her decision; and

'confront' me when my opinion differed from hers.

Authoritative interventions, when used in a therapeutic way can set safe boundaries and complement care (Fig. 8.2); when used in the defensive form described, they undergo degeneration.

In this phase of my illness, when I was attempting to rebuild myself and reorientate to the world, 'cathartic', 'catalytic' and 'supportive' interventions would have done much to release my emotional tensions, awareness, self esteem and worth.

Traditionally, nursing has evolved in the shadow of medicine and adopted a similar 'controlling stance' to care; such behaviour, if untempered by the self-enabling interventions, perpetuates dependence, depersonalisation, categorisation and emotional detachment. Therapeutic relations need to be mindful of this.

Perhaps at the time described I was splitting off the 'good' night staff from the 'bad' day staff, idealising one and rejecting the other; possibly this was regressive, emanating from an unconscious need to identify somebody to blame for my pain and distress (see 'Insights for carers (2)' and '(4)').

On supporting kin: humanistic values as a foundation for care

Anna and mother arrived later than usual the evening of my transfer. They had not been informed of my change of ward and had gone to the Intensive Care Unit. This aside, they did not seem at ease. Months later I heard the full story; they had initially sat outside the Intensive Care Unit hoping to catch sight of an available nurse.

AUTHORITATIVE INTERVENTIONS:

Prescriptive: gives advice to, recommends behaviour to the client.
(Practitioner is prescriptive in a way that enhances
self-determination in the client)

Informative: gives new knowledge and information to, interprets behaviour
to, the client.
(Practitioner is informative in a way that enhances informed
independent thinking in the client)

Confronting: challenges the restrictive attitudes, beliefs and behaviours of
the client.
(Practitioner is confronting in a way that enhances intentional
growth in the client)

FACILITATIVE INTERVENTIONS:

Cathartic: releases tensions in the client: elicits laughter, sobbing,
trembling, storming (the harmless and aware release of
anger).
(Practitioner is cathartic in a way that enhances aware release
of feelings in the client)

Catalytic: elicits information and opinion from, self-directed
problem-solving and self-discovery in the client.
(Practitioner is catalytic in a way that enhances self-insight in
the client)

Supportive: affirms the worth and value of, enhances the self image of the
client.
(Practitioner is supportive in a way that enhances a
celebration of self in the client.)

Heron, J. 'Behaviour Analysis in Education and Training'. Joint publication:
British Postgraduate Medical Foundation, University of London; and Human
Potential Research Project, University of Surrey; 1977.

Fig. 8.2 Six category intervention analysis (Heron, 1977).

Eventually they wandered in to be confronted by my empty bed. This
caused them to panic, from which they were just starting to descend
when they met me. It was some time before they found a nurse to tell
them where I was.

Insights for carers (8)

I am amazed that nurses could have overlooked informing my kin of my
transfer, thus leaving them to be confronted in Intensive Care by such a
potent symbol of death as my empty bed. Possibly the Ward Sister was
acting out an unconscious process of some kind (see 'Insight for carers
(4)') or was it that professional vision put more emphasis on the
performance of 'instrumental tasks' than 'interpersonal processes'?

As carers we need to realise and act on the premise that relatives suffer alongside clients. For example, Anna had much to contend with during my illness: she telephoned my workplace, friends and family, drove two hundred miles every couple of days to visit me, supported my son and counselled my mother; all the while meeting the demands of full time work and containing her own distress.

Next of kin are an integral part, once removed, of the therapeutic relationship. For instance, post-operatively, a singular act of kindness was performed by the surgeon who, following seven hours in theatre and within the first hour of Christmas Eve, telephoned my kin to report that the operation was over and had been successful; this did much to relieve distress and cement the emergent therapeutic relationship.

The therapeutic relationship, when isolated from the support of an appropriate value-base is at risk of degeneration. Throughout this chapter my own bias is one of 'humanism'; it is therefore only fair to alert the reader to what this implies, namely:

- that an individual's mind, intellectual and emotional being are indivisibly connected with their body;
- that given the resources, individuals have the potential to work towards resolution of their own problems;
- that it is important to maintain ongoing open-ended inquiry and to foster creative insight;
- that life experiences and relationships should be valued alongside freedom, growth and contentment as part of 'health'; and
- that there is a need to implement reason and the democratic processes into all social expression (Wilson and Kneisl, 1979).

Humanism puts the person at the centre of the care process, counters depersonalisation and instrumental task fixation and places the relational arts and humanistic philosophy alongside the medical sciences. It was missing from the Sister's actions and evident in the surgeon's.

On stress: the clinical environment as antagonistic to health and therapeutic relating

On entry to my new ward I had been given the option of being in a side room or the open dormitory. I chose the latter. After a few days this choice proved difficult to live with. I was in a twelve-bedded subdivision of the ward, at a period just prior to new year when only the most needy were retained. The nursing team was under-staffed with few seniors to guide them. They were constantly engaged in ongoing physical maintenance tasks with an ever present eye upon the clock as to what must be done next. Observations of temperature, pulse and respirations, and blood and dextrose infusions all had to be attended to 'on time', and emotionally nurses appeared as unsupported as the rest of us. It was rare to see a qualified nurse in the open ward. Everything seemed pressurised and 'jobs were done' rather than care carried out, and all the while the implied message behind ward activity was that 'time was running out'.

A poor soul to my left, demented, blind and deaf, regularly punctuated the night with loud tracts of disjointed dialogue. By the third day I asked if the offer of a side room was still available; it was, and I was glad to make my escape. Originally I hoped I might be distracted and enjoy the company of my fellows, but I had failed to realise how little energy I had or how sapping the pain was when the injections wore off.

My sleep pattern was disrupted. I would be alert until around 5 o'clock when I would then start to feel sleepy. From 6 o'clock on care staff performing and charting observations, issuing drinks and collecting samples of blood broke my rest.

The ward seemed most antagonistic to my rest or bio-psychological rhythms.

Insights for carers (9)
Stressors at any one time are patterned from three sources: our external environment, (physical/social) our internal environment, (psychological and emotional) and our physiological state or bodily needs. It is a sobering exercise to list those stressors at work in residential care settings.

Environmental stressors
- Sensory overload from constant noise, lights, people and constantly changing events
- Sensory deprivation due to chemical blurring and immobility
- Close proximity to others and the bustle of an ongoing working environment that never rests
- Loss of usual belongings and routines
- Sudden appearance of unknown others to take samples and perform various personal services
- Estrangement from home and usual life style
- The lack of choice and freedom

Psychological emotional stressors
- Constant fears of intrusion and/or being overwhelmed
- Fears of death and/or mutilation
- Depersonalisation and loss of self identity
- Inability to meet needs in socially acceptable or accustomed ways
- Fears of nakedness and psychic exposure
- Experience of powerlessness and pain
- Lack of privacy or potential for relaxed retreat
- Separation from supportive others and sexual and community relationships
- Having to adapt to strange new routines

Physiological stressors
- Being weakened through disease
- Suffering fever and/or metabolic changes
- Electrolyte imbalance

- The effects of anaesthesia and drugs
- Sleep deprivation
- Tensions/discomforts from investigative procedures
- An unfamiliar diet

To acclimatise to the clinical environment of the ward when healthy is challenge enough; to adjust to it when weakened through illness, let alone get well, is nigh impossible.

Nursing takes into itself and perpetuates much stress. The folklore and symbolism of the hospital felt by patients and their relations ('Insights for carers (2)') comes out in complicated ways. One moment a nurse may be venerated, showered with affection and gratitude, and the next receive resentment and anger from the self-same folk who now feel frustrated by dependence, jealous of professional esteem and resentful of the care nurses give to their loved ones:

'The hospital, particularly the nurses, must allow the projection into them of such feelings as depression and anxiety, fear of the patient and his illness and the necessary nursing tasks . . . Thus, to the nurse's own deep and intense anxieties are psychically added those of the other people concerned'

(Menzies, 1960)

Clinical environments may be made tolerable through sympathetic management, but healthy, never.

The nursing profession has long recognised the stress it takes into itself but has been resistant to facing up to and dealing with its own client-like parts. I believe a critique of nursing is called for here, for in its pursuit of professionalisation it has placed more attention on its 'status and tasks' than its 'role and processes'; consequentially, like a remote and defensive parent it has attempted to ignore and distance itself from its own emotional vulnerability. Such a charge falls squarely upon the shoulders of nursing education:

'Too often the nursing profession has bred in its practitioners an over strong degree of 'parenthood' along with such parental social fears as losing control, losing self respect and the respect of others. As a consequence, nurses have tended to conform too rigidly. They have not been prepared in a way where fears may be voiced and worked through; their preparation is nearer one of 'papering over the cracks'; their superficial veneer is shallow and prone to fracture.

Nurses are taught primarily to hide their vulnerabilities from others, and themselves, but in so doing they reduce their sensitivity.'

(Barber, 1989)

Burnout is thus let to continue unabated. Perhaps denial and displacement (see 'Insight for carers (4)') have become bonded to nursing's professional psyche? It is well to remember that when anxiety-motivated behaviours predominate over others burnout ensues. To survive such conditions patients need nurses trained as counsellors, and nurses require the support of supervision where they may be counselled and enjoy the benefits of a therapeutic relationship themselves.

On advocacy: acting out as a form of unconscious communication

By the start of my third week post operative depression commenced. Pain was still constant and I was attuned to sensation and had lost my emotional 'highs'. With abdominal discomfort increasing I felt an increased need to find out what had happened to me during surgery so that I might understand those strange sensations I felt inside me.

Doctors and nurses came and went and were unable/unwilling to explain the surgery performed. The nearest I got to an answer was from the consultant who said: 'You have had a fairly brutal operation, there is a lot of bruising inside and you will feel like you have been in the boxing ring for a few weeks; your diaphragm has now been stitched back together again and you are making a remarkably good recovery. You are also lucky to escape without any major complications.' It was impossible for me to extract any more information than this.

Normally self advocacy came easily to me, but the lack of energy I had available for any other than the basic functions of living at this time took it from me. Anna came to my aid at this time and served as an advocate for me. She queried nurses, consulted with the surgeons and fed back to me her findings. Her advocacy on my behalf helped me feel cherished and valued; it also nourished me with information I, as a patient, was denied. It was good to feel there was somebody on my side. As I had no key worker and no care plan had been instituted, there was no single professional to forge a therapeutic bond with.

On the wall of the staff bay a chart of Roper's (Roper *et al.*, 1980) model of nursing was exhibited. I never ever saw it put into practice.

As a practising nurse, Anna was perplexed at this lack of care planning. On one of her visits she brought a publication of mine on nursing models to the staff's attention, and gave them a copy to read. The effect of this was to sensitise staff to my potential to be a resource or a critic. Those who saw me as a resource made more contact and asked questions of me; those who saw me as a critic gave me a wide berth and made less contact than before. As I improved I too became critical, the more so over a couple days when:

- A staff nurse told me a friend had rung and sent me his best wishes but, yet again, she had forgotten the name of the person who rang!
- Two nurses on different days said they would make arrangements for my stitches to come out though these had been removed the week before!

- A doctor tried to remove my chest drain by pulling, before cutting the retaining stitch by which it was secured!
- I asked why I was syphoned daily of 10 mls of blood and was told because I was anaemic!
- I was informed I would have to stay on a gastric diet because of my ulcer repair!

Enough was enough. I walked down to the nursing bay, helped myself to my medical and nursing notes and sat down and read them.

My nursing notes made interesting reading:
- staff thought I was pain free, though they had not asked;
- because of the above I had routinely been given a minimal level of analgesia, even though I had occasionaly asked for more and it was indeed written up;
- though my blood haemoglobin was low no replacement therapy had begun and 10 mls of blood continued to be taken daily for testing;
- no care plan was in evidence.

This was a great blow to my trust. From this time on, I reasoned, I would have to pay more attention to what happened around me, and examine ways that I could take care of myself.

At root I was angry; after devoting so much of my work life to the nursing profession it felt so unfair that it could not be relied on to do a decent job now.

Insights for carers (10)

My invasion of my medical and nursing notes demonstrates that I was caught-up in behaviour symptomatic of 'acting out'. 'Acting out', in the context of mental health, relates to the discharging of tension through physical acts, fuelled by emotional energies an individual has failed to vent verbally. This may be due to:
- the impulse behind the acted out behaviour never having acquired verbal expression;
- the residual emotional energy being too intense for words;
- the individual concerned lacking the capacity for inhibition of his emotional energies (Rycroft, 1968).

'Acting out' has also been cited as the recreation of an individual's life experiences, an unconscious expression of their relationships with significant others, and as emanating from unresolved conflicts pertaining to their 'life script' or personal history (Wilson and Kneisl, 1983).

As a patient I had not been heard, I felt child-like and dismissed, and my emotional energy was at a level where words were insufficient; 'acting out', unconscious expression, was all that was left to me at the time.

Figure 8.3 illustrates the developmental phases of acting out; from the frustration of 'basic needs', the overwhelming of 'individual tolerance', through to a 'symbolic acting out of tensions'. At its extreme acting out may lead to acts of violence against self and others; it is thus in the carer's interest to establish a relationship with a client, of an

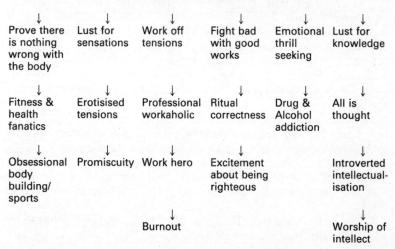

BASIC NEEDS
(To feel loved, trusted, a sense of belonging, autonomy and achievement)
↓
UNMET NEEDS
(Pain felt in the whole organism, and expressive outlets for sharing frustration blocked by parents, culture and fears of rejection)
↓
INDIVIDUAL TOLERANCE PASSED AND MIND OVERWHELMED
(Splitting of intellect and emotions from integrated action, and repression of painful experiences, with conflicts displaced into areas of sensation, emotion and relationships)

DISTRESSING SENSATIONS	PAINFUL EMOTIONS	RELATIONSHIP TENSIONS
(Anxious excitation, physical tensions banished to various organs)	(Emotional tensions sealed off & repressed or expressed via mental defences)	(Idealised relations projected upon others eg: idealised other can do no wrong; role becomes self)

SYMBOLIC ACTING OUT OF TENSIONS
(Tensions reappear in generalised form: 'mother hurt me' becomes 'women hurt me'; 'school crushed me' becomes 'life defeats me')

Prove there is nothing wrong with the body	Lust for sensations	Work off tensions	Fight bad with good works	Emotional thrill seeking	Lust for knowledge
Fitness & health fanatics	Erotisised tensions	Professional workaholic	Ritual correctness	Drug & Alcohol addiction	All is thought
Obsessional body building/ sports	Promiscuity	Work hero	Excitement about being righteous		Introverted intellectual-isation
		Burnout			Worship of intellect

(Adapted from Kilty J. 1989)

Fig. 8.3 Developmental phases of acting out (adapted from Kilty, 1989).

order where the energy behind acting out behaviour can be communicated.

Should this fail and acting out behaviours still be expressed, it is necessary to:

− bring the behaviour concerned to the client's attention;
− encourage the client to discuss their feelings and impulses;
− encourage the client to identify their feelings/needs prior to action;

- increase your frequency of contact with the client concerned;
- and, with repeated acting out, consider and state that you are considering withdrawing your support unless she or he sets limits on their behaviour (Carter, 1981).

Acting out is particularly destructive of the therapeutic relationship because it resists the building of rapport, and squanders energy, which might otherwise enrich carer-client interaction.

On post-operative depression and the quest for purpose: a research-minded examination of pain

Nights on the ward felt interminably long and encouraged the negatives within me to surface. In the early hours, with nothing to divert me, I would often question my state and my future. At my most despondent I would reflect 'Will the pain ever end'; 'Will I ever get near to the health I enjoyed before?'. When more hopeful, I would reflect on 'What is the usual amount of pain to have following an operation such as mine?'; and 'How might I facilitate my own advancement to a healthy recovery?'.

I also pondered my sexuality. I had no sex drive; 'Would it return?'; 'Would Anna ever find my scarred body sexually attractive?'; and, 'How much of a burden would I represent as a dependent, painfully preoccupied entity who could not care for himself let alone for her?'.

Depersonalisation and anomie were highly charged issues for me at this time. My life seemed purposeless and I felt myself slipping further into apathy. Anna broke through this with a simple intervention on her next visit; she brought along a note pad and pens. I was accustomed to writing and researching and now had tools for this. I had also begun to realise that I would have to self-facilitate myself to health.

Over the next few days I examined the major focus of my hospital life, 'pain', and kept a journal to this end. Every so often I would appraise my situation by attending to my 'thoughts', 'feelings', 'senses' and 'intuitions'. This tool, generated from Jungian concepts I had earlier forged in discussion (Kilty, 1989) and written for publication a little before my illness (Barber, 1988), now came into its own as a means of purging the remaining confusion within me.

Thoughts

As I start off this reflective process I'm aware of considering how best to make sense of my experiences and fit them into a cohesive structure I can understand. Intellectually, I am aware of housing a 'structure hunger' and a need for information so that I may work things out for myself. I am also aware of how hard I have to concentrate to move.

Feelings

Depressed and apathetic until aroused by fleeting bursts of thrill and emotional energy as my interest is mobilised by the immediacy of this task.

Senses

Special senses blurred by dull pain which motivates me to experiment with my postural alignment in an effort to achieve greater comfort. Aware of a sensation of stiffness in my thorax, the quickness of my eyes to spot potential hazards, the shallowness of my breath, and hic-coughs when changing posture, I note that tension and discomfort seem to be my present bodily norm. When I close my eyes I see colourful three-dimensional geometric patterns flickering about me.

Intuitions

Visualise myself as a balloon with a slow puncture gradually losing its buoyancy and air and needing to replenish itself with more energy. I suspect that as my energy returns I'll be able to screen my crushing sense of vulnerability with anger. I am aware of an intuition that I will survive this time no matter what it takes.

The more I engaged in the above exercise the more fluid my thinking became; I also improved my concentration span, self awareness and appreciation of my needs.

There was also another interesting discovery; when involved in activities which energised me with positive emotion, I felt less pain. Possibly 'involvement', 'love' and 'joy' countered pain? This was in some way confirmed for me in that I reported less pain during visiting and when engaged in humourous conversation.

As I continued to sift through my perceptions a five point pain scale emerged:

Level 1   +
Moderate discomfort, dull ache, attention can be displaced via concentration on sensory stimuli such as TV and renewed energy conquested.

Level 2   ++
Constant discomfort thwarts concentration, displaced attention helps but does not solicit more energy or over-ride residual feelings of dull heaviness, creativity lost, thinking an effort.

Level 3   +++
Greatly interferes with perception and continually drains energy and interferes with other activities, attention drawn inward, begins to consume consciousness, thinking impossible.

Level 4   ++++
Sharp focused pain overwhelms the individual's sense of self, little attention available for external world, fleeting glimpses of objective reality, disorientation and absorption in pain, responses instinctive.

Level 5   +++++
Individual powerless to communicate in grip of painful stimuli, no contact with external world as consciousness replaced by a twilight state attuned to pain inducing stimuli.

When in 'Level 1' I could still work, write and watch television with a degree of enjoyment; this was my base-line, a point at which I could doze, think, feel and fantasise. At 'Level 2', via concentrated effort, I could switch attention from pain to visual stimuli, that is, over-ride one sensory stimuli with another. At 'Level 3' my thoughts, feelings and imagination were drawn to the field of pain. At 'Level 4' painful sensation permeated the whole and perception of reality came only in fleeting glimpses. At 'Level 5' there was a non-appreciation of everything; it was as if pain filled the universe.

'Level 2' pain was tolerable, but if let develop to 'Level 3' life felt pointless. With this scale to hand I knew when it was necessary to request further pain-killers.

I speculated upon relaxation as a means by which pain might be reduced, and to this end experimented with prolonged hot baths. These I found relaxed the muscle spasms I associated with stimuli at 'Level 3' and above, and if persevered with could reverse the pain spiral and cause 'Level 3' pain to transmute back to 'Level 2'. With this information to hand my environment felt less muddled and helpless.

I had used my research-mindedness to provide me with purpose and power, and was beginning to exorcise the apathy within me.

Insights for carers (11)
My research freed me from the idiocy of ward life and gave me purpose and meaning; it also displaced my perception of pain and served as occupational therapy.

By keeping patients passively awaiting the next care intervention, clinicians retain much power. Ward life generally felt like one long wet Sunday when everything has closed down and when the only respite available was to read the papers or turn on the TV. Periodically into this sheltered climate someone dropped to perform tasks upon you and awaken your interest; less often your false sense of security is shattered by the sudden drama of an unforeseen crisis. Simply, clinical settings need to be normalised.

The 'Normalisation Principle' (Nirje, 1976) suggests individuals who are undergoing a crisis of living and/or state of ill health have the right to be treated as any other valued member of society and to receive care in an environment which preserves their dignity. If nurses are to act on this and preserve the dignity of those they care for, they will have to share their power base and avoid such devaluing responses as:

Dehumanisation   Treating clients as if they are less worthy than those who are healthy and gainfully employed; referring to clients as conditions; 'the dement in bed 10'; seeing clients as objects upon which instrumental tasks are performed, or paying so much attention to 'routines' that more care is lavished on the ward than the clients within.

Age inappropriate responses   Becoming over familiar with clients or calling them by nick-names such as 'Pops','Granny' or 'Grandad'; parenting and making decisions for patients so as to reinforce parent-child aspects of the nurse-patient relationship, or withholding information from them and acting on their behalf.

Fostering isolation   Attitudinally segregating patients from their civil rights and community; a legacy of the Victorian view of hospitals as places where the sick were to be isolated from the working well; keeping distant from clients and leaving them unsupported and unoccupied. (Adapted from Gunner, 1987; Tyne, 1978.)

Nurses need to pay attention to the space between 'what they believe they do' and 'what the consequences of their actions actually are'. They have great potential to serve as an advocate, to offer support and counsel, or to damage their clients by doing the reverse of these things. Interestingly, my account suggests when such positive feelings as humour, love and joy enter the care relationship its therapeutic potential grows. It might be well, therefore, if nurses as a norm in therapeutic relating:

– resisted entering into negative social collusions, such as exchanging gripes or feeding into such negative emotional games as 'nothing will change'; 'there's nothing anyone can do about it'; or 'you mustn't take life seriously';
– rewarded all positive behaviour, no matter how small or fleeting it may be;
– paid attention to their own emotional show, and how this has effects on clients and the feeling tone of the therapeutic relationship;
– acknowledged the role they have as culture carrier, and all this implies in terms of their influence on what they create around them.

Culture includes all those ideas and beliefs people hold about themselves, plus all those meanings which make life all the more worthwhile. In this context the nurse's clinical role as a 'culture carrier' and positive force for health is second to none.

On massage: the contribution of alternative therapies to nursing care

Since the operation my shoulders and thorax had remained rigid. It was as if I had armoured myself to protect the site of surgical intrusion. My shoulders were high, neck tight and I breathed shallowly. I looked and felt as if I was encased in metal.

Anna and I had always exchanged therapeutic massage and this now came into its own. We contracted that on each of her visits she would massage my back and neck.

The first time she massaged me it was difficult to take; my body had forgotten how to receive touch. In the night following this massage, I awoke to feel my whole body pulsating with a warm tingling sensation that bubbled up through my skin. It felt like life was flowing back into me. I also started to yawn. I evoked more yawns. The more I yawned, the easier my breathing became. Over the next few days my thoracic flexibility began to return. I now found I was able to stretch, breathe in deeply without coughing and, for the first time, could stand erect when walking. Trusting myself more to unconsciousness, I was now awoken less by sudden pain due to involuntary movements or coughs. As I now breathed and slept better, my energy returned and consequently my apathy began to lift.

Insights for carers (12)

Although alternative and body therapies are rarely taught in the formal curriculum, they have much to offer nurses. Note, the massage described above was the single most effective post-operative intervention I received.

As physiological organisms who psychologically determine their world and socially define it, clients need an approach to care which recognises and integrates all of these dimensions (see 'Insight for carers (6); (8)'). Alternative therapies do this. Some, such as Transactional Analysis and Gestalt, elicit how we make sense and relate to the world; others, such as the Alexander Method and Rolfing, help us to understand how postural integration can balance our internal and external energy flows; while Therapeutic Massage, Aroma Therapy and Bioenergetics provide us with modes of physical reintegration. Holistic approaches attend to the 'whole person' and experiential integration, areas of concern often missed by more orthodox systems of care.

The approaches below are recommended to nurses who wish to develop further their therapeutic potential.

Therapeutic massage Not to be confused with massage of the type associated with physiotherapy and sports, this form attempts holistically to reintegrate a client's body sense and to release feelings laid up through life in the various muscle groups. The effects of this are described in the text above.

Aroma therapy   Seeks to alleviate mental and emotional stresses via recourse to aromatic massage. Differing fragrancies are suggested to evoke differing reactions and are used to move a client in the direction of harmony and balance. Scented oils, incense and lotions are applied for the purposes described.

Aroma therapy combined with therapeutic massage was for me a very powerful relaxing agent post-operatively, at a time when my body was most resistant to relaxing.

Bioenergetics   After Alexander Lowen (1967; 1972), offers techniques for reducing muscular tension through the conscious release of feelings. Makes less use of direct body contact (therapist-client) than other therapies, in that it offers a series of exercises and verbal techniques, and sensor and releasor exercises in order to increase the client's appreciation of his body defences. Deep breathing, stretching, and rigorous movement may be used to break through muscle rigidity and to express feelings blocked and/or trapped in postural armouring which restricts the flow and free exchange of energy.

Gestalt therapy   As a practitioner of gestalt psychotherapy I must declare a bias to this approach. Gestalt is for me the quintessence of an integrated research-minded holistic therapy. Originally evolved by Perls (1969) and later refined by Zinker (1977) and Polster and Polster (1974), gestalt therapists invite us to join with them in a series of experiential experiments to evaluate that store of conflicting emotions, frustrated needs and false perceptions, which interfere with our ability to contact meaningfully ourselves and reality. In this sense the client is both a 'subject' and 'experimenter'. Via working through this bank of 'unfinished situations' we are enabled to assume responsibility for ourselves, appreciate the choices before us, and to experiment with living life as a self-regulating, contactful and aware being. 'In this way people can let themselves become totally what they already are, and what they potentially can become' (Clarkson, 1989a, b). Awareness is thus the process and the goal of a gestalt approach.

The Alexander method   Developed by F. A. Alexander (1976), focuses primarily upon incorrect alignments of the head, neck and shoulders which cause stress throughout the whole body. Intervention is mainly via massage, manipulation and postural re-education.

Transactional analysis (TA)   Originated by Eric Berne (1964) and developed by Harris (1973), presents a model for understanding socio-analytic influences within human development, role formation and interaction. Three ego states are commonly employed to explain personality and social functioning: the Parent – that part of ourselves formed by our own parents in childhood and the focus of 'world as we are socially taught it to be'; the Adult – which is a part of our personality that deals with the objective sensory world and facts, and gives us our orientation to 'the world as we have found it and checked it out to be'; the Child – the source of our free emotional energies, creativity and fantasies, and our reference for 'the world as we feel, intuitively create, or desire it to be'. Through analysis of our social 'scripts' and roles, TA enables us to understand ourselves and our conflicting social motivations. I have found TA an excellent vehicle for the transmission of relational insights.

Rolfing　Otherwise known as structural reintegration, it is based upon the premise that psychological conflicts are recorded and perpetuated in the body frame. Evolved by Ida Rolf (1977), Rolfing addresses the myofascia and connective tissue which supports the body weight; this, it cites, undergoes shortening and metabolic change that hampers energy flow and interferes with free movement. With age the body becomes a reflection of accumulated unresolved feelings. It is these that Rolfing attempts to undo.

Personally, I found increased energy, bodily awareness and the ability to unpack my own build up of physical and emotional stress emanated from my exposure to Rolfing.

The above approaches, through development of 'the person', serve to enhance interpersonal sensitivity. As a nurse's interpersonal awareness increases so does the professional skill which, in turn, enhances the ability to form therapeutic relationships.

On the clinical environment: the need for research-minded care

With the new lease of energy obtained from massage, I returned afresh to my role as researcher. I had 'looked within' to examine 'experientially' pain. Now I chose to 'look without' to evaluate 'objectively' the clinical environment.

In order to clarify progress to date, I set about reviewing 'progress markers', events that enriched my quality of life and/or restored hope and caused me to feel good to be alive:

1st day　–　Relief at being alive/seeing Marc and Anna/sucking ice
2nd day　–　First taste (a lemon stick)/talking with night staff
3rd day　–　My first recognisable catnap
4th day　–　First time standing up
5th day　–　First clear hour with visitors (no haze)/first hour's sleep/a taste of soup/first taste of orange barley squash
6th day　–　First comfortable time sitting in chair/walking without support/TV film appreciated/first bowel movement/ first day I can write a little/first yawn
7th day　–　First walk from ward/a short period of deep sleep
8th day　–　First transient painfree period/first painfree cough/first bath/a clear un-drug hazed day
10th day　–　First time I can take in what I read
14th day　–　Massage from Anna

15th day – Walked to hospital entrance
18th day – First day painkillers really relieve pain.

Such mundane events are very different from those medical nurses and doctors report in their notes.

After reviewing my past, I next turned my attention to what was happening 'now'.

Starting from the premise that a major nursing function is to nurture a safe environment in which clients may be observed and monitored, and speedily contacted when crises arise, I commenced one particularly sleepless night to check the time it took nurses to respond to the call bell over a twenty-four hour period.

A bell push operated in the 14-bedded section of the ward in which I was placed caused a red light to illuminate above the door of my room. Secure in the observation that nurses on answering a call had invariably in the past cancelled the summoning light before attending to clients, I used this light for the data collection of my survey. For brevity I chose to round up or down times of a minute or more to the nearest whole. Before this brief piece of research I thought 30 seconds to a minute would be the average time it took to answer a call. I was some way out in my estimation.

Time of call (light on)	Answer of call (light off)	Waiting time
8.38 pm	8.54 pm	16 minutes
9.45 pm	9.48 pm	3 minutes
10.07 pm	10.09 pm	2 minutes
10.20 pm	10.22 pm	2 minutes
10.23 pm	10.25 pm	2 minutes
10.37 pm	10.39 pm	2 minutes
11.26 pm	11.26 pm	½ minute
12.49 am	12.53 am	4 minutes
1.25 am	1.26 am	1 minute
1.26 am	1.26 am	½ minute
6.25 am	6.32 am	7 minutes
6.38 am	6.43 am	5 minutes
8.45 am	9.10 am	25 minutes
9.12 am	9.13 am	1 minute
9.15 am	9.20 am	5 minutes
11.10 am	11.12 am	2 minutes
11.20 am	11.23 am	3 minutes
3.20 pm	3.25 pm	5 minutes
4.47 pm	4.51 pm	4 minutes
5.30 pm	5.32 pm	2 minutes
6.15 pm	6.18 pm	3 minutes
6.25 pm	6.29 pm	4 minutes

Time of call (light on)	Answer of call (light off)	Waiting time
6.43 pm	6.49 pm	6 minutes
7.34 pm	7.36 pm	2 minutes
7.52 pm	7.53 pm	1 minute
8.20 pm	8.21 pm	1 minute
8.25 pm	8.28 pm	3 minutes

As a client I felt lucky to receive whatever I got; as a senior clinician my findings disturbed me. Out of every 27 calls I could expect to wait upwards of two minutes for some 14 and, of these, ten could be of four minutes' wait or more. On the outside I could expect a twenty-five minute wait.

In a crisis, a common occurrence on a surgical ward, a minute seems a very long time. I concluded from this that the ward was a very dangerous place indeed. I could be better served for the most part at home with a 'phone by my bed.'

Insights for carers (13)

At any one time the ward had an occupancy of 24 beds. Most of the workforce were students or pupils in training complemented by nursing auxiliaries. On an average night there was one senior student, one pupil nurse and one auxiliary, plus a roving night sister shared between other wards. During the days this tripartite workforce was supplemented by a ward sister or staff nurse who acted as team leader. Having worked as a student on the night and day shifts of a busy surgical ward, I can appreciate the work involved. As my sample represented one third of the ward population, during a twenty-four hour shift 70 to 80 calls might be expected. Besides these regular four hourly observations of pulse, temperature and respirations have also to be made, four hourly drinks to be given and input and output charts maintained, numerous drips and blood monitored, medication given and recorded, incumbent clients bathed, pressure areas rubbed, bowls for washing and drinks ferried around, and all this without the emergency admissions and pre-operation procedures that form a regular part of clinical life. As three to four staff are not always sufficient for this, it is little wonder crisis management thus becomes the norm.

Quality not quantity defines good care; but as successive governments apply profit and growth motives to the health service and ask hospitals in the public sector to run as if they were factories, care managers are driven to forsake qualitative aspects of care in favour of expediency. It is therefore essential that the effects of this are researched, for reduction of a ward's staff ratio may possibly correlate with higher levels of infection and other complications which necessitate an extended spell in hospital and in the long run cost more.

Nurses have little time, but ample data to research. As researchers they have potential to act as participant observers, to chronicle clinical events and to process record the interactions they engage in with their clients. The qualitative research tools for this have already been refined (see Reason and Rowan, 1981) and the skilful use of these can now be taught in nursing education.

Those simple research inquiries I performed could so easily be facilitated by a clinical manager, or a key worker alongside the client. The awareness that accrues from such activity would no doubt prove beneficial to clinician and client alike.

It is beyond the scope of this account to reiterate ways a nurse may perform research, but the point must be made that it is essential that research-minded care is enacted within the therapeutic relationship.

On professional relationships: research-mindedness and supervision

Besides the restrictions of staff and time, other factors appeared to contribute to 'crisis management' and the disruption of therapeutic relationships within the ward, namely, nurses seemed locked into person denying behavioural sets. Even when there were few patients within the ward, therapeutic relationships remained unformed. This awareness caused me to recollect a study some thirty years ago where Isabel Menzies (1960), researching into low morale, had identified ways nurses structured their professional relationships to protect themselves from stress. Such defences, which were noted to interfere with self and person perception, could, if linked to my present environment, do much to explain how seemingly conscientious and busy nurses could overlook their patients' needs. Initially I set about simplifying Menzies' findings; sifting through the main themes left me with seven categories.

1. Splitting up the nurse-patient relationship: tasks emphasised rather than personal processes, little opportunity provided for the development of one to one relationships.
2. Depersonalisation and categorisation: patients described by their medical conditions, individuality and creativity discouraged, and all patients treated the same.
3. Ritual task performance: instrumental activity encouraged and questioning discouraged; professionals let policies do their thinking for them.
4. Feelings denied and controlled: emotional expression discouraged and/or ignored, staff disciplined rather than counselled.
5. Avoidance of decisions – control pushed upwards to seniors and blame pushed downwards on juniors; personal and professional power unused.
6. Avoidance of change – problem confrontation avoided, and fear of facing new situations without prescribed procedures.
7. Checks and counter-checks – individual action discouraged, trust rare and fears of failure commonplace.

In order to evaluate the frequency of the above behaviours within the ward, I devised a five point scale:

Rare (+)   when a behaviour is rarely glimpsed;
Emerges (++)   when a behaviour draws my attention;
Frequent (+++)   when a behaviour is a usual feature of inter-action;
Very common (++++)   when a behaviour is a major characteristic;
Constant (+++++)   when a behaviour is ever present.

With the above constructs established, I now had an impressionable rating scale with which to profile clinical behaviour. As a participant observer, I attributed to nurses over an observational period of two weeks the following responses:

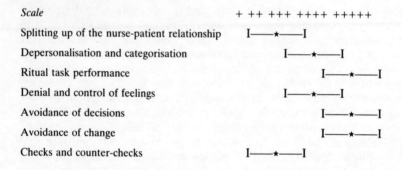

Scale   + ++ +++ ++++ +++++

Splitting up of the nurse-patient relationship   I——⋆——I

Depersonalisation and categorisation   I——⋆——I

Ritual task performance   I——⋆——I

Denial and control of feelings   I——⋆——I

Avoidance of decisions   I——⋆——I

Avoidance of change   I——⋆——I

Checks and counter-checks   I——⋆——I

Note   '⋆' shows the central position of my observations and 'I——I' the
range of variability in to which each behaviour fell.

Balancing my expertise as an experienced practitioner/researcher with the subjective nature and obvious limitations of my approach, the results give interesting cues to the clinical culture.

'Ritual task performance', 'Avoidance of decisions' and 'Avoidance of change' figured predominantly, with 'Depersonalisation and categorisation' and 'Denial and control of feelings' following closely behind. Surprisingly 'Splitting of the nurse-patient relationship', a central theme of this chapter, comes less to the fore than I expected, and as a patient I was less aware of 'checks and counter-checks'.

In sum, if this small sample – from the client's eye view – is in any way representative, it might be suggested that research-mindedness is still very much absent from practice and that feelings are still very much avoided. Certainly it appears those social defensive behaviours first identified some thirty years ago are very much alive and well in a modern provincial hospital.

Insight for carers (14)

My inquiry, first 'looking in' on my own condition, then 'looking out' to the clinical environment, suggests a frame from which clinical research-mindedness might emanate within the therapeutic relationship, namely:

Looking out (Sensing/Analysing)
Those external objects I sense: see, hear, taste, smell and touch, and use to intellectually structure reality with, my scientific biases.

Looking in (Feeling/Intuition)
Energies I feel emotionally within me, those creative meanings which intuitively arise from within, my ability to express and empathise.

Though models of nursing and knowledge of the 'care sciences' may be acquired by reading, facilitation skill and the 'caring arts' are only acquired via quality supervision and experiential reflection during practice.

The above diagram offers a frame for experiential reflection. It asks carers to be sensitive to and monitor their own internal processes, to attend to the 'emotional energy field' they share with a client and to pay attention to their biases and how they make sense of their clinical practice.

Figure 8.4 applies the above perceptual frame – 'Looking-in and Looking-out' to the observation of 'self' and 'other' within the therapeutic relationship, where internal and external reflections are shared in relation to the 'Examining social processes', 'Applying/sharing theoretical insights and models', and 'Owning emotional and intuitive meanings of relationship'.

When carers can witness themselves and their clients, without the clutter of intellectual and professional labels, they will have achieved one of the goals of this research-minded relational process.

On integrating the whole: insights into therapeutic relations in nursing care and professional supervision

As I finish this account I am eighteen months post surgery and am much healed. I also gained a great many insights from the trauma described. Much of my inquiry, post hospitalisation, was performed in psychotherapeutic settings in personal therapy. As a student and practitioner of gestalt psychotherapy, I had access to a therapy group and regular supervision (Clarkson, 1989; Parlett, 1989) in which to further inquire into my experience of the client's side of the therapeutic relationship; intuitive insights from this are shared below.

Precognition I am aware that at the end of the Autumn Term, prior to commencing my Christmas vacation, I was acutely aware of a strong desire to order my affairs and a sense that I would not return the following term. My intuition is that at an unconscious physiolo-

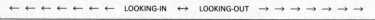

← ← ← ← ← ← ←   LOOKING-IN   ↔   LOOKING-OUT   → → → → → → → →

(Examining social processes)

Questioning self		Observing other
What am I experiencing now – my feelings/intuitions/thoughts?	↔	Observing the environment and the evidence of my senses, the other's response to me
How might I facilitate or be of use?	↔	Attending to what is asked of me, sharing information and expertise, experimenting with interventions
How do I feel in this relationship?	↔	Focusing upon how I am relating and being related to in return
How is this relationship like and different to a therapeutic one?	↔	Differentiating how I am meeting my needs and meeting the needs of others
How much empathy do I feel for the person before me?	↔	Examining what is mutually accepted and supported, and issues and ways in which we differ

(Applying/sharing theoretical insights and models)

Reflecting upon		Sharing/enacting
The therapeutic relationship	↔	The phase of our relationship
Therapeutic factors	↔	Reality orientation, trust building
Supervision strategies	↔	Forming a contract
Transactional analysis	↔	Ongoing analysis of the relationship process and transactions available
Models of care	↔	Care strategies & evaluation modes
Research approaches	↔	Illuminative/collaborative inquiries to assess effects of therapy
Mental defenses	↔	Exploring blocks to communication
Intervention analysis	↔	Testing appropriate interventions

(Owning emotional and intuitive meanings in relationship)

Examining own:		Speculating upon:
Emotions & fantasies received	↔	Projections onto other
Current awareness of self	↔	Current sensitivity to other
Memories evoked by relationship	↔	Projections acted upon by other
Staying sensitive to own defenses	↔	Attending to defenses of other
Own unsaid material	↔	Attending to what is unsaid by other
Personal fears	↔	Fears of other

Fig. 8.4 Research-mindedness in therapeutic relating.

gical level of functioning I was receiving biological cues to the internal physiological processes that were starting to come adrift. My dreams prior to illness were likewise disturbed with imagery of being stabbed in the abdomen.

Symbolic regression   With my academic year's work done, I started to relax, went back to my birth-place and, in a primitive symbolic way, returned to my mother to experience a life threatening illness. At an organismic level I suspect I may have chosen when to experience my illness, where to enact it and with whom.

Gestalt completion   Post surgery I feel in one way completed. As if nothing is left to instil such fear in me again, I know I can stand pain and work my way through it. Likewise I can rely on my own store of courage; I feel tested and somehow relieved. I am no longer the least bit afraid of death and, in my saying of this, conversely, feel I love life the more; as if this time 'I choose to be here' rather than 'find myself born'.

Personal gains   I know I can trust to my courage and no longer need to prove or test myself. As a consequence, I am more self caring. I have also gained a positive sense of vulnerability and feel more sensitive; and strangely stronger because of this.

In a Maslovian sense (Maslow, 1970) I feel I have stretched my boundaries and goals and integrated a new dimension of growth. The crisis of my illness plunged me from 'self confidence and self esteem' born of mastery of my environment and the affection of others towards consideration of 'how best to survive and get safe' again; see Fig. 8.5. (Note: In the context of Fig. 8.5, it occurs to me that the ward environment functioned very much at level 4.)

Reintegrating the whole   Reviewing my illness and convalescence, I am aware of having relived psychosocial crises of my childhood all over again; but this time, with a degree of consciousness and a sense of having been there before. Simply, I have gained greater reintegration. In a sense I have re-experienced crises of 'drive and hope' through to 'renunciation and wisdom' (Erikson, 1965); Fig. 8.6.

Interpersonally, Anna, Marc and myself have emerged from the experience closer, more loving and appreciative of one another. I am also more tolerant and at peace within myself.

Insights for carers (15)
A carer's ability to forge a successful therapeutic relationship relates directly to their own degree of self insight and understanding. Unaware carers give unaware care.

MASLOW	KOHLBERG	LOEVINGER
	6	
Self-actualisation: Being that self which I truly am and have it in me to be. Fully functioning person	Individual principles: True personal consciousness, universal principles fully internalised. Genuinely autonomous, selfishness (B)	Autonomous: integrated: Flexible and creative, internal conflicts faced and recognised. Ambiguity tolerated and feelings expressed
	5	
Self-esteem 2: Goals founded upon self evaluated standards, self confidence/respect	Social contract: Utilitarian lawmaking, principles of general welfare, long term goals	Conscientious: Bound by self-imposed rules, differential thinking, self aware
	4	
Self-esteem 1: Respect from others, social status, recognition	Law and order: Authority maintenance, fixed social rules – finds duty and does it	Conformist 2: Seeks general rules of social conformity, justifies conformity
	3	
Love and belonging: Wish for affection and a place in the group, tenderness	Personal concordance: Good-boy mentality, seeking social approval, majority as right	Conformist 1: Going along with the crowd, anxiety about rejection, needing support
	2	
Effectence: Mastery, personal power, imposed control, blame and retaliation, domination	Instrumental hedonism: Naive egocentrism, horse trading approach, profit and loss calculation, selfishness (A)	Self protective/ manipulative: Wary, exploitative, people are means to ends, competitive stance, fear of being caught, stereotypes ++
	1	
Safety: Defence against danger, flight or fight, fear – world as a scary place	Obedience/punishment: Deference to superior power, rules are external and eternal	Impulsive: Domination by immediate cue, body feelings, no reflection, retaliation fears

Fig. 8.5 Developmental spiral (adapted from Wright, 1974; as reported by Rowan, 1983).

The quality of the therapeutic relationship is dependent upon the degree a nurse is able to experience and positively use their own qualities of 'self' (Barber, 1989). Such awareness requires specialist facilitation. Clinical supervision can supply this level of development (Barber and Norman, 1988), and develop 'the self' when seeking to:

Age appropriate stages	Psychosocial crises	Significant relationship	Favourable outcome
Birth–first yr	Trust v Mistrust	Mother	Drive and hope
Second yr	Autonomy v-Shame	Parents	Self control and willpower
Third–fifth yr	Initiative v Guilt	Family	Direction and purpose
Six yr–puberty	Industry v Inferiority	Neighbourhood/ School	Method and competence
Adolescence	Identity v Diffusion	Peer groups/ Leadership	Devotion and fidelity
Early adulthood	Intimacy v Isolation	Partners/ Cooperation	Affiliation and love
Young-middle adulthood	Generativity v Self absorbtion	Divided labour/ Shared household	Production and care
Later adulthood	Integrity v Despair	'Mankind my kind'	Renunciation and wisdom

Fig. 8.6 Erikson's stages of psychosocial development (after Erikson, 1965; modified from original).

- combine personal with professional development;
- be attentive to the social dynamics that develop between the supervisor and supervisee;
- provide first hand experience of what it is like to be supported and cared for and enact a 'caring for carers';
- facilitate research aware practice and role model relational skills;
- work towards those higher levels of functioning described in Fig. 8.5 and 8.6.

Simply, the supervisor and supervisee, while remaining alert to the evolved behavioural levels of Fig. 8.5 and 8.6, and facilitating the research-mindedness of Fig. 8.4, can be managed in such a way as to illustrate social processes which are paralleled in carer-client relations. Supervision of this type sets up an experiential climate where practitioners can explore themselves along with their responses and skills. Supervisions of this kind can start in experiential groupwork via social analysis of the student-teacher relationship. Fears, social expectations, learner resistances and group defences are all present in the educational group and the resolution and working through of these may elicit immense personal and interpersonal learning; especially when approached in a psychodynamic way. Figure 8.7 illustrates what is available to a sensitive teacher in non-conspiratorial educational settings when the teacher/facilitator stops playing conventional classroom games (Barber, 1986a).

FEARS	LEARNER/CLIENT EXPECTATION	NON-COMPLIANT FACILITATIVE BEHAVIOUR	LEARNER RESISTANCES
Fears of being unable to control others	Facilitator will lead and initiate happenings		**Collusive resistances**
		Facilitator	Group conspires to be jocular and mildly cynical (cocktail party)
	Facilitator will adopt role of expert and impart information	resists	Retreat of two or more members into whispersemotional
Fears of losing control		collusion to	(subgroups/pairing)
			Passive resistances
		be a	
	Facilitator will act as authority figure to be blamed if things go wrong	parenting	'Lost' silence (please rescue us)
Fears of being rejected		figure and	Waiting to be led (dependency)
			Day-dreaming (fantasy)
	Facilitator will assume responsibility for group and learning process	structure	**Active resistances**
Fears of failing		reality for	Criticism and blame of persons or systems, authority chastised (scapegoating/ stereotyping)
		the group	
	Facilitator will acknowledge status barriers and stay emotionally remote		Teacher's credibility/contributions attacked (counter-dependency)
			Angry silence (rejection)

Fig. 8.7   Group fears – expectations and resistances.

In summary

I have attempted in this chapter to interweave client generated awarenesses and professional insights. To this end we have considered under respective headings of 'Insights for carers': (1) the nature of health, (2) symbolic interactionism, (3) nursing and reality orientation, (4) defence mechanisms, (5) spiritual meanings, (6) client-centred care, (7) intervention styles, (6) humanism, (9) clinical stressors, (10) acting out, (11) normalisation and clinical culture, (12) alternative therapies, (13) clinical research, (14) experiential reflection, (15) research-minded intervention and supervision. Finally, I will share how I weave my gestalt and psychodynamic vision to a conceptual frame where such insights can be therapeutically enacted.

Within the life of the therapeutic relationship, as described by Peplau (Fig. 8.1, p. 235), are acted through other cycles of therapeutic relating. These cycles, Fig. 8.8, demonstrate the application of a therapeutic experiential research process, where a nurse facilitates the awareness and resources of a client within the medium of a collaborative relationship. Many such cycles will be in operation at any time and proceed at differing speeds. The cycle relating to hospitalisation and recovery will obviously move at a slower pace than the cycle enacted by an investigation such as an electro-cardiogram.

As soon as one mini-cycle relating to something such as hunger is complete, another relating to physical or emotional comfort might arise. This goes a little way to explain burnout; when too many cycles are in operation and demand completion, unremitting stress will occur. A skilled intuitive nurse, by this same token, may be able to differentiate which cycle is on top for a client at any one time.

I am mindful, when enacting a therapeutic relationship and addressing a client's experiential cycle, of certain qualities – after Yalom (1970) – which facilitate the working through of unfinished gestalts and successful reintegration.

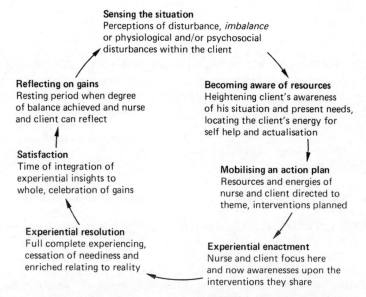

Sensing the situation
Perceptions of disturbance, *imbalance* or physiological and/or psychosocial disturbances within the client

Reflecting on gains
Resting period when degree of balance achieved and nurse and client can reflect

Becoming aware of resources
Heightening client's awareness of his situation and present needs, locating the client's energy for self help and actualisation

Satisfaction
Time of integration of experiential insights to whole, celebration of gains

Mobilising an action plan
Resources and energies of nurse and client directed to theme, interventions planned

Experiential resolution
Full complete experiencing, cessation of neediness and enriched relating to reality

Experiential enactment
Nurse and client focus here and now awarenesses upon the interventions they share

Fig. 8.8 Experiential research cycles. NB Healthy movement is in the direction described, though an individual may be at any stage in the cycle at any one time.

1. **Imparting of information** instruction, comments on psychodynamics, advice and suggestions about life problems.
2. **Instillation of hope** faith in the care givers and their approach.
3. **Universality** becoming aware of others feeling as you do, learning you are not alone and that others share your problem.
4. **Altruism** learning that you can help and be helped by others in return.
5. **Corrective recapitulation** being able to relive and rework old problems, and in so doing to discover new ways of coping.
6. **Development of socialising techniques** enhancing and learning new social skills and social behaviours.
7. **Imitative behaviour** role modelling, trying on the behaviours of others to find out if they can also work for you.
8. **Interpersonal learning** working through projections and correcting emotional experience.
9. **Group cohesiveness** being nourished via accurate empathy, non-possessive warmth and genuineness.
10. **Catharsis** the release of pent-up emotional energies.

As to how you enact the above, it is hoped after reading this chapter that they are no longer strangers to you and that you have sufficient insight to begin to enact them in your own therapeutic relationships.

Intuitively, I feel the cycle of this chapter is nearing completion and that it is time I moved to something else.

The way I make sense of the therapeutic relationship and those influences I blend into it might not be for you. Possibly you feel I have made too much use of psychotherapeutic and experiential material. I do not apologise for this; therapeutic relations are intensly personal things prone to the idiosyncracies of each carer. My way of relating is unique to me, a synthesis of sociological and psychotherapeutic biases, part forged by my client experience. It works for me. You must now find one which works for you.

References

Alexander, F. M. (1976). *The Resurrection of the Body*. Dell, New York:

Barber, P. (1986a). A process approach to education. *Nurse Educator*, **11(2)**, 40.

Barber, P. (1986b). The psychiatric nurses's failure therapeutically to nurture. *Nursing Practice*, **1(3)**, 138–41.

Barber, P. (1988). Learning to grow: the necessity for educational processing in therapeutic community practice. *International Journal of Therapeutic Communities*, **9(2)**, 101–8.

Barber, P. (1989). Developing the 'person' of the professional carer.

In *Nursing Practice and Health Care*, S. M. Hinchliff, S. E. Norman and J. E. Schober (Eds), pp. 702–27. Edward Arnold, London.

Barber, P. and Norman, I. (1987). An eclectic model of staff development: supervision techniques to prepare nurses for a process approach – a social perspective. In *Mental Handicap: Facilitating Holistic Care*, P. Barber (Ed.), pp. 80–90. Hodder & Stoughton, London.

Barber, P. and Norman, I. (1989). Preparing teachers for the performance and evaluation of gaming-simulation in experiential learning climates. *Journal of Advanced Nursing*, **14(2)**, 146–51.

Berne, E. (1964). *Games People Play*. Penguin, Harmondsworth.

Blumer, H. (1969). *Symbolic Interactionism: Perspective and Method*. Prentice-Hall, Englewood Cliffs.

Carter, F. M. (1981). *Psychosocial Nursing*. Macmillan, New York.

Clarkson, P. (1989a). *Gestalt Counselling in Action*. Sage, London.

Clarkson, P. (1989b). Personal communication.

Erikson, E. (1965). *Childhood and Society*. Penguin, Harmondsworth.

Glasser, W. (1965). *Reality Therapy*. Harper & Row, New York.

Gunner, A. (1987). Putting community care together: a rationale for nursing interventions using Henderson's model – a community perspective. In *Mental Handicap: Facilitating Holistic Care*, P. Barber (Ed.), pp. 12–24. Hodder & Stoughton, London.

Harris, T. (1973). *I'm OK – You're OK*. Pan, London.

Henderson, V. (1969). *Basic Principles of Nursing Care*, revised edition. Karger, Basel.

Heron, J. (1977). *Behaviour Analysis in Education and Training*. British Postgraduate Medical Foundation and University of Surrey, London.

Jackins, H. (1965). *The Human Side of Human Beings: the Theory of Re-evaluation Counselling*. Rational Island Press, Seattle.

Kilty, J. (1982). *Experiential Learning*. Human Potential Research Project, University of Surrey, Guildford.

Kilty, J. (1989). Personal communication.

Kroeber, T. (1963). The coping functions of the ego mechanisms. In *The Study of Lives*, R. White (Ed.). Atherton, New York.

Lowen, A.(1967). *The Betrayal of the Body*. Macmillan, New York.

Lowen, A. (1972). *Depression and the Body*. Penguin, Baltimore.

Maslow, A. (1970). *Motivation and Personality*, 2nd edition. Harper & Row, New York.

Menzies, I. (1960). *The Functioning of Social Systems as a Defence Against Anxiety*. Tavistock, London.

Nirje, B. (1976). The normalisation principle. In *Changing Patterns of Residential Services for the Mentally Retarded*, R. Kugel and A. Shearer (Eds). President's Committee for the Mentally Retarded, Washington.

Oakes, A. R. (1981). Near-death events and critical care nursing. *Topics in Clinical Nursing*, **3(3)**, 61–78.

Orem, D. (1980). *Nursing: Concepts of Practice*, 2nd edition. McGraw-Hill, New York.

Orne, R. M. (1986). Nurses' views of NDEs. *American Journal of Nursing*, **86(4)**, 419–20.

Parlett, M. (1989). Personal communciation.

Peplau, H. (1952). *Interpersonal Relations in Nursing*. Putnam, New York.

Perls, F. (1969). *Ego, Hunger and Aggression*. Vintage Books, New York.

Polster, I. and Polster, M. (1974). *Gestalt Therapy Integrated*. Vintage Books, New York.

Reason, P. and Rowan, J. (Eds) (1981). *Human Inquiry: a Sourcebook of New Paradigm Research*. Wiley, Chichester.

Rogers, C. (1983). *Freedom to Learn for the 80s*. Merrill, Columbus.

Rogers, M. (1970). *An Introduction to the Theoretical Basis of Nursing*. Davis, Philadelphia.

Rolf, I. (1977). *Rolfing: the Structural Integration of the Human Structure*. Rolf Institute, Boulder.

Roper, N., Logan, W. W. and Tierney, A. J. (1980). *The Elements of Nursing*. Churchill Livingstone, Edinburgh.

Rowan, J. (1983). *The Reality Game*. Routledge & Kegan Paul, London.

Roy, C. (1979). Relating nursing theory to education: a new era. *Nurse Educator*, **4(2)**, 16–21.

Rycroft, C. (1968). *A Critical Dictionary of Psychoanalysis*. Penguin, Harmondsworth.

Trevelyan, J. (1989). Near-death experiences. *Nursing Times and Nursing Mirror*, **85(28)**, 39–41.

Tyne, A. (1978). *'Looking at Life' – in Hospitals, Hostels, Homes and Units for Adults who are Mentally Handicapped*. Campaign for the Mentally Handicapped, London.

Wilson, H. and Kneisl, C. (1979). *Psychiatric Nursing*. Addison-Wesley, Menlo Park.

Wilson, H. S. and Kneisl, C. R. (1983). *Psychiatric Nursing*, 2nd edition. Addison-Wesley, Menlo Park.

Yalom, I. (1970). *The Theory and Practice of Group Psychotherapy*. Basic Books, London.

Zinker, J. (1977). *Creative Process in Gestalt Therapy*. Vintage Books, New York.

9 Power, politics and policy analysis in nursing

'The word "politics" is enlisted here when speaking of the sexes primarily because such a word is eminently useful in outlining the real nature of their relative status, historically and at the present. It is opportune, perhaps today even mandatory, that we develop a more relative psychology and philosophy of power relationships beyond the simple conceptual framework provided by our traditional formal politics. Indeed, it may be imperative that we give some attention to defining a theory of politics which treats power relationships on grounds less conventional than those to which we are accustomed. I have therefore found it pertinent to define them on grounds of personal contact and interaction between members of well-defined and coherent groups; races, castes, classes and sexes. For it is precisely because certain groups have no representation in a number of recognised political structures that their position tends to be stable, their oppression so continuous.'

(Millett, 1977; p. 24)

A personal note to begin

The approach to politics and policy analysis presented in this chapter represents an airing of some of the ideas which have been fermenting for most of the past fifteen years. Entry in 1977 into the (part-time) world of academia to study for an MA by research began the slow and often painful process of consolidation of previously disjointed ideas and experiences. The process can be compared to peering down the tube of a kaleidoscope and seeing at first only a jumble of assorted shapes and colours. Shake the tube gently and suddenly a coherent pattern emerges; turn it again and the colours and images present in sharply different focus. The contents of the kaleidoscope are unchanged but there is a constant stream of opportunities to see them in different profiles and orderings of significance. The process of conceptual clarification is always demanding higher levels of refinement. Hence the drive to clarify one's ideas is never complete for they are being tested and re-tested continuously by various means. Publication is one vital stage in this testing process, and looking back over the years certain themes recur in my tentative attempts to

271

express in public the issues which concerned me greatly. Questions of power and oppression are never far from the surface, especially in relation to women; women as either the recipients of health care services or women as part of the health care delivery system. And women in these situations are often divided on two sides of a fence instead of pressing together for the recognition of their problems as valid policy issues in the public, political world of men. I wrote on these themes concerning women in Jolley and Allan's book *Current Issues in Nursing* (1989) with which this chapter could usefully be read in conjunction. Here I am beginning to locate the study of nursing political issues within a developing critical policy analysis tradition. It draws on many different sources of literature and beginning to make sense of its jumble of origins takes us back to the unshaken kaleidoscope. Nevertheless it is a beginning and in the first part of the chapter I set out some basic definitions, supported by certain key references. In the second much longer part, I begin to construct an analysis of several of the most well known recently published works on nursing politics. The re-working of other people's ideas is another important way of moving conceptual analysis further. The reader is left to draw his or her own conclusions as to whether the product 'fits' the experience of his or her own 'life world'. Whether it does, or not, readers are invited to participate themselves in taking up the challenge and to refute or refine the ideas so presented. The creation of knowledge is not some elite form of occupation for the chosen few, it is something with which we should all be concerned and in which we should actively participate.

Introduction

The 1980s have seen an upsurge of interest in what may be termed 'the politics of nursing'. A succession of books, all with nursing and politics in their titles, have been published (Salvage, 1985; Clay, 1987; White, 1985; 1986a; 1988) and speakers urging nurses to become more political have become a familiar aspect of the Nursing Conference circuit. Yet, despite all the *talk* of politics and political consciousness in nursing, there has been little theoretical development derived from the now fairly substantial case study literature on nurses' experiences of unequal power relationships and the welcome awakening of interest in a subject previously considered taboo by the professional nurse. We are able to describe but not yet to *explain* the phenomenon. This is not at all surprising – the discourse of public policy is the discourse of *men*. Feminist theorists (with whom nurse theorists share much in common but also some important differences; Robinson, 1989) have recognised and struggled with this problem. The quotation taken from Kate Millett's book *Sexual Politics* with which this chapter began illustrates how the very basis of 'taken for granted' assumptions about the nature of special relationships has to be questioned in order to begin to understand the *unquestioning* acceptance of oppression by certain social groups.

Part One: The development of a critical approach to politics and policy analysis in nursing

To begin to understand political issues in nursing in terms of unequal power relationships requires the study of a complex web of social interactions. They are complex because they involve nursing's relation to both specific and general government policies on health and welfare; and also to its own internal policies. These are developed against the backdrop of the social and economic circumstances in which the activity of nursing is practised – so these too should inform the debates. This contextualisation of issues proved crucial in the four year study of the management of nursing following the implementation of general management in the National Health Service (Robinson and Strong, 1987; Strong and Robinson, 1988 and 1990; Robinson *et al.*, 1989) for without the analysis of the broad picture it would not have been possible to illuminate how relatively unimportant nursing is to government and to managers in comparison with medicine. This insight led us to conclude that nursing remains in the social equivalent of an astronomical Black Hole. It appeared from our empirical evidence that even when nurses themselves were trying actively to break free from the negative gravitational force of tradition, and not all of them were, others on the outside showed little interest in trying to harness, or even to understand, the frustrated energies locked deep within the occupation of nursing. And this was not, apparently, a temporary aberration in policy matters; for the process whereby many senior nurses were sidestepped and stripped of their power during the structural changes in the NHS following the Griffiths Report (NHS Management Inquiry Team, 1983) appears to be continuing unabated with the recent resignation of one of the most formidable Regional Nursing Officers in the country (Nursing Times, and Nursing Mirror, 1989).

Perspectives on power, politics, policy and decision–making

Before going further with this particular line of critical policy analysis it is important to stand back and to set it within more conventional definitions of politics and policy studies. Pollitt *et al.* (1979) and Ham and Hill (1986) argue that because the terms politics and policy have evolved untidily writers should avoid the intellectual imperialism of insisting upon tight, stipulative definitions. Indeed, as Millet argues, the unquestioning acceptance of imposed definitions can lock us into accepting the very assumptions we ought to be questioning. At first sight definitions *appear* nevertheless to be relatively straightforward. The Greek word *polis* is the root for both English words *policy* and *politics* which, according to the Shorter Oxford English Dictionary, refers to issues concerned with citizenship, government and the state. Hence political *theory* has been concerned traditionally with the science and art of Government, and in particular with the form, organisation and administration of the whole, or some part, of the state. Things are less straightforward however, when we return to the *applied* aspects of policy and politics. First, it is important to recognise that the terms policy analysis, policy studies and public administration have often been used inter-changeably. Second, such studies are *multidisciplinary* and may draw on the insights of disciplines as varied as economics, psychology, sociology, history and anthropology. Third, they consist of two main approaches, used either simply or in conjunction with one another:

- the description, evaluation and solution of practical problems
- the analysis of the way societies go about these same tasks

In other words, policy studies involve *both* the acquisition of knowledge and the development of theories about problems *and* an understanding of the political issues involved in solving them. These issues turn centrally on the question of *power* and how it is mediated in the policy process. Policy studies in nursing can help therefore not only to clarify some of the political issues involved in providing a nursing service within a health care system, but also to unravel some more general aspects of power in the policy-making process.

The substantive *area* of nursing is, of course, the subject matter of nursing policy studies. There may however be many different *topics* within it. For example, policy may be analysed in respect of clinical nursing, nurse education, nurses' pay or the management of nursing. The study of each of these policies involves, as mentioned above, *many different modes of thinking*: sociological; economic; historical; political theory; psychological and so forth. Hence the claim that policy studies is a multidisciplinary activity. Thus collections such as *Readings in the Sociology of Nursing* (Dingwall and McIntosh, 1978), *Re-writing Nursing History* (Davies, 1980a) and *Understanding Nurses; the social psychology of nursing* (Skevington, 1984) all help to illuminate in some way political issues in nursing.

The impossibility of merely *describing* events without seeking to draw policy lessons from them is also increasingly acknowledged. Hence the analysis *of* policy becomes almost invariably a case *for* policy. In this sense the activity can never be value-neutral. Rein

(1976) challenges researchers to acknowledge this situation. However, as he notes, this does not mean abandoning scholarly values. Rein also urges the importance of a sceptical approach and the need to develop a value-critical stance to policy issues. This requires the analyst to question his or her own values as well as those he or she seeks to study. Nurses, in particular, need to take this lesson to heart or their writing on policy issues can become barely concealed polemic.

Policy studies implies then not just the gathering of facts about an issue, but also the analysis of how and why the issue becomes, or does not become, 'a problem' worthy of public attention and solution. It follows that one of the central topics of policy studies is how and why some issues get selected as a serious problem for public concern while others, potentially no less important, are neglected. The how and why crucially concern matters of power and influence. Nursing, with little of either, is rarely an issue in public policy. An important topic for research must therefore be when, and about what, nursing issues become matters for public concern.

Two important inter-related issues arise from the above discussion for nursing policy studies. First, where is nursing placed in relation to the location and exercise of power, power both external and internal to the profession? Second, where does nursing stand in relation to particular institutional frameworks for health and social welfare? In order to move forward on these issues it is important to investigate further the nature of power and decision-making.

Power and decision-making

There are many theoretical analyses of the nature of power and of its distribution within society. Ham and Hill (1986) group the major studies which examine the relationship of power to decision-making into three broad categories which theorists have developed over the past fifteen years. First, there are those which study the power to make key, concrete policy decisions. These are generally focused on actual decision-making behaviour. They analyse whether the power to make decisions is concentrated within one or several elite groups or, alternatively, through a pluralistic system in which various regulatory mechanisms ensure that ultimately the majority view prevails. This approach embodies the notion of an ultimate rationality in decision-making and the power to ensure a consensus in policy terms in order to achieve that goal. It tends to focus therefore on studying those who already hold a considerable measure of power to shape events!

The second group of studies originates from the critiques of the nature of power portrayed in the first. They are concerned with analysing the power to keep key issues *off* the policy agenda – and involve the nature of non decision-making. Bachrach and Baratz (1962) were amongst the first to develop an argument for this approach to policy studies and their original article remains highly relevant. This perspective has, in turn, been criticised because of the empirical difficulty of demonstrating the nature of a non decision. Nevertheless writers such as Crenson (1971) have illustrated, for example, the indirect influence of the economic power of a major industrial monopoly in preventing the passage of clean air legislation.

The third dimension of power (as developed by Lukes, 1975) is the product of more than a decade of debate over the validity of the first two perspectives. Lukes' position, which is developed from, and loosely related to the second, argues (despite the even greater problems of empirical validation) that power concerns the subtle and complex ways in which 'the sheer weight of institutions – political, industrial and education' (p. 38) serve to shape people's cognitions, perceptions and preferences. As a result:

'. . . they accept their role in the existing order of things, either because they can see or imagine no alternative to it, or because they see it as natural and unchangeable, or because they value it as divinely ordained and beneficial. To assume that the absence of grievance equals genuine consensus is simply to rule out the possibility of false or manipulated consensus by definitional fiat.'

(Lukes, 1986; p. 24)

Other authors have explored similar ideas, and the study of policy in the field of health care provides rich examples of his view that power is sustained through the values of dominant belief systems. Alford (1975) argues that the politics of health care are governed by dominant, challenging and repressed structural interests. He sees the sustaining of the medical model of health and illness as being of fundamental importance to the maintenance of the dominant structural interests and therefore the power of the doctors. Certainly the events observed in the four year study of the management of nursing after the implementation of Griffiths, referred to above, could be explained as a fundamental struggle by the government, represented by general managers, to challenge the dominant power of medicine. The invisibility of nursing in this struggle merely confirms its status as a repressed policy interest. (See Chapter 6.)

Ideology, politics and health care

The position so far arrived at suggests that politics may be seen as the possession of power to ensure that:

- certain issues become defined as valid for policy concern and therefore receive a place on the public policy agenda; or
- certain issues are kept off the public policy agenda whether deliberately, or by default.

Women's issues, of which nursing may be seen as one subset, are rarely counted as matters of valid policy concern except in time of national emergency such as war. Even then the issues tend to be defined in ways which ensure that they can be removed from the agenda as soon as the emergency is over. Child care facilities, for instance, are seen as important in order to release women to contribute to the national work effort rather than to enable them to pursue careers and fulfil their individual potential. Clearly, a third crucial aspect of power must then concern *the ability to define issues in such a way that they can meet certain chosen means and ends*. Means and ends imply values and values involve an underlying ideology. Hence policy is never value-neutral, but is always founded on an implicit or explict belief system (see Chapter 7). For example, if women's first obligation is to their home and children it follows, according to this particular value system, that child care facilities are unnecessary unless a greater obligation (the national good) intervenes, when the first may take a lower priority to the second.

Describing issues in this way may sound emotive and it is crucial to emphasise that the underlying system of ideas *is* neutral. It is only when the ideas are put into practice and, as a result, some people's interests suffer at the expense of others that feelings and emotions come into play. The Shorter Oxford English Dictionary defines Ideology in two ways:

- the science of ideas; the study of the origin and nature of ideas;
- a system of ideas concerning phenomena, especially those of social life; the manner of thinking characteristic of a class or an individual.

It is the incorporation of ideas into a system which can command the power to define goods and services according to their *value* which translates ideology into a political belief system. Hence, in a detailed study of welfare work, Cousins (1987) sees contradictions in the values applied to caring work such as nursing. On the one hand there is a 'factory-like logic' where welfare labour is subjected to wage pressure and de-skilling similar to that applied in the private sector; reflecting Marx's ideas of an *exchange value* for labour. On the other hand Cousins argues that welfare services are produced also in terms of alternative moral values:

'These services (also) provide a material resource for labour that mitigates to some extent the exploitative relation of capital and labour, especially for women and ethnic minority groups. The state sector can provide progressive employment and labour relations practices – for instance equal opportunities practices, contract compliance policies, or health and safety procedures – practices which advance the public interest although these may not be the agencies' specific policy objectives.'

(Cousins, 1987; p. 185)

The move during the 1970s from a political consensus over the provision of state welfare to one which emphasises the rights and obligations of individuals within a market economy is documented by Deakin (1987), and Klein (1983 and 1989) and the range of different systems of ideas involved in what has come to be called 'The New Right' is described by Green (1987). In summarising the relationship between markets and morality Green describes a set of beliefs which are almost completely at variance with those set out by Cousins above:

'It is frequently said that markets promote selfishness . . . that there can be little doubt that the market fosters personal attributes, such as greed and a lack of concern for one's neighbour . . . What truth is there in such claims? The new liberals have typically argued, not that selfishness is a good thing, but that selfishness exists whether we like it or not, and they have urged that we must therefore strive towards institutions which prevent selfishness from doing too much harm. Competition is said to be the chief safeguard available . . . The case for liberty rests only in part on the value of competition in channelling the efforts of possibly selfish individuals into the service of their fellows. It also rests on the belief that there are any number of alternative ways of meeting human wants – some like charity and mutual aid the very antithesis of profit seeking – and that only in a free society can such alternatives flourish.'

(Green, 1987; p. 217)

The task of the policy analyst is to tease out the concepts and values which underpin statements such as these and then to evaluate the consequences of their application for different groups of people involved in the system. Feminists would argue, for example, that charity and mutual aid usually involve the exploitation of women somewhere in the process while state welfare too has depended on the cheap use of women's labour. The latter has had the benefit however of providing a sense of identity with health care as a moral enterprise; an identity which is fast becoming alienated as welfare work is transformed into a market economy through contracting out and other mechanisms (Tonkin and Hart, 1989).

Part Two: Politics and policy analysis in nursing: some examples from the literature

Thinking about the issues to be discussed in the second part of this chapter began in 1987 when four of the five books on nursing politics cited at the beginning of the introduction had been recently published. Asked at that time to review one of them (White, 1986) I found myself struggling to identify a conceptual framework which would provide a structure for analysis across the wide range of nursing topics which were being called *political*. It was very difficult. White's two extant publications contained a range of fascinating case study material but one was hard put to discover a unifying political theme running through them. Indeed, while the notion of power was always implicit, the mechanisms through which it is mediated in nursing were rarely discussed. Similarly, Salvage and Clay, while arguing very strongly for consciousness-raising and political awareness amongst nurses, seemed to be coming at the problem from different positions.

In examining White's work at that time I tentatively identified five broad categories within which the subject matter of her 1985 and 1986 edited collections could be discussed. These were:

1. The case for unity in nursing: a false premise?
2. The divisive effects on nursing of cost-containment and other contemporary policy initiatives.
3. The marginalisation of nursing arising from the implicit value conflicts in health policy.
4. The structural effects of class and gender on nursing.
5. The power of nurses as oppressors.

In writing this current chapter in 1989 I returned to my earlier (unpublished) paper to try to identify how well White's further (1988) collection could be fitted together with Clay's and Salvage's work into the framework provisionally developed for the two earlier volumes. Even with subsequent modification it is still not perfect for conceptual analysis. One particular problem is that there is considerable overlap between the categories. Nevertheless it is a beginning. Setting out the discussion which follows within this modified structure I am conscious of writing for a textbook on the knowledge base for nursing practice. This seems be an excellent forum in which to achieve the following important goals: to declare the provisional state of our knowledge on nursing politics; to demonstrate the very different perspectives which are already emanating from this embryonic conceptual debate; to challenge students to continue the process of clarification through their projects and essays; and to plead with them for *publication* so that our knowledge base can be developed and refined. What follows is no definitive state of the art; it is put forward for challenge and refutation.

The framework in current use

Returning to the analysis referred to above after a two year breathing space I was struck by the need for a greater sense of balance in the proposed framework. Subjects did not appear as black and white as when I had reviewed them earlier. Nurses were putting forward varied perspectives on the same subject. The framework was therefore modified as follows:

1. Nursing as a force for challenge and change; the costs and benefits of unity.
2. Contemporary health policy initiatives; the potential and the risks for nurses and their clients.
3. The structure of nursing: its constraints and its potential for development.
4. Class, gender and race in nursing.
5. Nurses as oppressors or enablers; power for or against each other and the client?

The following discussion sets some of the contents of the five books cited in the introduction within the above framework. Surprisingly, given nurses' increasing challenge to the medical model, the five volumes contain relatively little about nursing's relationship with medicine. They do however contain rich empirical evidence on nursing's place within different welfare systems. Also strongly implicit is the idea of conflicting values and the pressures to which these subject different groups of nurses. This leads naturally to the issues concerning power and value systems described in Part One. Hopefully this process moves us slowly but closer to an underlying theory, or theories, of politics in nursing.

Nursing as a force for challenge and change; the costs and benefits of unity

Two conflicting issues dominate much of the material in the five books:
- the contribution made to its powerlessness by the historic divisions within nursing;
- nursing as a potential force for challenge and change in health care.

The authors all have very different ideas about how to resolve the first in order to achieve the second. Trevor Clay, writing as General Secretary of The Royal College of Nursing, put forward a powerful argument for unity within one umbrella staff organisation:

> 'This diversity, currently a weakness, could, if unified, be the profession's greatest strength. Of course, it is the RCN's belief that the profession will be stronger and serve society better if there is only one organisation for nurses called the RCN . . .'
>
> (Clay, 1987; p. 29)

He disagrees vehemently with Rosemary White's (1985) account of nursing as a pluralistic society and her argument that 'the enforcement of a unitary policy, of consensus, inhibits change,' (Clay, 1987; p. 33). White, in her turn, is equally convinced of the power of diversity – although there is little doubt that her sympathies lie with the professionalist group of nurses who look for their authority to 'higher education and a specialized knowledge base' (White, 1988; p. 19). In describing three distinguishable groups White identifies two, the managers and the professionals, who, by virtue of identifying with the value systems of their respective peer groups, are locked within inevitable conflict. The remainder, the 'generalists', are in White's terminology 'the task workers . . . content to work within the hierarchy, supervised by the nurse managers' (p. 19). It is this third group with whom Jane Salvage in a book which 'strongly reflects the author's own feminist and socialist beliefs' (Dunn 1985) apparently identifies. Her belief that the personal is political and that nurses at *all* levels should be aware of, and react to, policy initiatives which constrain their practice also brings its own sharp rebuff from Trevor Clay. He only agrees on one level with Salvage's argument that 'nurses must confront the consequences of political and policy decisions as they affect them in work and in their personal experience of those decisions . . .' (p. 2). He supports nurses in 'a little personal confrontation' (with the hierarchy, doctors or general managers) but when it comes to threatening patients' welfare 'there is another way' (p. 3). Unsurprisingly, the route lies, in Clay's terms, through organising as a profession and as a trade union.

Here, in simplified terms, we see some of the fundamental roots of disagreement within nursing over ways of overcoming its powerlessness. Each of these highly credited authors puts forward the values derived from his or her system of ideas; we hear the views of the professional trade union; the representative of a professional elite; and the voice of the worker on the ward. It is fascinating to reflect that the third, proletarian, view is expressed by a nurse who entered nursing after a Cambridge degree, went on after working as a staff nurse to become a highly respected nurse journalist and eventually a supporter of nursing development units – a true grass roots movement. Already it is possible to see from this brief outline of the different systems expressed that we do not need to look outside nursing in order to begin to appreciate the location and exercise of power. We may guess but don't yet understand how different career patterns may influence individual perceptions of power and change. Hardy in White (1986) begins to explore the politics of the career histories of senior nurses but there is, as yet, no systematic attempt to explain the relationship between biography and ideology.

It is possible, however, to tease out the importance of historical and cultural contexts to nursing developments from other authors in White's collections. Larsen (White, 1988) argues for nursing leaders to understand the politics of public policy-making and to act appropriately. Unsupported by reference to empirical evidence her case verges on the polemic. Perhaps in Canada (of which she writes) nurses are more able to become politically assertive but we should not assume that this form of action is feasible in every culture. Davies (1980b) develops an extremely useful international comparative perspective on nurse education in Britain and the USA up to 1939 which helps us to understand the importance and complexity of cultural variation. She concludes that American nurses had far greater self confidence than the British. In addition, there were differences in the legislative framework, the educational system and the patterns of employment available to them. Asking why such arrangements were available in the USA and not in Britain, Davies states that the answer would require:

'. . . a consideration of how economic, political and social forms are deeply intertwined. The point of the present argument, however, is to show that a different matrix of institutions gives different experiences and different opportunities for compromise and struggle for an occupational group such as nurses.'

(Davies, 1980b; p. 115)

Davies' lesson is that the defining and achievement of policy goals cannot be understood divorced from the cultural context in which they are formulated.

Zwanger's (White 1986) account of Jewish nursing education in Palestine between 1914–1948 provides a national comparative perspective. There was, it seems, a striking difference between the content of the syllabi in the British colonial schools of nursing in Palestine and those in Jewish national nursing schools. The British were committed to traditional forms of training; the Jewish to wider educational values. Regrettably Zwanger's description excludes any analysis of the respective political ideologies involved. Nevertheless one detects the implicit notion of higher values being placed on nurse education by national interest groups than by the resident colonial

power. Is this, we may enquire, characteristic of nationalist movements everywhere and, if so, what part do women play in these drives
for self-determination? If, as may be hypothesised, their contribution
is more highly valued during periods of intense pro-nationalist
activity does nursing, by association, stand to benefit? Alternatively,
are women naturally more assertive during these periods of historical
development?

Further international comparisons may be made from White's
collections. For example, can a parallel be drawn between the
situation described in Palestine and the account of nursing's move to
higher education in Australia described by Parkes (White, 1986)? She
attributes the successful outcome of the struggle for educational
reform in Australia during the thirty years following the Second
World War to her belief that the education movement amongst
nurses served as a massive consciousness-raising activity and as a
focus for unity. This unity, Parkes argues, together with the increased
political participation which followed was both a necessary and a
sufficient condition for change. Her analysis in this respect does not
ring fully true. She does not account for *party* political influence in
Australia at that time and the national commitment to increase
female participation in higher education. This may have been the
sufficient condition required before nurses' *necessary* activity in
campaigning for higher education produced results.

Fondiller (White, 1986) is less idealistic than Parkes about the idea
of unity. She describes how, paradoxically, the perceived need for a
unified nursing profession led to the policies which had exactly the
opposite effect. The American Nurses' Association (ANA) and the
National League for Nursing (NLN) were originally created in 1952
in order to function in a complementary fashion. (The ANA as a
professional nurses' association; the NLN focused on organised
community service and the educational standards and facilities
necessary to provide a good nursing service to the public.) The two
organisations subsequently found themselves representing different
groups and different interests. Concentrated to a large extent on the
level, location, and entry requirements for nurse education these
conflicts have a familiar ring. The recently achieved concensus in the
USA on the educational preparation of professional baccalaureate
nurses and technical nurses, as described by Fondiller, reflected more
the proportionate strength of the respective memberships of these
two organisations, than the achievement of any substantial unity
between them. Fondiller's detailed account of these political
manoeuvrings is an object lesson for anyone who subscribes to the
utopian ideal of unity. She is realistic and concludes that with the rise
of the clinical specialisation movement nursing groups will continue
to evolve and multiply. She strongly advocates therefore the logical
development of coalitions, arguing that if nurses are to deliver a

collective clout to national policy-making then a common voice on key issues will be essential.

The ways in which nurses have sought, perhaps unwittingly or perhaps deliberately, to strengthen the power of one group to the detriment of others is part of the subject of Campbell's chapter (White, 1988) reviewed later for its account of the social construction of nursing documentation. It contains a telling account of how the Canadian Nurses' Association's commitment to an all graduate profession has worked *against* the career interest of non-graduate nurses. The talk of unity becomes an empty vessel unless nurses are prepared to address the claims of challenging and repressed interest groups within nursing.

It is from examples such as these that nurses may come to realise the crucial importance of cultural context to the presence of nursing issues on a policy agenda in a particular place at a particular moment in time. Furthermore, consensus does not necessarily mean the absence of conflict. Instead, faced with supra-ordinate goals, nurses may have to address the question of internal negotiation more realistically in order for their collective activities to be meaningfully directed.

Contemporary health policy initiatives; the potential and risk for nurses and their clients

Two chapters in White's most recent volume (1988), one from the United Kingdom and one from Canada, take up the theme of the effects of wider contemporary health policy initiatives on nursing which in her two earlier volumes was left to North American nurses to explore. Their chapters centre on cost-containment policies in the USA and because there are important general political lessons to be learnt from the phenomena which they describe their work will be summarised in some depth.

Gray (1984) points out that the phenomenon of cost-containment in health care is now a matter of international concern and, as a result, particular aspects of the North American health care system are slowly being extrapolated to other cultures. One of these – the introduction of Diagnostic Related Groups (DRGs) and their effects on nursing – is the subject matter of the three chapters from North American authors, Milio on *Nursing within the ecology of public policy: a case in point* (White, 1985), Melosh on *Nursing and Reagnomics: cost containment in the United States* (White, 1986) and Beatrice and Philip Kalisch on *Nurses on strike; labour management conflict in US hospitals and the role of the press* (White, 1985).

Melosh and Milio both argue that DRGs are part and parcel of an overall fiscal policy which aims to reduce a huge government deficit by cutting social programmes. By providing a fixed pre-determined payment for the health services given within each of the 467 DRGs, providers are forced to operate within a traditional market economy model. If the service they provide exceeds the allowable cost then the shortfall must be found by cost-cutting within other sections of their budget. If, on the other hand, the service can be provided for less then providers are given the incentive of keeping at least a proportion of the saving made. Proponents of the system argue that DRGs not only provide essential controls over individual professional (medical) profligacy but also that it gives those same professionals real motivation in seeking 'value for money'. If they are encouraged to manage their own budgets in this way, then the power to ensure the availability of resources for new developments lies firmly in their hands.

All of this now has a familiar ring in the United Kingdom but, nevertheless, in considering the possible extrapolation of these ideas to other cultures, it is critically important to keep in mind the key background to these developments. Health care costs in the USA had rocketed from the 1960s onwards (Gray, 1984). The introduction of state-sponsored Medicare and Medicaid had led to a 'blank cheque' approach to medical care in a system which 'traditionally included little structure or incentive for controlling costs' (Melosh in White, 1986; p.146). There was therefore an urgent need to address congressional concern about resultant over-treatment and at the same time to work through the complexities of the American health care billing system. Certainly this *could* mean that DRGs are less appropriate in other settings but the evidence needs to be systematically assessed. The various implications of this policy for nursing also need to be thought through carefully and the lessons from the American experience noted. All of these three North American authors offer analyses of cost-containment policies which fall into three broad categories:

– The opportunity which they provide for enhancing the professional power and status of some nurses.
– The increased workload which they bring for some nurses, accompanied by the impoverishment of others.
– The possible benefits (and potentially adverse consequences) which can be identified for patients and their families.

Thus they argue that a policy initiative such as cost-containment, introduced through the medium of DRGs, can result in some costs and some benefits for different groups. Not only may certain sections of nursing find their interests at odds with others but also those same interests may coincide, or conflict, with those of the patients. A summary of their evidence, under the three broad headings, follows.

Opportunities for enhancing nurses' power and status

Melosh describes the conflicting perspectives on DRGs which can be found from her reading of nursing journals since 1983. Nursing proponents of the system are to be found mainly amongst nurse managers who display a guarded optimism. The DRG hospital is portrayed as an arena of opportunity, the system is accepted as given and the discussion centres on strategies for negotiating its risks and benefits. She argues that this cautiously optimistic view rests on the hope of using the DRG system as a device to support nursing's historical struggle for professional autonomy; nurses being urged to establish their own productivity measures in order to demonstrate their cost-effectiveness *vis-à-vis* the doctors.

Nurses' major grievance is undoubtedly that nursing costs are merely collapsed into the daily DRG room rate giving no account of the nursing acuity of individual patients; illustrating in a specific way the general principle outlined in Part One that nursing issues are frequently excluded from the policy agenda. American nurses have therefore challenged the validity of the DRG indicator as an adequate predictor of the *real* costs of patient care. Such challenges call for a major revision of the categories used in calculating DRGs and offer a variety of instruments for calculating nursing costs. In turn, nurses' claims for a pivotal managerial role for nursing are enhanced and nurses are exhorted to become computer-literate and to learn cost-accounting as an essential management tool. In this context primary nursing is promoted as a cost-effective pattern of practice, but Melosh cautions nurses to consider dangerous historical precedents when extrapolating from this argument to the suggestion that nursing might in future be based on fee-for-service practice. She summarises nursing's optimistic view of DRGs by locating its search for more independent nursing arrangments within the cost-containment system. Nevertheless, in justifying their loosening of dependence on the doctors by pointing to their cost effectiveness nurses also have to look to threats emerging from below. In the USA medical technicians emerge as potential substitutes for higher-paid nurses and Melosh cites examples where nurses' associations have sought to confine the activities of these lower-paid competitors.

The increased workload and impoverishment of some nurses

Milio summarises a variety of hospital administrative strategies which were introduced in order to deal with the economic and competitive problems exacerbated by the attempts of Congress to contain Medicare and Medicaid which included the introduction of DRGs. She suggests that the overall effects on hospital services were likely to include:

- computerization of jobs;
- reduction in the lesser-reimbursed services, for example, maternity care;
- increase in admissions and intensity of care;
- increase in too early discharges, of the long-term and severely ill . . .;
- avoidance of the severely ill who do not have maximum private insurance or payment capacity (White, 1985; p. 92).

Milio describes this as the language of 'skim and dump'. The system skims the least risky, paying patients like cream from the milk. The rest, the low payers and the high risk patients are either refused, transferred, or released into public sector hospitals.

The effects on nursing are several-fold. First, for hospital-employed nurses, nurse managers match patient 'case-mix' with nursing 'skills-mix'. The results include:

- reducing the proportion of registered nurses;
- hiring nurses on a seasonal or part-time basis, avoiding fringe benefits and job security;
- increasing the intensity of workload with nurses caring for sicker patients with shorter hospital stays.

Second, and hypothetically, nurses working in community-based care are likely to be more involved with a sickness-remedial perspective than with a wellness-preventive point of view. In addition, nurses are called upon to try to remedy the adverse effects of premature discharge upon sick patients sent home without adequate informal systems of care.

The Kalischs, in their turn, describe the impact of such policies on *industrial relations* in nursing. Closures and lower utilisation rates were one consequence of attempts to minimise hospital expenditure. When hospitals in Minneapolis found themselves in competition for patients they turned to cutting labour costs, their biggest item of financial outlay. Nurses being the largest labour group took the worst toll (in 1984 30 per cent of Registered Nurses (RNs) were employed full time compared with 50 per cent in 1980). Senior, more expensive, nurses were laid off in preference to cheaper, junior staff. Part-time positions became obligatory, and working hours were cut. This situation led, in 1984, to the largest strike of nurses in the history of the USA. The Kalischs' case study thus provides empirical support for Melosh's analysis of nursing in a DRG future:

'Hospitals are likely to work their staffs harder, retain fewer full-time workers and rely on temporaries to cover the busiest times . . . In this unfavourable climate, nurses will not easily be able to defend or extend improvements in wages and working conditions.

Already hospitals are economizing by cutting health benefits and resisting pay rises . . .'

(White, 1985; pp. 160–1)

The consequences for patients and their families

Milio describes the effect of cost-containment policies in health care alongside broader cuts in income maintenance; food stamps; subsidies for heating-fuel and housing and in the enforcement of environmental and health standards. She cites evidence that up to 10 per cent more people were impoverished in 1983 than in 1979 and claims that this became a particularly acute economic and health-threatening problem for children. She concludes:

'Thus the accumulating weight of recession, the withdrawal of supportive Federal social policies and the DRG-induced pressures on already-limited public health services carry high risks to the health of those who are already most vulnerable: the poor, who are disproportionately children, elders, women and racial minorities.'

(White, 1985; p. 95)

Thus, in describing the effects of specific health policy within the overall context of public policy she highlights the probable long-term health consequences for the sick and especially the sick poor. She argues that there will be an increase in preventable health problems which will bring in train an unintended *increase* in total health care costs. Her arguments bear close resemblance to those of the British Black Report (Department of Health and Social Security, Research Working Group, 1980) and The Health Divide (Whitehead, 1987).

These three studies of the effects of cost-containment policies in the USA illustrate the complexity of the relationship between the values of a dominant political ideology and the policy initiatives which it generates. Nursing, in reacting to the costs and/or benefits of such policies, becomes divided as the various sub-groups within it identify with either dominant, challenging or repressed interests. At the time that they were written these case studies described the impact of a policy on nursing which functioned within a very different health and welfare system to that of many other countries. The extrapolation of similar ideologies to other cultures has led nurses in other countries to begin to examine their implications for nursing; although not specifically within cost-containment policies. The two authors in White's most recent volume (1988) explore the following contemporary issues: Campbell on *Accounting for care: a framework for analysing change in Canadian nursing*; and MacGuire on *Dependency Matters: an issue in the care of elderly people.*

They describe various ways in which nurses are attempting to improve nursing practice through the development of scientific or quasi-scientific methods for delivering or auditing nursing care. Their observations, in line with many of the analyses referred to in this review, demonstrate that for every apparently rational human act there are unintended consequences which carry costs and benefits.

Campbell's Canadian account of the social organisation of nursing documentation demonstrates how the development of tools such as Care Plans, Patient Classification Systems and Nursing Audits tends to lead to their taking precedence over nurses' primary task – that of caring for people. The production of information becomes the focus around which nurses' work is oriented. She observes:

'What I have described is not an aberration; but the contemporary method of knowing objectively, designed for efficient and effective management of an enterprise.'

(White, 1988; p. 65)

This outcome conflicts with the original intention of documentation which is to account for nursing's 'ideal representations' of their work through various models for practice. Instead, the paper work not only assumes a life of its own but also becomes recruited into the service of management as a tool for implementing budget cuts and justifying efficiency drives. Nurses find themselves in this situation struggling to maintain their own levels of excellence under difficult conditions. Campbell sees the problem of how nursing can *shape* its practice without being coerced into *adapting* practice to the corporatisation of health care as the major challenge facing nurses today.

MacGuire's detailed review of the concept of dependency contains similar challenges. She suggests, amongst a wealth of other information, that major shifts in the definition of the category of old age are taking place with a postponement of entry into official old age. She concludes that it is tempting to suggest that 'a restructuring of reality' is taking place 'akin to the bases for redefining the unemployed' (White, 1988; p. 73). Geriatric beds in the NHS have declined and the rate of provision per 1000 population in local authorities has gone down sharply, meanwhile the number of beds in private nursing homes has doubled. MacGuire argues, in the light of all these changes, that dependency is a crucial variable on which information is essential when assessing admission and discharge policies; nurse staffing establishments; and quality assurance issues. Hence she sees the *proper* management of documentation on dependency as vital to the success of auditing both individual patient care *and* organisational performance over time. Dependency information can give nursing staff the power to argue for changes in policy relating to patient admissions and length of stay, including the provision of adequate discharge facilities; and for staffing levels appropriate to identified, real time, patient needs. Here we see the crucial role of nursing information in order to argue a proper case in the face of cost-containment issues. Yet MacGuire observes that dependency data are rarely collected routinely and that many nurses are either unaware that such systems exist or, alternatively, believe that they run 'counter to the principle that every patient is unique and care must be tailored to meet his specific requirements,' (p. 79). Meanwhile, the statistical indicator of patients per occupied bed is widely utilised whilst ignoring the fact that the patients in the beds may be getting sicker and that the numbers of nursing staff may be going into relative decline.

Both of these authors highlight the crucial importance to the policy agenda of how social reality is constructed, defined and documented. Nurses are encouraged to participate in the development of scientific management techniques by various inducements such as greater autonomy for nursing or a more rational basis for planning staffing in relation to patient need. Whilst the benefits of such strategies appear to be undeniable, the North American experience of cost-containment policies suggests that a whole range of hidden costs may be incurred. Perhaps one answer is for nurses to insist that they must retain the control and ownership of the data and that its utility must be demonstrated in routine formal audits on the quality of care. This may be just a pious hope unless the ideological positions subscribed to by nurses in various organisational positions and the divisions within nursing which result are seriously addressed.

The structure of nursing: its constraints and potential for development

This section summarises the work of six authors (five chapters) each of whom tries to encapsulate the effects on nursing of more diffuse and less explicit ideologies. It may not be coincidental that three – McIntosh on *District Nursing: a case of political marginality*, Robinson on *Health visiting and health* (White, 1985) and Hennessy on *The restrictive and wanting policies affecting health visitors' work in the field of emotional health* (White, 1986) – write about community nursing within the British NHS, while Storch and Stinson on *Concepts of deprofessionalization with applications to nursing* (White, 1988) work in a University Department of Community Medicine in Canada. It is in non-institutional care that the broader, inter-sectoral aspects of welfare policy are most apparent and often the most difficult to address. Keyzer (White, 1988) is something of an exception to this rule. His chapter on *Challenging role boundaries: conceptual frameworks for understanding the conflict arising from implementation of the nursing process in practice* is based on empirical research in a community hospital, geriatric, psycho-geriatric and psychiatric rehabilitation units; areas which are nevertheless marginal in many debates about nursing power and politics. (See Chapter 10.)

McIntosh describes the marginalisation of district nursing during the historic process of change in the years following the introduction of the NHS in 1948. She claims that this was an effect of 'policy drift' which arises because health policy is determined as much by interest groups outside parliament as by governmental dictat. In describing groups contending for power amongst themselves and who, as a result, successfully block government initiatives for resource reallocation McIntosh, like White herself, subscribes implicitly to the theory of a power elite in health care. She believes that the inability of district nursing to compete successfully for the status which would ensure a greater share of resources originates from a number of historical events. First, in 1948, district nursing was catapulted from the arena of voluntary sector provision into the statutory framework of the NHS. The requirement at that time that local health authorities should provide home nursing care resulted in the nursing voice being suppressed by the managerial authority of the Medical Oficer of Health. This had long term implications for district nurse training which reverberate today.

Second, the ultimate managerial control of community nursing by nurses recommended by the Mayston Report (Department of Health and Social Security *et al.*, 1969) proved a mixed blessing. On the one hand, divisions where several groups of community nurses were managed under one head tended to have a health visitor as director of nursing services. On the other, these managerial changes also coincided with the 1974 reorganisation of the NHS which not only abolished the former local authority control but also introduced a 'centrally controlled techno-bureaucracy' (White, 1985; p. 49). One outcome was that community nursing divisions were integrated into hospital management structures, with the further loss of district nursing input into crucial policy-making groups. McIntosh argues, in familiar terms, that a second outcome of this change was for district nurse managers to identify with managerial instead of nursing reference groups. However the most crucial implication of all these managerial changes for district nursing was its distancing from any direct influence over the total budget. Thus despite government policies intended during the 1970s to bring about a reallocation of resources to the district nursing service, and to the priority groups which formed a large part of its clientele, other powerful forces were able successfully to obstruct their implementation. This was particularly true of the attempt to redistribute any substantial amount of resources from the hospital to the community sectors. Fifteen years later community nurses in the United Kingdom fear that this situation may worsen following the implementation of two White Papers on health and welfare service provision (Department of Health, 1989a and 1989b).

Third, policies for the attachment of district nurses to primary health care teams, which were being implemented concurrently with the 1970s managerial change, often proved divisive in terms of leadership, authority and control of district nursing. The empirical evidence of district nurses being perceived to be merely handmaidens of the doctors contrasted vividly with the rhetoric of egalitarianism in team relationships. This not only reinforced district nurses' subservient position but also prevented their managers from organising and allocating their scarce resources in order to meet wider needs than a general practice population might require.

McIntosh does not subscribe explicitly to any specific welfare ideology. Yet she clearly feels strongly that district nursing has been marginalised along with the needs of those groups, such as the elderly, disabled, chronic sick, who form its focus of concern. This outcome can be usefully compared with the results of cost-containment policies described above, MacGuire's work on dependency in the elderly and with Hennessy's account of policies affecting health visitors' work in emotional health which follows. It appears that the power to exclude nursing issues from policy agendas is exercised in many and subtle ways. Nurses, it seems, can often be the victims of the *rhetoric* of policy change. On the one hand they are encouraged to believe that if they comply with certain policy initiatives then their concerns will become more dominant. On the other, nothing changes because of the failure of policy-makers to address underlying power and resource issues.

Hennessy describes the ambiguous nature of the policy objectives and guidelines for health visitors when working in the field of maternal emotional health. She states:

'. . . health visitors have to be flexible. In one situation they must respond to health needs defined by the family and, in the next, they must note health needs of the family, as defined by professionals, the district health authority, local social service policies and national guidelines. Health visitors are therefore in a very difficult situation with conflicting guidelines and policies. The result of a health visitor not searching for the professionally defined needs of an abused child leads to public criticism, whereas the impact is not quite the same when health visitors do not search for those needs that the patient identifies, such as the depressed mother. This does not help the health visitor's dilemma.'

(Hennessy, 1986; p. 89)

Hennessy claims that despite their growing awareness of emotional problems health visitors do not recognise all postnatally depressed mothers. She suggests a number of factors which may account for this failure. First, many women who are distressed in the postnatal period do not experience sufficiently severe symptoms to need referral to a psychiatrist. As a result, health visitors are searching for a set of criteria which do not merit a *medical* diagnostic label. Indeed the diagnosis of moderate distress depends on how the mother says she feels as compared with how she felt before she had her baby.

Second, individual general practitioners react idiosyncratically to postnatal depression. Many will not be interested if the syndrome is not deemed worthy of the 'medical' label. This places the health visitor in an invidious position if she has identified a need but can find no collaborative professional network in which a care strategy could be planned.

Third, the situation may be exacerbated by the organisation of community psychiatric care. Many community psychiatric nurses, considered to be an outreach of institutional psychiatric care, only accept referrals from a consultant psychiatrist. Hence the one nursing colleague with whom the health visitor might confer is frequently out of reach.

Fourth, professional help for moderately distressed postnatal mothers usually involves the provision of a 'listening ear', and possibly the organisation of community support systems. Hennessy points however to the anomalous organisational position in which health visitors find themselves: despite exhortations to work with the whole family, the health visitor's workload is defined statistically only in terms of the children; 'listening' is not deemed officially to constitute skilled professional work, especially if no medical diagnosis is involved; and finally, community development work by health visitors is frequently discouraged by their own nurse managers.

Thus from the point of view of both district nursing and health visiting those client needs and issues which appeal to concepts of health and sickness outside the frame of reference of the dominant medical model, with associated lower priority ratings in a needs hierarchy, tend to be excluded from the day to day policy agenda. They may feature grandiloquently in strategic plans but nurses may find their actions obliquely diverted when they make serious attempts to address the needs in practice. These are examples of the repressed issues described by Alford and Lukes cited in Part One. The nursing care which is performed in relation to these client needs lacks status as important 'work', and may be dismissed as 'work' at all, partly on the grounds that it is carried out invisibly in the home, and partly because it defies evaluation and quantification.

The two remaining chapters in this group of four describe policy concerns in more abstract, conceptual terms. Robinson focuses on an analysis of the vulnerable basis which the abstract ideal of 'health as a value' provides for legitimated health visiting activity and touches on several of the philosophical and ideological questions which underpin some of these issues. She argues in line with Stacey's (1976) position that the generalisation of value subscription to *one* concept of health throughout society is a highly questionable proposition. Health in western society is conceived along several dimensions:

(*a*)   individual or collective;

(*b*)   functional fitness or welfare (care);

(*c*)   preventive or curative or ameliorative.

Robinson notes that the dominant interests of medicine have ensured that the predominant model in health care is based on the concept of individual functional fitness, and curative service objectives. This marginalises on the one hand the concerns of district nurses who are likely to be more concerned with care and amelioration than with cure and on the other, health visitors who are educated to see their role as involving collective as well as individual prevention.

Robinson believes that many health visitors, faced with the ideological dilemmas which underpin these different conceptual approaches, rationalise their claims to effectiveness through the use of quasi-scientific evaluation techniques. In the process they ignore some of the fundamental distinctions between positivist and interpretive paradigms for understanding and interpreting the behaviour of both health care providers, and their clients. Nursing, although she does not describe the phenomenon in these terms, is once again divided into those who seek to identify with the values of the dominant interest groups, a challenging minority, and a repressed majority.

Storch and Stinson's Canadian perspective on concepts of deprofessionalisation might equally be included in the preceding section on contemporary health policy initiatives. It is discussed here only because their conceptual analysis relates to the more abstract idea of structure than to concrete examples drawn from empirical research, although they relate their observations to 'real world' situations currently affecting mental health professionals. Deprofessionalisation, they argue, is a contemporary phenomenon in many health care occupations which previously sought full professional status. The concept itself has been described however in the literature in three different ways: as deskilling; as proletarianisation; and as the erosion of professional knowledge and trust. Their clarification of these perspectives is invaluable.

Deprofessionalisation as *de-skilling* arises from a combination of circumstances which include a general anti-professional bias and management pressures for increased efficiency. This 'attack on two fronts' is related to Braverman's (1974) thesis that the labour process is shaped by the accumulation of capital and that a dominant goal in profit-making is to purchase labour as cheaply as possible. As a result, workers who aspired to professional status by the possession of unique knowledge and skills and autonomy of action become subjected to the principles of 'scientific management'. Job analysis leads to its break up into component parts, the sum of which becomes divorced from the whole. The worker becomes divorced from control of the totality of the labour process. Storch and Stinson believe that nursing is faced with increased pressure to comply with scientific management. The measurement of patient acuity levels, nursing workload etc. (all commendable activities if they enhance decision-making) can, if used as means to the end of cost-containment, lead to 'cheaper and less effective levels of care, and become instruments of the deskilling of nurses because the craft and creativity of nursing is destroyed' (Storch and Stinson, 1988; p. 36). Deprofessionalisation as *proletarianisation* occurs when applied to professional occupations. First, advances in technology lead to huge capital investment in complex machines rather than in people; the control of this investment is centralised by various means. Second, although certain professional services may expand in order to meet the needs of large numbers of clients, the professionals themselves tend to become controlled by a central administration. Third, professional markets for clients are invaded by public and private capital. The result is that professionals have become subordinate employees within the control of centralised bureaucracies.

It may be argued that nurses in the NHS have always been subjected to bureaucratic control and that nursing has therefore always been proletarian by nature. The arguments put forward by Storch and Stinson suggest however that full proletarianisation may not yet have run its full course. For example, the progressive fragmentation of work leads to a situation where knowledge about the *whole* task is separated from the execution of its component parts. Indeed, the tasks may be allocated to different groups of workers outside the control of nursing – a form of *technical* proletarianisation. There is another form however – *ideological* proletarianisation – where the very values, goals and social purposes of the work are taken over by others. If nurses cannot maintain control of a nursing system which defines nursing work in acceptable terms for them, then they are rendered truly powerless by the process of alienation.

Storch and Stinson's summary of this situation is very telling:

'The proletarianization of professionals has commonly been discussed in the context of unionization and the use of union tactics by professionals. Perhaps a better understanding of the proletarianization theses can sensitize us to the frustrations many nurses experience when they feel they have lost control over the social purpose of their work (ideological proletarianization) and when they are denied the satisfaction of conceptualizing their nursing tasks but are instead directed to execute their tasks as prescribed by management (technical proletarianization)'

(Storch and Stinson, 1988; p. 37)

Deprofessionalisation as *erosion of professional knowledge and trust* is an extension of the consequences of the two former categories. As tasks are fragmented and controlled by others the whole notion of a coherent, professional, public service ethos becomes dissipated and de-mystified. In terms of meeting client need in non-hierarchical ways this may indeed represent a beneficial and humanising process rather than the reverse, but only if occupational disintegration can be prevented. Otherwise, nursing as a *human* service agency will be denied its own coherent value system, nursing tasks will merely exist as isolated interventions in a vacuum created by the principles of scientific management.

Keyzer's chapter on the conflicts arising from implementing the nursing process (White, 1988) represents an intriguing analysis of the structural constraints on implementing change. Just as McIntosh observes in the case of district nursing, so the official rhetoric of policy objectives appeared to support overtly a change in nursing practice. The reality was somewhat different. The power of entrenched interest groups was so great that, whether deliberately or by default, the *real* process of changing nursing practice was continually obstructed. For, as Keyzer explains in detail, the introduction of the nursing process implies a revolution in power structures and attitudes to practice:

'A true patient-centred model for nursing practice, which imbues the client with the power over decision-making, would be a direct challenge to the tightly controlled boundaries . . . between the roles of the doctor, the nurse and the woman in her own home . . . It is unlikely that such a model for practice would be welcomed by those whose power it seeks to remove.'

(White, 1988; p. 105)

Keyzer sees nursing's structural relationship with medicine as the key obstacle to reform in clinical nursing practice. All other structural constraints are seen as secondary to this: the emphasis on nurses as managers rather than autonomous clinical practitioners; and the denial of adequate continuing education in order to assume that clinical role merely serve to confirm the status quo.

Each of the five chapters discussed in this section has illustrated the constraining power of existing structures in society against which nurses have to struggle if they are serious about effecting change. All of them, at their root, express concerns about nurses' powerlessness to help their clients *effectively* because of these constraints. It is at once both depressing and exciting to realise just how many nurses are beginning to identify the relatively obscure sources of power in society. (But then, if you have the power there isn't any need to publicise the fact.) It is depressing because challenging the status quo is extraordinarily difficult. Those in existing positions of authority can isolate, ignore, ridicule and make those challenging them feel guilty and unworthy. It is not surprising that many nurses give up in the attempt. It is also exciting because the published evidence now demonstrates that nurses are coming politically of age. What is needed now is the will to take the issues forward.

Class, gender and race in nursing

In the earlier version of this paper I commented that it was disappointing that relatively little empirical evidence on class and gender emerged from the first two volumes on *Political issues in nursing*. Once again it is encouraging to note that White's more recent volume re-dresses the balance. In addition to the two exceptions in White (1986) – Hardy in *Career politics: the case of career histories of selected leading female and male nurses in England and Scotland*, and Simnett in *The pursuit of respectability: women and the nursing profession, 1860–1900*, Orr and Thompson in White (1988) address respectively women as receivers of care and nursing in South Africa.

Hardy documents the great dissimilarities between the career histories of thirty six females and thirteen male nursing leaders. The women in the group were older, and came from middle class backgrounds, while the men were younger and had working class origins. Most of the women, unlike their brothers, and despite their social advantage and scholastic ability had not been encouraged to think seriously about a career. Nursing embodied the notion of 'worthwhile work' but even so most of the women, like the men, entered nursing by accident.

Once in nursing striking differences emerged. The women made more horizontal career moves between different specialisms whereas the men demonstrated an orderly swift move up the vertical nursing hierarchy. The women therefore took much longer to reach senior positions. This pattern appeared to stem partly from different career aspirations – the men had longer-term ambitions – and partly from irrational expectations within nursing. The women felt that gaining other certificates was expected, and every change of direction brought a return to the bottom of the career ladder. Hence they achieved an average of five qualifications, compared with 3.5 for the men who were more concerned anyway with higher educational achievements than with nursing certificates. (This observation was not supported in a recent national survey of Chief Nurses at District Health Authority level, Robinson *et al.*, 1989, where the female nurses had more general education.)

Hardy found that the availability of mentors was an important factor in helping both men and women to break out of traditional career patterns. Even so the men experienced more help of this kind and earlier in their careers. She concludes that the domination of top posts in nursing by men arises from the complex and different socialisation process which men and women experience. It is partly the product of self image, with women expecting to serve others, not themselves, and partly the effect of direct influence by others. Both aspects intermesh and illustrate how gender, even in a predominantly female profession, can still substantially determine who enters its dominant interest groups.

Simnett, using a relatively rare historical perspective, examines the social origins of women entering nursing in Billericay Poor Law Union Workhouse, and St. Bartholomew's Hospital between 1860–1900. She concludes that despite the apparent differences in these institutions' ability to recruit in the first place, nursing during the early part of the period was not a solidly middle class occupation even in the London hospital. The middle class women who did enter St. Bartholomew's appear often to have been driven by the economic necessity of family circumstances into making provision for themselves.

Nevertheless, the status of nursing as an occupation was raised, albeit relatively, in both institutions during the period studied. The policy of the Local Government Board eventually forced the Boards of Guardians to employ trained nurses as supervisors, whilst the propaganda effects of the 'lady' probationer image led to improved recruitment and attempts to improve standards in the London teaching hospital. The situation in the workhouse was nevertheless, by contrast, bleak. Most of the nursing care during the early part of the period was carried out by the able-bodied paupers themselves.

Both of these accounts are interesting vignettes of the impact of class and gender on nursing in different contexts and at different times. Gender works two ways in nursing. It is usually women who *deliver* care but women are also frequently the *recipients* of care and discrimination can work so that both categories are divided against each other (Robinson, 1989). In a chapter which takes a sophisticated view of the mediation of power in health care Orr, writing on *Women's health: a nursing perspective*, describes four main themes. First, the medicalisation of life experiences from birth to death ensures that neither women as patients nor as nurses find it possible to challenge doctors' claims to intervention. By defining situations as pathological any other interpretation is ruled out. Hence women's mental health problems get treated with tranquillisers and their social origins become relegated as unimportant. Thus the power of governments, drug companies and doctors goes unchallenged.

Second, the increased use of technology alienates people from their bodies and conveys a sense of mystery and power to those in control of the machines. Hence the progressive medicalisation of child bearing has resulted in pregnancy and birth being treated as disease processes instead of altered states of health. Women's knowledge and experience of their bodies is discounted.

Third, the division in health care labour reflects the sexual division of labour in all other areas of life. Thus doctors are male and identified with high status 'scientific' knowledge, nurses are female and concerned with 'caring' which is considered low status, women's work.

Finally feminists, at least, see that the existing ways in which health care is provided perpetuates the structure of power in society and acts as a powerful mechanism of social control. Nurses as doctors' handmaidens are often seen in this context as oppressors rather than supporters of other women. (In this sense Orr's chapter could have been included in the final section.)

All of the issues described in this section illustrate Lukes' third face of power. The socialisation of women into 'knowing their place' is achieved through the sheer weight of institutions – family, education, nursing careers, the prevailing definition of 'Science' – shaping their expectations and leading them to adopt certain attitudes and roles. Orr does see a way out of the impasse through her experience of the women's health movement. But this involves an enormous shift in attitudes and challenge to the status quo. If nurses are to play a key role in influencing health care policies for women they will need first to become aware of the structures which oppress *all* women. Only then can they work *with* women as equal partners, helping them to define their problems and solutions for themselves. In doing this it is inevitable that nurses will find themselves challenging existing value systems, something which does not come easily to a group for whom the unequal experience of power is so deeply entrenched.

The final part of this section touches on the structural issue of race, although Thompson's *The development of nursing in South Africa* (White, 1988) refers only obliquely to the subject. Race, in general, remains a sadly neglected area in the study of the politics of nursing. One concludes that Thompson's chapter was written with the constraints of the South African political regime very much in mind, for although it contains a wealth of statistical information on demography and the labour force participation in nursing by different racial groups, the reader is left very much to draw her or his own conclusions as to the practical effects. Hence we are told that with a population in which 72.2 per cent is black, just 0.23 per cent of that population received a university or college education in 1985.

The black population has a high birth rate and high mortality rates at all ages resulting in a population pyramid characteristic of an underdeveloped country. The white population pyramid, by contrast, resembles the developed world with a low birth rate and a large proportion of elderly people. Yet Thompson shows that in 1985 the blacks had a ratio of 1 qualified nurse to 721 total black population compared to 1:157 for whites. Commenting on the World Health Organisation's recommendation that 1 registered nurse to 500 of population is required to deliver a basic comprehensive health service in a Third World Country, Thompson claims that the number of black nurses admitted to the profession would need almost to double in order to achieve this ratio by the year 2000. Economic factors make this an enormous task. There are shortages of teaching posts *and* shortages of teaching staff. Yet the blacks experience patterns of disease which are most amenable to basic primary and secondary health care – infective and nutritional diseases predominate.

Compared with accounts of nurse education elsewhere, South Africa appears historically to have been remarkably progressive in some areas. South Africa was the first country in the world to achieve state registration for nurses and midwives in 1891 and university diploma courses for nurse tutors began in 1937. The first Chair of Nursing was established in 1967 although a degree programme had been established in 1956. Nevertheless Thompson is clear that progress has been limited to very small numbers and that much remains to be done. Not least, one concludes, for the black nurses who must experience multiple forms of discrimination through race, gender and class and yet are so desperately needed. The experience of apartheid leads us to conclude that meeting the nursing needs of the different populations within that country remains as two separate and unequal agendas for action.

Nurses as oppressors or enablers: power for or against the client?

Discussion until now has concentrated upon the diverse ways in which nursing issues may be affected by policy and politics. By extension, it is claimed that the concerns of the patient, client or consumer become sucked into the consequences of the power to define certain issues in certain ways. Only Orr, of the authors considered so far, has openly claimed that nurses are ever anything but on the same side as the patient. Several other chapters contain the suggestion that nurses in pursuing certain policy objectives may indeed work against the interests of their clients. On the whole, however, nurses are portrayed as 'on the side of the angels'. Only Hawker in *Gatekeeping: a traditional and contemporary function of the nurse* (White, 1985) has the temerity to make this dark aspect of nursing policy the central focus of her enquiry. She does so by describing a historical role for nurses – that of keeping patients' visitors at bay. Admittedly it may be argued that nurses merely carried out the rules. Yet Hawker shows that over a period of years many policy initiatives designed to open access for the families of patients have been successfully obstructed by nurses and by doctors. (See Chapter 8.)

Some nurses, it seems, while becoming more aware of their own powerlessness in the policy arena, have additionally begun to systematically evaluate the even greater powerlessness of their clients, and their own potential contribution to this situation. The World Health Organisation's current initiatives in seeking Health for All by year 2000 emphasise not only the crucial role that nurses can play, but also stress that success will be dependent upon enabling customers actively to control the factors which contribute to their health. It is encouraging that many of the authors reviewed in these collections have begun to analyse the powerlessness of patients from a variety of perspectives. Nevertheless it is essential that in raising their own awareness nurses remain conscious of their considerable power to act against the best interest of their clients. Future analyses of nursing policy and politics must keep the relationship of nurses' to consumers' power firmly on the agenda.

Conclusion

The contents of the second part of this chapter reveal a heightened awareness amongst nurses (and other authors) of the relevance of understanding the nature of politics and power to the practice of nursing. They also demonstrate how elusive in general terms these concepts can sometimes prove to be and that teasing them out of a mass of empirical data is no easy matter. Five provisional categories have been suggested within which most of the subject matter reviewed could be subsumed: problems of unity in nursing and nursing as a force for challenge and change; the potential and the risks for nurses and clients of contemporary health policy initiatives; the structure of nursing – its constraints and its potential for development; class, gender and race in nursing; and nurses as oppressors or enablers, power for or against the client. What this analysis has begun to show is how different systems of value and belief can impinge in different ways upon a range of health policy issues which have important bearings on nursing practice. As a result different groups of nurses and clients frequently find themselves subjected to conflicting pressures. Unpacking the various dimensions of any one situation requires first and foremost a crucial awareness of the social, political and economic culture within which particular health policy initiatives take place. There is then a need to see whether any common themes can be traced across the diverse subject areas and cultures in order to identify where general principles pertaining to power and politics can be applied to nursing.

What then, if any, are the general lessons that we can learn from this exercise? First, on the basis of the evidence reviewed it appears that nursing is virtually never ever primary in policy terms. This reinforces the messages from the first part of the chapter regarding the hidden face of power; the power to keep issues *off* the policy agenda; or the power to ensure that issues are defined only in certain ways. It appears that policy in relation to nursing almost invariably develops second-hand as a consequence of other actors' responses to health and welfare initiatives which, in turn, are developed elsewhere. Second, in the process of trying to adapt to various initiatives, nursing becomes sub-divided as certain sub-groups seek to gain the maximum advantage from policy change. Nursing is almost always therefore an example of a divided issue only parts of which succeed in obtaining a place on the public, policy agenda. Claims for reform in the delivery of nursing care; for developing methods of providing a more cost-effective service; for paying attention to people's *real* health needs (as opposed to medically defined areas) almost invariably fall on deaf ears. Why should this be? Presumably because suggesting to those who currently hold the power to determine the nature of health care and the way that it is provided that there could be a better, cheaper, or more effective way of delivering a service is to admit to the real power of a challenge to the status quo. As nurses struggle to gain a hearing for their claims there are a great many losers who may, or may not, be aware of their experience of oppression. The effects of class, race and gender on this unequal state of affairs has been touched upon but, as yet, these are imperfectly explored in relation to nursing. That nurses are not agreed on a way to move forward is exemplified by the different positons adopted by Clay, Salvage and White, all key authors on the subject of nursing and politics.

Understanding this oppressive state of affairs could nevertheless be a liberating experience for nurses. If gaining an advantage invariably means the exploitation of someone else in the system then nurses everywhere could begin to see that their real power lies in solidarity with their weaker members and, above all, with their client groups. Nurses have to ask 'if I gain a benefit, who stands to lose and am I content with that state of affairs'? If the answer is 'No' then they have to decide what they are prepared to do about the situation.

In this review of the available evidence an attempt has been made to push the debate along; to begin to identify the issues which could be used in order to develop some broader generalisations. It is one small step in what must be an enormous and continuing task.

End notes

1. I am indebted to Culyer (1983) for his discussion of the development of the study of Health Indicators and, in particular, for clarification of concepts such as 'area, topic of study' and 'mode of thinking'.

2. Other authors who have produced categorisations within health policy and management research include Hunter (1986) and Pettigrew *et al.* (1987).

3. White's idea of pluralism is open to debate. The system she describes as pluralistic could more acurately be termed elitist for it consists of: nurse managers who identify with the values of a dominant, managerial class; a challenging but small minority intelligentsia; and a repressed proletariat. Pluralism in political theory describes a concept which embodies inbuilt societal checks and balances (usually through a democratic voting system) which then ensure a consensus where the majority view prevails. Clearly this rarely happens in nursing (and, according to Lukes' thesis, doesn't occur in reality anywhere else).

4. Melosh differs from the Kalischs' analysis of the effects of cost-containment on RNs. She claims that it was Licensed Practical Nurses (LPNs) who lost their jobs, leaving RNs as a greater proportion of the labour force.

5. Carpenter first described the proletarianisation of nurses at the same time as the 1974 reorganisation of the NHS, with its emphasis on managerial values (Carpenter, 1977). In a more recent study he finds that however militant they may have been in 1972 by 1984/5 a new realism had taken its toll. Their attitudes to unions and professional associations had become less to do with their perceived potential for collective action than with their role of protection and indemnity against the risk of making mistakes (Carpenter, *et al.*, 1987).

References

Alford, R. R. (1975). *Health Care Politics: Ideological and Interest Group Barriers to Reform*. University of Chicago Press, Chicago.
Bachrach, P. and Baratz, M. S. (1962). The two faces of power. *American Political Science Review*, **56**, 947–52.
Braverman, H.(1974). *Labor and Monopoly Capital: the Degradation of Work in the Twentieth Century*. Monthly Review, New York.

Campbell, M. L. (1988). Accounting for care: a framework for analysing change in Canadian nursing. In *Political Issues in Nursing: Past, Present and Future. Volume three*, R. White (Ed.), pp. 45–70. Wiley, Chichester.

Carpenter, M. (1977). The new managerialism and professionalism in nursing. In *Health and the Division of Labour*, M. Stacey, M. Reid, C. Heath and R. Dingwall (Eds), pp. 165–93. Croom Helm, London.

Carpenter, M., Elkan, R., Leonard, P. and Munro, A. (1987). *Professionalism and Unionism in Nursing and Social Work*. Department of Applied Social Studies, University of Warwick, Coventry.

Clay, T. (1987). *Nurses: Power and Politics*. Heinemann, London.

Cousins, C. (1987). *Controlling Social Welfare: a Sociology of State Welfare and Work Organisations*. Wheatsheaf, Brighton.

Crenson, M. A. (1971). *The Unpolitics of Air Pollution*. Johns Hopkins, Baltimore.

Culyer, A. J. (1983). *Health Indicators*. Martin Robertson, Oxford.

Davies, C. (Ed.) (1980a). *Rewriting Nursing History*. Croom Helm, London.

Davies, C. (1980b). A constant casualty: nurse education in Britain and the USA to 1939. In *Rewriting Nursing History*, C. Davies (Ed.), pp. 102–22. Croom Helm, London.

Deakin, N. (1987). *The Politics of Welfare*. Methuen, London.

Department of Health (1989a). *Working for Patients: the Health Service: Caring for the 1990s*. HMSO, London (Cmnd 555).

Department of Health (1989b). *Caring for People: Community Care in the Next Decade and Beyond*. HMSO, London (Cmnd 849).

Department of Health and Social Security, Scottish Home and Health Department and the Welsh Office (1969). *Report of the Working Party on Management Structures in the Local Authority Nursing Services*. DHSS, London.(Chairman E. Mayston.)

Department of Health and Social Security, Research Working Group (1980). *Inequalities in Health: Report*. DHSS, London. (Chairman D. Black.)

Dingwall, R. and McIntosh, J. (Eds) (1978). *Readings in the Sociology of Nursing*. Churchill Livingstone, Edinburgh.

Dunn, A. (1985). Foreword. In *The Politics of Nursing*, J. Salvage, pp. vii–viii. Heinemann, London.

Fondiller, S. H. (1986). The American Nurses' Association and National League for Nursing: political relationships and realities. In *Political issues in Nursing: Past, Present and Future. Volume two*, R. White (Ed.), pp. 119–43. Wiley, Chichester.

Gray, A. (1984). European health care costs. *Social Policy and Administration*, **18(3)**, 213–28.

Green, D. G. (1987). *The New Right: the Counter Revolution in Political, Economic and Social Thought.* Wheatsheaf, Brighton.

Ham, C. and Hill, M. (1986). *The Policy Process in the Modern Capitalist State.* Wheatsheaf, Brighton.

Hardy, L. K. (1986). Career politics: the case of career histories of selected leading female and male nurses in England and Scotland. In *Political Issues in Nursing: Past, Present and Future. Volume two*, R. White (Ed.) pp. 69–82. Wiley, Chichester.

Hawker, R. J. (1985). Gatekeeping: a traditional and contemporary function of the nurse. In *Political Issues in Nursing: Past, Present and Future, Volume one*, R. White (Ed.), pp. 1–17. Wiley, Chichester.

Hennessy, D. A. (1986). The restrictive and wanting policies affecting health visitors' work in the field of emotional health. In *Political Issues in Nursing: Past, Present and Future, Volume two.* R. White (Ed.) pp. 83–100. Wiley, Chichester.

Hunter, D. J. (1986). *Managing the National Health Service in Scotland: Review and Assessment of Research Methods.* Scottish Home and Health Department, Edinburgh. (Scottish Health Service Studies No. 45).

Jolley, M. and Allan, P. (Eds) (1989). *Current Issues in Nursing.* Chapman & Hall, London.

Kalisch, B. and Kalisch, P. (1985). Nurses on strike: labour-management conflict in US hospitals and the role of the press. In *Political Issues in Nursing: Past, Present and Future. Volume one*, R. White (Ed.), pp. 105–51. Wiley, Chichester.

Keyzer, D. M. (1988). Challenging role boundaries: conceptual frameworks for understanding the conflict arising from the implementation of the nursing process in practice. In *Political Issues in Nursing: Past, Present and Future. Volume three*, R. White (Ed.), pp. 95–119. Wiley, Chichester.

Klein, R. (1983). *The Politics of the National Health Service.* Longman, London.

Klein, R. (1989). *The Politics of the National Health Service*, 2nd edition. Longman, Harlow.

Larsen, J. (1988). Being powerful: from talk into action. In *Political Issues in Nursing: Past, Present and Future, Volume three*, R. White (Ed.), pp. 1–13. Wiley, Chichester.

Lukes, S. (1986). *Power: a Radical View.* Macmillan, London.

McGuire, J. M. (1988). Dependency matters: an issue in the care of elderly people. In *Political Issues in Nursing: Past, Present and Future. Volume three*, R. White (Ed.), pp. 71–94. Wiley, Chichester.

McIntosh, J. B. (1985). District nursing: a case of political marginality. In *Political Issues in Nursing: Past, Present and Future.*

Volume one, R. White (Ed.), pp. 45–66. Wiley, Chichester.

Melosh, B. (1986). Nursing and Reaganomics: cost containment in the United States. In *Political Issues in Nursing: Past, Present and Future. Volume two*, R. White (Ed.), pp. 145–70. Wiley, Chichester.

Milio, N. B. (1985). Nursing within the ecology of public policy: a case in point. In *Political Issues in Nursing: Past, Present and Future. Volume one*, R. White (Ed.), pp. 87–104. Wiley, Chichester.

Millett, K. (1977). *Sexual Politics*. Virago, London.

NHS Management Inquiry Team (1983). *NHS Management Inquiry*. The Team, London. (Team leader E. R. Griffiths.)

Nursing Times and Nursing Mirror (1989). Regional CNO resigns. *Nursing Times and Nursing Mirror*, **85(45)**, 5.

Orr, J. (1988). Women's health; a nursing perspective. In *Political Issues in Nursing: Past, Present and Future. Volume three*, R. White (Ed.), pp. 121–37. Wiley, Chichester.

Parkes, M. E. (1986). Through politics to professionalism. In *Political Issues in Nursing: Past, Present and Future. Volume two*, R. White (Ed.), pp. 101–18. Wiley, Chichester.

Pettigrew, A., McKee, L. and Ferlie, E. (1987). *Understanding Change in the NHS: a Review and Research Agenda*. Centre for Corporate Strategy and Change, University of Warwick, Coventry.

Pollitt, C., Lewis, L., Negro, J. and Patten, J. (Eds) (1979). *Public Policy in Theory and Practice*. Hodder & Stoughton, London.

Rein, M. (1976). *Social Science and Public Policy*. Penguin, Harmondsworth.

Robinson, J. (1985). Health visiting and health. In *Political issues in Nursing: Past, Present and Future. Volume one*, R. White (Ed.), pp. 67–86. Wiley, Chichester.

Robinson, J. (1989). Nursing in the future: a cause for concern. In *Current Issues in Nursing*, M. Jolley and P. Allan (Eds), pp. 151–78. Chapman & Hall, London.

Robinson, J. and Strong, P. (1987). *Professional Nursing Advice After Griffiths: an Interim Report*. Nursing Policy Studies Centre, University of Warwick, Coventry. (Nursing Policy Studies 1.)

Robinson, J., Strong, P. and Elkan, R. (1989). *Griffiths and the Nurses: a National Survey of CNAs*. Nursing Policy Studies Centre, University of Warwick, Coventry. (Nursing Policy Studies 4.)

Salvage, J. (1985). *The Politics of Nursing*. Heinemann, London.

Simnett, A. (1986). The pursuit of respectability: women and the nursing profession, 1860–1900. In *Political Issues in Nursing: Past, Present and Future. Volume two*, R. White (Ed.), pp. 1–23, Wiley, Chichester.

Skevington, S. (Ed.) (1984). *Understanding Nurses: the Social Psychology of Nursing*. Wiley, Chichester.

Stacey, M. (1976). *Concepts of Health and Illness: a Working Paper on the Concepts and Their Relevance for Research.* Department of Sociology, Unversity of Warwick, Coventry. (Paper produced for the Health and Health Policy Panel of the SSRC.)

Storch, J. L. and Stinson, S. M. (1988). Concepts of deprofessionalisation with applications to nursing. In *Political Issues in Nursing: Past, Present and Future. Volume three*, R. White (Ed.), pp. 33–44. Wiley, Chichester.

Strong, P. and Robinson, J. (1988). *New Model Management: Griffiths and the NHS.* Nursing Policy Studies Centre, University of Warwick, Coventry. (Nursing Policy Studies 3.)

Strong, P. and Robinson, J. (1990). *The NHS under new management.* Open University Press, Milton Keynes.

Thompson, R. (1988). The development of nursing in South Africa. In *Political Issues in Nursing: Past, Present and Future. Volume three*, R. White (Ed.), pp. 163–202. Wiley, Chichester.

Tonkin, E. and Hart, E. (1989). *I Love My Work, I Hate My Job: a Study of Hospital Domestics.* Department of Sociology, University of Birmingham, Birmingham. (Report prepared for the ESRC.)

White, R. (Ed.) (1985). *Political Issues in Nursing: Past, Present and Future. Volume one.* Wiley, Chichester.

White, R. (Ed.) (1986). *Political Issues in Nursing: Past, Present and Future. Volume two.* Wiley, Chichester.

White, R. (1986). From matron to manager: the political construction of reality. In *Political Issues in Nursing: Past, Present and Future. Volume two*, R. White (Ed.), pp. 45–68. Wiley, Chichester.

White, R. (Ed.) (1988). *Political Issues in Nursing: Past, Present and Future. Volume three.* Wiley, Chichester.

Whitehead, M. (1987). *The Health Divide.* Health Education Council, London.

Zwanger, L. (1986). Jewish nursing education in Palestine 1918–1948. In *Political Issues in Nursing: Past, Present and Future. Volume two*, R. White (Ed.), pp. 25–44. Wiley, Chichester.

10 Nursing knowledge – ultimate objectives

Definitions of knowledge and nursing

Knowledge is defined in several ways including 'the range of information, perception or understanding enjoyed by an individual or group' and 'the fact or condition of knowing something through experience or association' (Longman, 1984). These two definitions seem particularly pertinent to nursing as together they embrace the concepts of 'a group having knowledge', that knowledge can be developed 'through experience' and thirdly that having knowledge can be 'enjoyable'! Nursing is more difficult to define especially if one turns to nursing textbooks where complex explanations of nursing include:

'Nursing is a process of human interactions between nurse and client whereby each perceives the other and the situation and through communication, they set goals, explore means, and agree on means to achieve goals'.

(King, 1981; p. 144)

'Nursing is a science and the application of knowledge from that science to the practice of nursing'.

(Andrews and Roy, 1986; p. 8)

'Nursing as a learned profession is both a science and an art. A science may be defined as an organized body of abstract knowledge arrived at by scientific research and logical analysis. The art of nursing is the imaginative and creative use of this knowledge in human service'.

(Rogers, 1980)

At first glance all three of the above explanations may seem wordy and irrelevant to the practising nurse who is inclined to see nurse theorist's work as 'out of touch' with the clinical nurse's role (Miller, 1985b). Yet on close examination all the definitions have useful concepts to offer, namely that nursing involves individual perception and communication between nurse and client (King, 1981), the application of knowledge in practice (Andrews and Roy, 1986) and the imaginative use of knowledge to assist others (Rogers, 1983). Different concepts of nursing are present in Henderson's (1960) definition which states:

'Nursing is primarily assisting the individual (sick or well) in the performance of those activities contributing to health, or its recovery that he would perform unaided if he had the necessary strength, will or knowledge. It is likewise the unique contribution of nursing to help the individual to be independent as soon as possible.'

The main advantage of Henderson's (1960) definition above the others referred to is that it is easily understandable. This quality, together with the fact that the role of the nurse and the aim of nursing (i.e. helping people gain independence) are clearly identified, is presumably the reason for its adoption by the International Council of Nursing. It is interesting to note, however, that the universally accepted definition does not allude to the need for nurses to have a sound knowledge base from which to plan imaginative individualised nursing care.

Knowledge for practice?

It could be argued that it is irrelevant whether or not 'knowledge' is referred to in the International Council of Nurses' definition of nursing, yet the inclusion does seem important to many nurses – especially to nurse theorists and the argument for its inclusion is not just an academic one. The United Kingdom Central Council for Nursing, Midwifery and Health Visiting (UKCC) code of conduct (1984) states that nurses should 'act always in such a way as to promote and safeguard the wellbeing and interests of patients and clients' while Rule 18 of the Nurses Midwives and Health Visitors Act (Statutory Instrument, 1983) places a responsibility on first level nurses to assess, plan, implement and evaluate care. McFarlane (1977) believes that it is impossible for nurses to make decisions regarding the prescription of nursing care and ways of safeguarding patients without having a sound understanding of theory on which to base those decisions.

While there is clearly evidence to suggest that nurses require knowledge for practice, the question must be asked 'what knowledge do they require?' and 'what characteristics do nurses need to select and apply relevant knowledge?'.

The knowledgeable practitioner

The aim of Project 2000, the document which outlines a framework for nursing education in the United Kingdom over the next twenty years, suggests that tomorrow's first level nurses need to be knowledgeable doers. The effective 'knowledgeable doer' will presumably be a reflective decision maker who uses relevant theory to underpin practice. Such nurses will require a clear understanding of nursing, health, people and the effects of society, the environment and the politics of health care from which to problem solve. In order to practise effectively, nurses in the future will need to have an understanding of theory from the social sciences, including sociology, psychology and biology, in addition to specific nursing knowledge (UKCC, 1986). There is an implication that the use of knowledge from these sciences is new; in fact nurse theorists have developed conceptual frameworks for practice over the last century which have incorporated similar knowledge. Several nurse academics suggest that it is necessary to be explicit about the nature of man, nursing, health and society in order to depict nursing as an entity (Stevens, 1984).

Nightingale (1859) reported the importance of clean air, rest, quiet and good food for patients while more recently nurse theorists have described the need to encourage patient independence (Orem, 1985; Henderson, 1960) and to extend patients' coping abilities through teaching, counselling (Peplau, 1952) or altering those stimuli which are known to contribute to disability (Roy, 1984). Most clinical nurses incorporate knowledge, related to the concepts described by these theorists, into practice.

For example, a nurse on a medical ward will ensure that a patient who has just been diagnosed as suffering from diabetes understands the nature of diabetes, the need for an appropriate diet and regular mealtimes, the effects of prolonged exercise, the signs of hypo and hyperglycaemia, the actions to take in the event of hypo/hyperglycaemia commencing and, if necessary, how to self administer insulin prior to discharge. Such a nurse will apply knowledge concerning teaching, counselling, diabetes, the pancreas, diet and the nature of anxiety, in order to help the patient extend their own ability to cope with the actual and potential problems of diabetes. When planning the best way of intervening for this kind of patient, the nurse will also consider their social conditions, financial position and family support. If relevant the nurse will then assist the patient in applying for financial help, or in teaching other family members about the disease. Many nurses reading this paragraph may feel that what is written is just common sense. That is precisely where nurses have denigrated their own knowledge in the past, frequently implying that nursing is 'common sense' rather than recognising it as a complex human task which involves the application of theory in practice (Stevens, 1984; Benner, 1984).

Present practice – knowledge and ritual?

Accepting the hypothesis that nurses do underpin much of their practice with knowledge – do they, as has been reported, also resort to ritual (Menzies, 1960; Chapman, 1983)? There is little doubt that nursing is a stressful occupation where relatively young people come into contact with the horrifying realities of disease, disability and death. Psychological theory suggests that humans try to avoid stress by utilising defence mechanisms to protect themselves from reality (Hilgard *et al.*, 1975). It is hardly surprising, therefore, that Menzies (1960) reports nurses using rituals to distance themselves from the reality of human suffering. A more recent work hypothesises that some of the rituals Menzies described as a defence against anxiety are, in fact, concerned with conveying social meaning (Chapman, 1983). Chapman (1983) cites Max Weber who described four types of actions – traditional, those determined by habit; 'Zweckrational', purposely rational actions which involve assessing the probable results of a given act based on empirical evidence; 'Vertrational actions' where the means and ends of an action are based on a systematic set of ideas and beliefs which are not empirically proven; and fourthly, 'affective actions' which are carried out under emotive impulses. The fourth named action roughly equates with Menzies observations but the other three involve different interpretations of ritual. Taking temperatures may be a 'Zweckrational' action when the result will influence care, but to some extent it becomes a non-rational ritual or traditional action when the patient is well. Alternatively it may be that taking a temperature at this time is perceived by the nurse as a reassuring measure to the patient (a Vertrational action).

Both authors infer that ritual actions in nursing inhibit the delivery of psychosocial patient care yet any solution to enhance practice will clearly be dependent on which interpretation of the defined problem, sociological (Chapman, 1983) or psychoanalytic (Menzies, 1960), is accepted.

At least two interpretations of ritual actions in nursing can be made and it is probable that they both contain truth, yet neither can be proven in the empirical scientific sense. This is because social science theory is developmentally in infancy (Jacox, 1974). Chapman (1976) suggests that this is doubly so for nursing which is such a new discipline in the academic sense.

It is only by accepting a level of uncertainty in nursing knowledge and relevant theory from the social sciences that nursing is likely to develop and grow. The clinical nurse can be respected for her cynicism of nursing theory if her desire is to have concrete prescriptive theory from which to practice. In the absence of being told what is right and therefore how to act by nurse theorists, clinical nurses must have the ability to be reflective decision makers who are prepared to choose the 'best option' when delivering care rather than the 'correct one.' The 'best option' today, may well not be the best tomorrow. For example in the early seventies, I, along with many other nurses used egg white and oxygen to treat superficial pressure sores. This action worked and I asked a senior sister how this happened. She gave me a complex description which involved oxygenation of the tissues combined with the protein in albumin. I remained convinced of this action for some years until reading Norton *et al.*'s (1962) work on pressure sores. It was difficult to change my practice in the light of this new (to me) knowledge because I had adopted a set of actions to prevent and treat pressure sores into my repertoire, based, it seems now, on ritual rather than theory! Imagine then, the horror at subsequently finding a patient, who did not score highly enough on the Norton scale to warrant preventative care, developing a sore. It took some time for me to 'problem solve' how this had happened. The patient was on steroids and no calculation was made for this on the Norton scale, yet the patient's skin was papery thin. The penny dropped and I now consider steroids when using the tool; however, the point of revealing my inadequacies is to note:

(*i*)   That steroids were not commonly given to elderly people when Norton undertook her work, and the pressure area assessment tool was valid and reliable when produced.

(*ii*) Advances in medical care and the use of steroids reduced the reliability of a nursing instrument.

(*iii*) I ignored the evidence of papery skin and just used the scale.

(*iv*) Nurses need to continually update their knowledge, to adapt patient assessment prescriptions for care as necessary.

(*v*)   I had begun to use Norton's scale in a ritualistic manner rather than in a thoughtful proactive manner.

Clearly tomorrow's individual accountable practitioner needs to constantly evaluate practice, read research, judge the relevance of research and instigate useful findings into practice if the decisions they make about care are to be based on a sound level of theory (McFarlane, 1977) and reduce unnecessary ritual. If nurses have the common objective of enhancing client care through the application of knowledge as suggested in the code of conduct (UKCC, 1984) it is necessary to have formal methods of evaluating the efficiency and effectiveness of nursing care.

Evaluating nursing care

Bailey and Clause (1975) believe that if evaluation of nursing is to be effective it should be conducted in accordance with accepted and proven principles. The American Nurses' Association (ANA, 1977) has developed a mode of quality assurance which is widely used and proven in practice. It is cyclical in nature, demonstrating that the quality assurance process involves not only identifying standards and evaluating care given but also striving to enhance nursing care by changing standards as necessary (see Fig. 10.1).

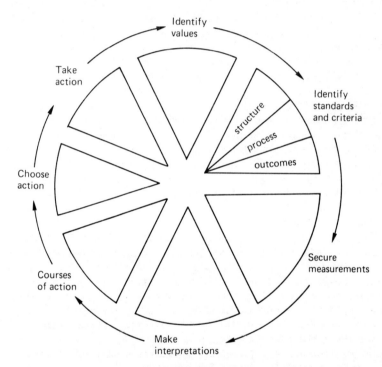

Fig. 10.1   American Nurses' Association Quality Assurance Cycle (American Nurses' Association, 1977).

Standard setting

The first step in the development of standards involves value clarification (ANA, 1975) and defining nursing (Van Maanen, 1984; Wright, 1984). At this stage the use of a nursing model may help nurses to define their values and beliefs about nursing (Wright,

1984). The purposes and values of nursing will vary according to the practice setting of care delivery and the selection or development of an appropriate model will be dependent on these factors. For example, psychiatric nurses involved in caring for clients suffering from clinical depression may value the concept of 'nursing being an interpersonal process through which clients develop and grow' (Peplau, 1952). While nurses involved with clients who have a mental handicap may wish to adopt the values of Orem (1985) whose model emphasises the need to motivate and educate people to their maximum ability to self care. Well recognised models are sometimes considered restricted and for this reason Wright (1990) describes the development of a model specifically for care of elderly people while Watkins (1988) has adapted two models – the activities of living nursing model (Roper *et al.*, 1980) and a stress adaptation model (Zarit *et al.*, 1985) – to encompass care of elderly people who are primarily supported at home by carers. These latter models embrace the values of small nursing teams involved with care. Although this can be regarded as a strength because models developed in this way tend to be 'client group specific', they can also be less useful in terms of value clarification for nursing in a broader sense. Mega-models such as Roy's (1984) stress adaptation and Roper's *et al.* (1980) 'activities of living' models have been shown to be applicable in many nursing settings and may therefore be more useful in terms of value clarification where quality assurance standards are to be agreed across several types of nursing within one hospital or community care setting.

Having identified professional nursing values the second stage of value clarification commences. This is a complex procedure because nurses must attempt to arrive at a consensus between the values of the nursing profession, the public, government, general managers and other health care workers. Lang and Clinton (1984) acknowledge that this can be especially difficult when cost containment of a service conflicts with professional values. A simple example of this would be when the nursing team of a surgical day patient unit values having time to communicate on a one-to-one basis with patients, which can be costly in nursing time, while management favours fast patient throughput and cost containment of the nursing budget. If nurses are to be able to debate these kind of issues with health care professionals and politicians, and present their case for consideration, it is vital that they apply knowledge from the study of ethics and relevant nursing research (DHSS, 1989).

Once a group of nurses completes the formidable task of defining values of care which are consistent with both their professional values and the constraints of their working environment, the remaining steps of the quality assurance cycle are relatively simple.

The next step is to develop 'standards' and 'criteria' with which to assess nursing (Wright, 1984). It is suggested that the terms can be used interchangeably but in fact a standard evolves from a criterion (Bloch, 1980). 'A criterion is the value-free name of a variable believed or known to be a relative indicator of the quality of patient care' (Bloch, 1977; p. 22). Thus a nurse may decide that one *criterion* for measuring nursing is 'the level of knowledge a patient has about the side effects of medication he takes'. With this criteria established, an acceptable standard can be set against which to indicate nursing performance. A standard can be defined as 'being the desired and achievable level (or range of performance) corresponding with a criterion, against which performance is compared' (Bloch, 1977; p. 22). The standard for the patient's knowledge about the side effects of his medication may be as high as 100 per cent or, if the nurse believes a range of 80–100 per cent is acceptable, then this can be indicated (Bloch, 1977; Wright, 1984). Crow (1981) noted that the term 'standards of care' is often used synonymously with effectiveness, although this is not necessarily true. A 'good standard' of terminal nursing care can be achieved yet the patient outcome will still be death. Thus measures which indicate a 'quality of life' standard for patients must be developed as well as more traditional 'outcome measures'.

Three types of standard will emerge; those of structure, process and outcome. Structural standards involve factors within the care system such as staffing, styles of supervision, organisational, environment, and physical resources (Block, 1977; Lang and Clinton, 1984). Process standards involve defining the activities expected of nurses when care-giving. This will include, amongst other processes, methods of assessment, planning, implementation and evaluation of care delivery. Outcome standards are concerned with changes in the patient's health status, feelings, knowledge and satisfaction; thus the standard referring to patient knowledge is an 'outcome standard'. Standards will, of necessity, vary to some extent between different nursing teams and if, as Hockey (1979) suggests, most evaluation takes place within the boundaries of one hospital or health care centre, standard setting may best be done at a local level. Several authors note the need for standard setting groups to consist of experts in their own clinical fields who have access to, and examine, relevant literature to ensure standards are based on the best available scientific knowledge (Wright, 1984; Crow, 1981).

Whenever possible nurses should incorporate research based knowledge into their standards; for example Hayward's (1975) research demonstrated the need for trained staff to have sufficient time to explain the nature of post-operative pain, pre-operatively, in order to reduce such pain. Thus the number of trained staff on a surgical ward (structural standard) needs to reflect such research (Bloch, 1980) and the process standards need to incorporate the action of pre-op preparation. Unfortunately, the extent of nursing knowledge available today is insufficient to ensure that all nursing standards can incorporate empirically developed theory in this way. However, in the long term, accurate quality assurance programmes may demonstrate new relationships between nursing processes and patient outcomes which, in turn, could provide theory on which to develop future standards (Henney, 1984).

The study of process-outcome

Bloch (1975) believes that it is possible to establish new nursing theory by observing the relationships between current nursing practice and patient outcomes and suggests that this is the most important evaluative work for nurses. As relationships between variables are found and acknowledged, grounded theory which has a clear base in practice should emerge. This kind of research could be very exciting in that it may reveal and explain some of the nursing practices which have evolved through experience without having been subjected to scientific scrutiny.

A recent work by Benner (1984) attempts to uncover the knowledge embedded in clinical nursing practice by systematic observation and interpretation not only by the researcher but also by clinical nurses themselves. To understand the study it is necessary to acknowledge that there are differences between practical and theoretical knowledge. She refers to the work of Kuhn (1970) and Polanyi (1958) who observe that 'knowing that' and 'knowing how' are two different kinds of knowledge; the former being the scientific or theoretical knowledge which is established by identifying the relationships between variables while 'knowing how' is practical knowledge which 'may elude such scientific formulations' (Benner, 1984; p. 2).

Benner (1984) uses the Drefus model of skill acquisition to explain the development of the clinical nursing expert. This model outlines five stages of performance, those of novice, advanced beginner, competent, proficient and expert practitioner. The novice must be given rules for behaviour to guide performance due to the fact that they have no experience, yet those very rules legitimate against success because the rules do not 'Tell them the most relevant task to perform in a given situation' (Benner, 1984; p. 20).

For example, a novice nurse may be taking a patient's temperature and fail to see that the patient's situation is rapidly changing, their skin becoming cold and clammy, pulse weak and thready and respirations low and shallow. Conversely, the expert nurse operates from a deep understanding of a total situation, taking a holistic view and presumably using a 'gestalt', makes an accurate assessment and intervenes; in this situation giving oxygen and alerting the cardiac team all within the space of seconds. Ways in which nurses move from being novices to experts are outlined by Benner (1984) although she is unable to explain in a prescriptive manner the step by step process by which 'knowing how' develops. She suggests that nurses acrue clinical knowledge and lose track of what they have learned although they recognise that their clinical judgement becomes more refined and acute 'over time'. It is probable that as individual clinical nurses observe that a certain action works in terms of patient outcome they begin to incorporate that action into their repertoire. In this way expertise is developed but not always adequately understood or explained. It is this lack of explanation which often makes 'knowing how' undervalued in comparison to the scientifically developed 'knowing that' knowledge.

One way of increasing the respectability of clinical nursing knowledge would be to study the relationships between acknowledged 'expertise' and patient outcome. If it could be demonstrated that the experienced expert nurse positively affects patient outcome through the use of skilled nursing imagine the power of the 'know how' theory. The fact that one could not fully interpret the 'know how' would be of secondary importance if the practical knowledge could be found to be cost-effective in terms of patient care. Indeed Benner (1984) cautions researchers to remember that some of the richness of 'know how' theory could be lost by trying to break it down into sub-sets of knowledge in a reductionist fashion and reminds us that nursing is essentially a rich humanistic practice which lends itself to synthesis rather than analysis. This interpretive approach relies on understanding the context of any situation in which particular actions occur. It is demonstrated that by such interpretation the concepts and principles underlying practical knowledge can frequently be extrapolated and that expertise which is based on experience can at least be partly explained. This work (Benner, 1984) suggests that some nursing actions may, as Chapman (1983) hypothesises, be 'vertriactional actions' based on systematic sets of ideas which are not yet empirically proven. Benner (1984) has shown that the 'know how' of clinical nursing can be partly explained. The next stage of research in this area needs to examine the relationships between 'know how' knowledge and patient outcome.

An experimental research design approach can also be used to identify differences in terms of patient outcome between two nursing structures or processes intended for similar patient care situations. It is, however, sometimes difficult from an ethical perspective to deny 'control groups' a specific nursing action which is currently accepted practice, in order to compare their outcomes with those of patients who receive the same action. Yet, when it is believed that a new type of nursing action may be better than current practice, there is rarely an ethical problem and an 'experimental' process-outcome design can be used. For example, the use of this method by Miller (1985a) demonstrated experimentally that individualised nursing care was more effective in terms of preventing nurse induced patient dependence in elderly people than was task allocation. Similar approaches have been used in several studies where single variables could be controlled although results cannot necessarily be explained in an empirical fashion because of the complexity of human nature (Patel *et al.*, 1985).

Clearly the case for process-outcome research in practical nursing knowledge development is strong (Bloch, 1975; Benner, 1984) yet, until recently, little of this kind of work has been undertaken in either general (Goodman, 1989) or psychiatric nursing (Davis, 1981). The reluctance to evaluate currently practiced nursing actions may be due to several factors including lack of finance, education and perhaps, more importantly, the fear of finding out how ineffectual some actions may actually be in terms of patient outcome. In many respects the path of process-outcome research could be bumpy for investigators who need to accept that the results will show up the weaknesses of nursing actions as well as the strengths. The rewards of process-outcome research are, however, likely to outweigh the disadvantages in that the very nature of this kind of research brings clinicians and theorists closer together which can only help to dispel the current gap between the two groups' philosophies (Miller, 1985b). Similarly, it is through the development of 'know how' knowledge that nurses may begin not only to understand the complexity of their practice but also to '*enjoy*' having knowledge which is developed from experience.

Interdependence of nurse clinicians, researchers, managers and educators in quality assurance and process-outcome research development

The topics of quality assurance and process-outcome research demonstrate the interdependence of the four groups of nurses alluded to. In particular, clinicians require the theory developed by researchers to identify suitable standards of care while, in turn, researchers need to develop theory from practice if 'know how' knowledge is to be understood. Benner's (1984) work has clear implications for nurse education in that she suggests knowledge is gained from experience and therefore curricula need to reflect this with sufficient time being given to gain practical experience during training.

The two processes of quality assurance and process-outcome research are symbiotic in that they feed one another in order to enhance practice and produce new theory. Inevitably, therefore, standards of care will need to be adapted as the results of quality assurance programmes are produced and new knowledge developed. Nurse managers have an essential part to play in ensuring that relevant change in practice is both resourced and implemented when quality assurance programmes demonstrate new ways of enhancing care.

Nurse managers, clinicians and researchers need to work together to help develop suitable standards for care which are based on sound theory. This will involve altering and adapting recognised quality assurance tools such as Monitor (Goldstone, *et al.*, 1982) and Qualpacs (Wandelt and Stewart, 1975) if new research demonstrates the need to update their validity. The validity of such broad tools must inevitably be questioned when it is recognised that nursing values will vary within differing practice settings. For this reason the recent development of specialist editions of Monitor for psychiatry and paediatrics must be applauded.

Communication between nurse clinicians, managers and researchers needs to be open, so that in addition to researchers informing clinicians and managers of theory development the latter two groups can commission research to investigate particular problems or questions concerning structure, process and outcome standard setting as necessary. Figure 10.2 demonstrates how this has been conducted in the Mental Health Unit at West Lambeth Authority. In this instance a nurse researcher identified the need for night hospital care for elderly confused people following a process-outcome study of the existing provision. Nurse Management wished to know whether night hospital nursing care would actually work in terms of patient and carer outcome. As a result a research study was commissioned, with money for the project being provided from both research trust and nursing budgets. Structure and process standards for care were set jointly by the research leader, managers and clinicians, as can be seen in Appendix 10.1. These were based on relevant theoretical knowledge and elements of 'know how' practical expertise.

Patient outcomes are being measured using a dependency tool (Morrison, 1983) designed to measure changes in elderly patients' behaviour and by asking carers' opinions of the service in interviews. It is hoped that the results will demonstrate the value of the service in terms of carer and patient outcome so that Nurse Management can make decisions with regard to future provision. It is part of the Mental Health Unit's philosophy that future care provision should be based on clients' perceptions of value as well as professional opinions and, for this reason, the research design is considered pertinent.

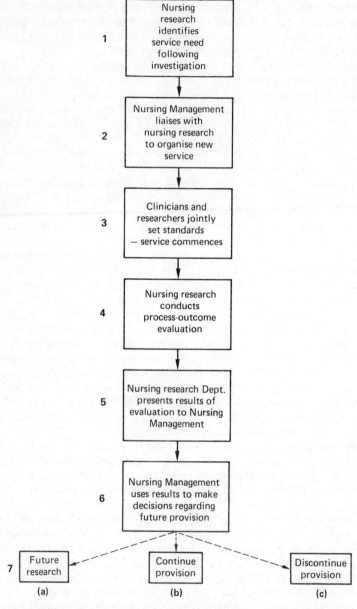

Fig. 10.2 Model of research-based service provision. Mental Health Unit, West Lambeth Health Authority.

While it is accepted that nurses from all fields of the profession have to work closely together to monitor and improve standards of care through the use and development of knowledge, their paths will sometimes be disparate. This is because nurse managers, practitioners, educators and researchers inevitably have differing motivations for and goals of nursing knowledge.

Knowledge for practice

'All clinical practice should be founded on up-to-date information and research findings; practitioners should be encouraged to identify the needs and opportunities for research presented by their work'.

(DOH, 1989)

This statement, extracted from the recent report *A Strategy for Nursing* reinforces the fact that clinical nurses require not only a sound theoretical base from which to practice but also an understanding of the research process in order to identify areas for future investigation. The same report acknowledges the necessity to set achievable standards of nursing care based on relevant research findings, as previously discussed. The additional targets state that practising nurses should be accountable for care delivery, encourage primary nursing, and use health education. They should also consider the views of consumers, contribute to the work of ethical committees, computerise procedures where possible, be trained in the use of information technology and develop the role of specialist practitioners. These targets, developed by senior members of the profession following extensive consultation with nurses at all levels, embrace quite clearly the objectives for knowledge in the practice area.

All the goals outlined involve enhancing patient care through the application of knowledge in practice, which must surely be the ultimate goal of knowledge for practising nurses (McFarlane, 1977). What is important is the breadth and depth of knowledge which clinical nurses will be required to have if these targets are to be achieved. In particular, the extent of knowledge required in order to be truly accountable is indicated in the UKCC (1989) paper outlining ethical aspects of professional practice. This paper acknowledges the need for collaboration between all health care workers as well as patients and their relatives when considering the best method of provision or improvement of services. Therefore clinical nurses require not only a sound knowledge base from which to practice, but also the skills necessary to communicate research based findings and 'know how' knowledge to other professional groups when decisions concerning client care are made within multidisciplinary teams.

The strategy document (DOH, 1989) highlights the need for clinicians to indicate areas of practice which require further investigation and also encourage the use of primary nursing. Advantages of primary nursing have been demonstrated over short periods of time, with both nurses and patients, reporting satisfaction with the system (Sellick *et al.*, 1987). It has also been shown to be cost effective (Marram, 1976). Yet this method of care delivery requires great commitment on behalf of the nurse, demanding close involvement with individual patients (Pearson, 1988) which can be stressful (Menzies, 1960). Further work needs to be undertaken to establish the extent to which primary nursing can be conducted with long term clients without causing the adverse effects of burn out in nurses. This kind of research is very time consuming in that a longitudinal study is the only way of establishing sound results. If, however, clinical nurses are to be accountable not only for the care they deliver but also their own health promotion, they must be provided with sufficient knowledge from which to decide appropriate methods of care delivery for long term, as well as short term, clients. There are several other areas for investigation, but perhaps Bloch (1975) is correct in believing that the most vital work for clinical nurses, in terms of theory development, is to discover the relationships between current nursing actions and patient outcome. Nursing actions in this context could include not only 'nursing processes' but also the 'structural standards' currently employed in terms of staffing, skill mix and the environment of care delivery. The results of structure-outcome, and process-outcome evaluation studies should produce useful theory which clinical nurses could then employ in practice.

The literature suggests that clinical nurses need to use theory in order to problem solve the 'best' way of delivering care, yet it must be recognised that many research findings have not, as yet, been fully incorporated into practice (Miller, 1985b). There is a debate as to whose responsibility this is. Some suggest that it is because nurses do not read and evaluate published research (Wells, 1980), while others imply it is because nurse researchers fail to fully explain their findings in a clear, concise manner (Hockey, 1987). There is little to be gained from arguing whose fault the problem really is, but much from finding methods of ensuring current knowledge is incorporated into practice in addition to developing new practice based theory.

Knowledge for education

The Committee on Nursing (Briggs report) (1972) stated that nurse educationalists should incorporate research findings into their teaching and this seems doubly pertinent today when clearly knowledge is not always used by clinical nurses. If 'education is today's great enabler' (DOH, 1989; p. 23) then nurse education must use knowledge derived from adult education theories to assist nurses in developing the skills of critical thinking, decision making and the delivery of individualised patient care. This implies that nurse educators must themselves have those skills at a high level, in addition to teaching skills and sound academic backgrounds (UKCC, 1986; DOH, 1989).

The main objective for knowledge in nurse education is to facilitate the development of able practitioners in all spheres of nursing, at basic and advanced levels of practice. This is a complex task when one considers that Benner (1984) acknowledges the difficulty of explaining how nurses move through various levels of competency from novice to expert. One way of enhancing nursing education is outlined by Dolan (1984) who believes that the use of a *'preceptor system'* and *'clinical judgement seminars'* is useful in developing 'know how' knowledge amongst both undergraduate and postgraduate student nurses. If nurse educators are to work in this way there is clearly a need for them to be clinically credible in the area of practice which they teach (DOH, 1989); in other words they too must be able to apply knowledge in practice.

Theory derived from the social sciences needs to be incorporated into the curriculum (UKCC, 1986) in order that tomorrow's nurses have a sound theoretical base from which to practice. The increase in time made available within the new Project 2000 training for theoretical teaching should allow for time to be given to these subjects. The ultimate goal for knowledge from a nurse teacher's perspective must be to develop a curriculum which allows both basic and advanced nursing students to become 'knowledgeable doers' who are reflective decision makers. It may be useful for nurse educators to remember Merlin's adage in 'Sword in the Stone', that 'education is experience and the essence of experience is self reliance'. Thus curriculum planning should be orientated to developing self reliant nurses who enjoy using theory, read research and are willing and able to be accountable for care.

Knowledge for management

Nurse managers require knowledge derived from the study of leadership, organisations and management if they are to provide 'managerial leadership' in addition to the theory necessary for 'professional leadership'. The DOH (1989) details the complex role of today's nurse manager; identifying some nine targets for manpower planning and seven for leadership and management. The manpower planning goals indicate the need for nurse managers to conduct skill mix exercises, find methods for encouraging practitioners taking a career break to re-enter nursing, and to use systematic methods to ensure that staff appointed to posts have the relevant skills for such jobs.

Nurse managers are also expected to 'encourage and enable practitioners to function at their highest level of ability' (DOH, 1989; p. 39) and it is suggested that personal appraisal systems should be used to achieve this end.

It is clear that nurse managers are required to apply managerial theory in practice in order to ensure that appropriate structural standards, in terms of staff, are agreed and employed in the clinical area. In addition, they need to be able to conduct 'managerial processes' aimed at developing individual nurses and care assistants to their maximum potential (Vaughan and Pillmoor, 1989).

Since its inception the NHS has consumed steadily increased resources and it now uses approximately 6 per cent of our gross national product (Patel *et al.*, 1985). It is hardly surprising, therefore, that there is an increasing emphasis on resource management and auditing in health care within the system (DOH, 1989). Nurse managers require an understanding of, and the ability to measure, care in terms of both efficiency and effectiveness (Butler and Vaile, 1984) so that the policies, practices, and procedure agreed within a nursing team meet the objectives of the organisation within which the team operates. The current demographic changes in society will result in a shortage of nursing manpower in the future. Nurse managers need to use information technology to assist nurses in their work, particularly where this can be demonstrated to be cost effective. For example, computerisation of care plans could save nursing time (Sovie, 1989). There may be other advantages in this approach: for example, meta analysis studies of nursing process outcome revealed that patients who receive research-based nursing interventions can expect significantly better outcomes than those who receive standard nursing care (Heater *et al.*, 1988). If research-based interventions were programmed into a computer this could aid clinical nurses in their practice, for up-to-date care plans would be available as a response to the identification of patients' problems. Clearly the nurse manager has a vital role both in agreeing research-based standards with staff and providing the resources in terms of structure to ensure that those standards can be achieved.

The alteration of skill mix and introduction of information technology are just two examples of change which nurse managers may be expected to facilitate. Change is both disturbing and exciting and often causes emotional responses in those expected to change. The skilled nurse manager will prepare staff for, and assist them in, the process of introducing change by applying relevant change theory (Bailey and Claus, 1975). Change should not be introduced for its own sake but because it is believed that it will be innovative in terms of improving performance. Enhancing performance through the use of quality assurance programmes, the application of research and the development of staff are the main tasks of nurse managers. Their ultimate goal, in terms of the application of knowledge, therefore involves balancing the efficiency and effectiveness of nursing care. As nurses well know, faster throughput does not necessarily mean 'better care'. Alternatively 'better care' for a few may not be just if others are left to suffer without any access to nursing care. If nurse managers apply knowledge developed from both managerial and professional studies it may soon be possible to identify the most cost-effective methods of nursing care delivery.

Knowledge for research

This chapter has discussed at some length the advantages of process-outcome research, and has indicated that this may well be the most important work for both researchers and clinicians (Bloch, 1975). It is vital, however, to acknowledge that theory must be developed both inductively and deductively if nursing is to develop in an academic sense. The advantages of nursing developing in this way should include both an improvement in patient care through the application of research based theory (Heater *et al.*, 1988) and an enhancement in the quality of research undertaken (Treece and Treece, 1982). Most theory produced by researchers is questionable and subject to change (McFarlane, 1977) and nurse theorists must explain to those they give research results to that theories are generally open to conjecture (Rines and Montag, 1976). It is by explaining the difference between descriptive and explanatory theory to all nurses in the profession that researchers can help nurses to choose how best to select and apply theory. Descriptive theory looks at phenomenon and identifies its major elements or events; it involves a basic level of conceptualisation including

(*i*)   factor isolating theories which classify and label, and
(*ii*) factor relating theories which depict and relate a single factor to another (Stevens, 1984; Dickoff and James, 1968).

Explanatory theories include situation relating theory which is predictive in nature and situation producing theories which have status of a law or principle (McFarlane, 1977).

'The test of explanatory theory is whether it holds true of a prediction of future interactions of the same constituents in that phenomenon'.

(Stevens, 1984; p. 4)

While researchers should seek to develop explanatory theory, wherever possible, this is not always achievable in the complex human world of nursing where each individual is another variable! This concept is an essential one for all nurses to comprehend in order that it can be accepted that an individual patient may react differently to other patients in response to a certain 'nursing action'.

A wide spectrum of research methods, including experimental designs, case studies, action research and surveys, need to be employed by researchers to ensure that eclectic new theory is developed (Treece and Treece, 1982).

The debate about qualitative versus quantitative research approaches continues and is well outlined in Leddy and Pepper (1989) who suggest that it is essential for nursing to use both types. In future nurse researchers need to remember that there is a danger that nursing research could become too introspective, that much nursing activity is complementary to, and interdependent with, medicine and other complementary disciplines, and that the development of multi-professional research needs more attention (Goodman, 1989). Although many nurse theorists are criticised for being removed from practice (Miller, 1985b) this may sometimes be essential. If nursing is to develop and grow it requires an academic body of nurses who take time out to have ideas and be imaginative, for it is from imagination that truly exciting theories are sometimes developed. For example, it is very difficult to believe that at one point we knew absolutely nothing about aeroplanes, insulin and psychoanalysis yet it was by man's imaginative thought that these things were developed. It is interesting to note that fifty years ago the terms computer, megabyte, nuclear energy, echo-cardiograph and allograft were unknown. It was due to research that theories concerning these phenomena were developed and it is vital that nursing encourages and values original thinkers today. It is currently fashionable to criticise Rogers' 'unitary fields of nursing theory' yet one cannot help but wonder whether in a hundred years we will look back on her new words 'integrality and helicy' (Rogers, 1980), understand their meaning and, more importantly perhaps, that the role of the nurse may encompass therapeutic touch and the moving of magnetic fields around a patient's body in order to improve patient health status. It certainly seems essential to acknowledge that visionary thought has its place in nursing and that nurse researchers should be allowed and expected to develop and investigate radical ideas.

Chapman (1989) outlines the aims for nursing research over the next twenty-five years which include the need to maintain high quality work, use multiple methods, increase replication studies and improve dissemination of results in addition to increasing the application of theory in practice. These aims are challenging but clearly essential if it is accepted that changes in nursing cannot occur without the use of theories, principles and concepts (Rines and Montage, 1976). Nursing researchers, it seems, have a duty not only to analyse current practice but also to develop new theories which will provide the building blocks for change within the profession.

Conclusion

The way forward for knowledge in nursing must be to both *value* and *enjoy* developing and applying theory. There is a need to recognise the vast body of experience and expertise within clinical nursing teams and try to identify the relationships within the 'know how' of nursing (Benner, 1984). In addition more traditional theory derived from scientific investigation, commonly referred to as 'know that' knowledge, needs to be both applied and developed. It has been argued that nurse researchers, managers and educators have interdependent roles in developing quality patient care through the use of quality assurance cycles and the study of process-outcome research. This is because nursing is perceived as a practice discipline and therefore any theory of nursing or theory applied to nursing must be intimately related to practice (McFarlane, 1977).

A theory practice gap exists and it is evident that clinicians do not readily use theory in practice. When attempting to disseminate findings researchers must avoid the JIDS (jargon induced drivel syndrome) from which many suffer and write up their results in a manner that is readily understood by most colleagues if their aim is to encourage others to use the findings in practice (Miller, 1985; Chapman, 1989). It is vital that *nursing knowledge is applied in practice* because research demonstrates that this can positively affect patient outcome (Hayward, 1975; Miller, 1985b; Heater *et al.*, 1988). The ultimate objective for nursing knowledge must therefore be the enhancement of care through the application of knowledge. If nursing is to develop and grow then new concepts and theories must be produced so that change can occur (Rines and Montag, 1976). Researchers must be encouraged to investigate not only present practice but also to test imaginative ideas in order that the development of new theory is not restrictive in the sense of rejecting originality of thought.

Although nurse managers, researchers, clinicians and educators have a common purpose in improving care through the use of knowledge, the path they follow to achieve this end will inevitably differ due to varying motivations. Orem (1985) describes three levels of objectives for care – short, intermediate and long term. It may be useful to conceptualise the long term goal for nursing knowledge as enhancement of care delivery, with each of the four groups of nurses described having differing short and intermediate goals in order to achieve the ultimate goal. The intermediate goals for each group are outlined in Table 10.1.

It is interesting to note that each group has highly complex objectives to achieve but through the use of knowledge this should be possible. Indeed Baroness Warnock (1986) recently wrote 'if we can't follow knowledge where it leads us, we are unlikely to be able to lead

Table 10.1   Intermediate goals to achieve long term goal – enhancement
of care through application of theory.

Education
Enabling basic and advanced nurses to develop the skills of critical thinking,
analysis of research, decision making and the application of theory in
practice.

Research
To have original thoughts, respond to requests from clinicians to investigate
problems; produce and disseminate theory for application and standard
setting.

Management
Provide adequate resources to achieve agreed standards of care and facilitate
quality assurance progress, develop staff to their maximum potential.
Conduct manpower planning exercises to ensure relevant skill mix.
Commission research as appropriate. Minimise stress of change through the
use of appropriate principles.

Clinicians
Apply theory in practice using the skills outlined in education goals, conduct
quality assurance cycles and introduce change into practice as appropriate.

ourselves or others.' It is hypothesised that if nurses do follow
knowledge we will become truly accountable practitioners who work
in partnership in care with patients to maximise their health status.
This could just be enjoyable!

Appendix 10.1a

Operational policy – night hospital elderly care

1.   Background

Nurses involved in caring for elderly people are looking towards
the future and trying to provide facilities which meet the needs of
the community they serve.

This innovative service aims to offer nursing support for elderly
people at night on weekdays – Monday to Thursday. It is envisaged
that the users will be individuals who have difficulty sleeping at
night, who may be noisy and disrupt their carer's sleep. At present,
these people are frequently admitted to in-patient care to give
carers relief rather than for formal intervention. It is hoped that the
Night Hospital will provide sufficient relief to carers without
warranting full admission.

Sitting services for elderly confused people have been shown to be effective, in particular with those too frail to travel. A sitter service does, however, have the dual disadvantages of a stranger going into the home for long periods denying carers privacy, and in small homes the noisy confused individual may continue to disrupt carers' sleep. The Night Hospital service may, in many instances, therefore have advantages over a sitter service.

2. Aims

2.1 To provide, as part of the comprehensive community, orientated mental health services support for elderly mentally confused people and their families at night.

2.2 To provide relief for relatives who are caring for elderly mentally infirm people at home. The Night Hospital will give the opportunity to relatives to have a night free, allowing them to rest or socialise undisturbed.

2.3 To provide, for each client at night, individualised programmes of care which are orientated towards facilitating clients' independence and dignity.

2.4 To provide a service which supports informal carers by working in partnership with them to deliver quality care to clients.

3. Philosophy of the service

3.1 That clients should be able to remain in their own homes for as long as possible cared for by relatives and friends who are, in turn, supported by the statutory health services.

3.2 Where a sitter service would be deemed more appropriate, due to a client's frailty, the Night Hospital staff will arrange appropriate referrals to voluntary and statutory agencies.

3.3 The service will be developed around the individual needs of clients and their families. Each client will have an individualised treatment programme using a nursing intervention approach (p. 337). The key objective of the service being to meet clients needs.

Nursing staff will be committed to taking a truly realistic approach to clients' needs and be aware of the contribution both statutory and voluntary services can make to their clients' health.

3.4 Clients will receive care and treatment in the least restrictive setting with as much freedom as possible.

3.5 Clients will have the right to personal privacy.

3.6 They will have the right to be addressed with courtesy and respect at all times, and to be addressed as they choose.

4. Referral procedure

4.1 The service will be open to all residents of the AHA.

4.2 An open referral procedure will be adopted. Referral will be accepted from:
Patients' relatives
Community nursing staff
Hospital nursing staff
Community Physicians – GPs
Consultant Psychiatrists
Social Services
Voluntary Services

4.3 A formal system of assessment will be used to find out which professionals or volunteers are also involved so that liaison can take place.

4.4 Each referred client will be visited at home by a member of the team to assess suitability for attendance. Assessment will normally be conducted in conjunction with other members of the community multidisciplinary team.

4.5 In emergency situations clients may attend the Night Hospital prior to liaison with other members of the health care team involved in their care, although consultation should take place as soon as possible.

4.6 Referrals will only be accepted from the Day Hospital on the basis of attendance at the Night Hospital being an alternative not in addition to attendance during the day.

4.7 Referrals should normally be in writing and addressed to the Charge Nurse.

4.8 The Community Psychiatric Nursing Department Secretary will receive referrals during the day.

5. Attendance periods

5.1 The service will run four nights a week – Monday to Thursday inclusive.

5.2 The Hospital will cater for a maximum of 15 per night giving a maximum of 60 places per week.

5.3 Clients will be collected by sitting ambulance with a nurse escort between 8.00pm and 9.00pm. They will be returned home the following day between 8.00am and 9.30am.

5.4 Clients may be delivered to the Hospital between 8.00pm and 9.00pm and collected by 9.30am by relatives/friends.

5.5 Clients will attend for a minimum of one night a week and a maximum of four nights.

5.6 Clients progress will be reviewed on a regular basis. Where the prime aim of attendance is respite care a thorough reassessment after three months attendance will be made in conjunction with the multidisciplinary team and relatives.

6. Programme

6.1 Individual assessments will be completed after four nights attendance using a Stress Management/Activities of Living Model of Nursing.

6.2 Individual programmes will be drawn up based on clients' assessment. Most programmes will be aimed at at least one of the following:
(*a*) Facilitating independence through social activities
(*b*) Promoting continence
(*c*) Reducing nocturnal restlessness and promoting sleep
(*d*) Providing respite care to the carer

6.3 Individual programmes will be reviewed with the minimum frequencies of:
(*a*) Two weekly for those aimed at promoting continence.
(*b*) Four weekly for those aimed at facilitating independence through social activity and/or reducing nocturnal restlessness and promoting sleep.
(*c*) Four weekly for those aimed at providing respite care. Where the aim is largely orientated towards the carer, attendance will not normally exceed three months.

6.4 Light entertainment will be provided for clients eg. use of video, television, games, reading material. A hot drink and light snack will be provided before 11.00pm. Hot drinks and snacks will be available throughout the night.

6.5 Between 11.00pm and midnight depending on individual programmes, clients will either be encouraged to prepare for sleep or involved in appropriate activities.

6.6 Most clients will be woken at 7.00am to promote regular sleeping patterns and to ensure that the clients are returned home in time for the hospital to accept day patients. When deemed necessary for an individual, a client will be left to sleep on until 8.00am. If clients can be collected by a relative/friend they may be left to sleep until 9.30am.

6.7 A light breakfast will be prepared and served by nursing staff, for clients in the morning.

7. Managerial organisation

7.1 The Community Nursing Manager (Mental Health Unit), will be managerially responsible for the Unit.

8. Staffing

8.1 The service will be run by nursing staff comprising:
1 C/N Full Time
2 S/N Full Time
2 SENs Full Time
2 Part Time Qualified Nurses
1 Helper

9. Medical supervision

9.1 Carried out by the Consultant Psychogeriatrician.

9.2 Clients will be asked to visit their General Practitioner for non-emergency medical care.

9.3 Clients will be referred for psychological medical assessment to the Consultant Psychiatrist (Elderly Mental Health) from the service when appropriate.

10. Admission and discharge

10.1 This will be the responsibility of the clinical nursing team.

11. Evaluation of the night hospital

11.1 A part time project evaluator has been appointed for a two year period.

11.2 A comprehensive evaluation of the service will be conducted and a report of the findings presented to the Health Authority in Spring 1991.

11.3 Interim reports will be presented to the project team at six monthly intervals.

11.4 The evaluator will receive research supervision from the Department of Nursing Institute of Psychiatry.

11.5 The evaluator is responsible to the Director of Nursing Services, Mental Health Unit.

Stress management/activities of living model

Although a trained nurse can rapidly assess a patient's nursing requirements using an activities of living model of nursing, to do this in isolation from the caregiver would be insensitive and irresponsible.

One method of identifying priority problems for the family unit and planning support for informal caregivers is the dementia stress management model (Zarit *et al.*, 1985).

The dementia stress management model

This is a two stage model that aims to minimise stress of the caregiver:

Stage 1   Information giving
Stage 2   Problem solving

In **stage 1** the nurse gives carers information about the patients' disease and the availability of resources to support them.

Stage 2   The problem solving cycle can be broken down into a series of steps and used to help resolve problems caused by a person with Alzheimer's disease in any family unit (see Fig. 10.1A).

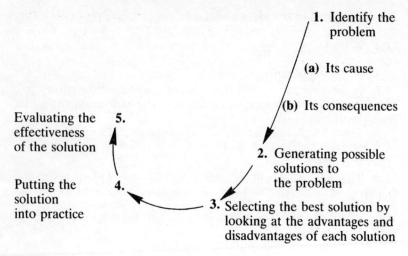

Fig. 10.1A   Problem solving cycle

Patient-orientated needs identification using an activities of living model

The activities of living model can be used by the nurse and carer to assess the patients' ability to carry out their activities of living and patients' actual problems are defined:

Maintaining a safe environment including memory and orientation
Communicating
Breathing
Eating and drinking
Eliminating
Personal cleansing and dressing
Controlling body temperature
Mobilising
Working and playing
Expressing sexuality
Sleeping
Dying
Memorising
Perceiving

(Watkins, 1987 after Roper *et al.*, 1980)

Carers can be facilitated to express which patient behaviours' cause them most distress. The majority of caregivers report finding certain problems more difficult to cope with than others. For example, most carers can tolerate a patient's inability to dress and to walk unaided, but 60 per cent find it difficult to cope with inappropriate urination and verbal abuse from the sick person. (Argyle *et al.*, 1985.)

Aims of nursing/selection of solution

Having identified the clients' problems care can then be organised with the aim of nursing being to:
– maintain/increase patients' independence; while ensuring patient comfort.
– reduce carers' stress.
It is important that both the nurse and carer are involved in the selection of a solution as frequently the carer will be involved in its implementation. For example with a continence promotion programme.

Implementation

The selected solution is then implemented by the nurse in the Night Hospital and in some cases concurrently at home by the carer.

Evaluation

Finally, the nurse and caregiver evaluate the outcome of the chosen solution. If the strategy is successful, it should continue, if not, the problem solving cycle is recommenced.

References

Watkins, M. J. (1987). *In and Day patient care for elderly people.* Unpublished MN Thesis. University of Wales.
Zarit, S. H., Orr, N. K. and Zarit, S. M. (1985). *The Hidden Victims of Alzheimers Disease.* New York University Press, New York.

Appendix 10.1b

Nursing standards

1. All nurses working in the night hospital are aware of the standards of nursing care, have read them, and been given their own copies.

Assessment

2. Each client referred to our service is visited at home, by a member of the nursing team, to assess suitability for attendance prior to admission.

3. Assessment is normally conducted in conjunction with all members of the community multidisciplinary team involved in the care of the client. Where admission is deemed to be necessary immediately, and liaison with all members of the multidisciplinary team has not been possible prior to admission, liaison takes place as soon as possible afterwards.

4. Each client is asked during assessment what he or she wishes to be called. If he or she is unable to make his or her wishes known, his or her carer is asked. The name decided upon is recorded and adhered to.

Primary nursing

5. Each client has a primary nurse who is responsible together with associate nurses, for planning and delivering his or her care.

6. The primary or associate nurse, responsible for the delivery of care to an individual, introduces him or herself to that client at the beginning of his or her span of duty, and at intervals throughout.

7. In the absence of the primary and associate nurses for an individual client, any nurse may attend to any client. This applies for a whole span of duty, for part of a span of duty, e.g. during a meal break, or simply when the client's own nurse is occupied with another client.

Care planning

8. Each client has his or her own individualised care plan which is in operation by the fourth night attendance at the latest.

9. Individual assessments are completed using a Stress Management/Activities of Living Model of Nursing, in cooperation with the clients' carers.

10. Clear goals are known and recorded on the care plan for each client.

11. Each individualised care plan is evaluated at least once every four weeks, or by the eighth night attendance, whichever is the sooner. Evaluations are carried out in consultation with carers.

Management of incontinence

12. Incontinence is not regarded as the inevitable consequence of ageing.

13. If the General Practitioner has not already investigated the causes of incontinence this is requested prior to admission, or as soon as possible after admission.

14. Appropriate medical treatment for problems related to incontinence is given when prescribed, in conjunction with the carer.

15. When medical treatment is not prescribed, or is completed, and incontinence persists, this is treated by nursing measures.

16. Each client has his or her incontinence needs assessed during care planning, and appropriate nursing measures are prescribed by the primary nurse.

17. All clients who are incontinent have clear nursing orders in their care plan for the treatment and/or management of this problem.

Prevention of pressure sores

18. On admission every client is assessed on the Norton Scale for susceptibility to pressure sores.

19. Reassessment on the Norton Scale takes place every time the care plan is evaluated, and at the onset of physical illness, and at any time that the client's health is considered to have deteriorated.

20. Every at-risk client has an individualised care plan for the prevention of pressure sores.

21. Pressure relieving aids are always available, and are used on all at-risk clients who are assessed as being in need of them by their primary nurses.

Personal hygiene

22. The personal hygiene needs of each client are discussed with the client and the carer prior to admission.

23. Whenever possible the client looks after his or her own personal hygiene needs with a minimum of help from nursing staff.

24. All clients are bathed while in the night hospital, at least once a week, unless the client and carer prefer to make their own arrangements.

25. Each client decides when and how he or she is bathed.

26. Each client who is incapable of looking after his or her own personal hygiene needs is washed thoroughly, or bathed, every morning unless he or she refuses.

27. Carers are always informed if clients refuse to be washed.

Freedom of movement

28. Clients are allowed to decide when they wish to go to bed, and are never awoken before 7am.

29. When it is impossible to persuade a client to go to bed, he or she is allowed to spend the night reclining in a chair. Blankets and pillows are provided for warmth and comfort.

Reality orientation

30. Twenty-four hour reality orientation is practiced. All staff understand the full implications of Reality Orientation and participate in its practice.

31. Formal sessions of Reality Orientation and Reminiscence Therapy are available for any patient requiring them, but no-one is forced to participate.

General

32. Every effort is made to maintain the dignity and privacy of each client in our care.

33. The cultural and religious needs of all clients are monitored and planned for.

34. Diversional therapy is available for any patient who requires it, but no-one is compelled to join in.

Acknowledgements to the Mental Health Team, West Lambeth Health Authority for content of Appendices.

References

American Nursing Association. (1975). *The American Health Care System*. ANA, Chicago.

American Nurses' Association. (1977). *Guidelines for Review of Nursing Care at the Local Level*. ANA, Kansas City.

Andrews, H. A. and Roy, C. (1986). *Essentials of the Roy Adaptation Model*. Appleton-Century-Crofts, Norwalk.

Bailey, J. T. and Claus, K. E. (1975). *Decision Making in Nursing: Tools for Change*. Mosby, St. Louis.

Benner, P. (Ed.) (1984). *From Novice to Expert*. Addison-Wesley, Menlo Park.

Bloch, D. (1975). Evaluation of nursing care in terms of process and outcome: issues in research and quality assurance. *Nursing Research*, **24(4)**, 256–63.

Bloch, D. (1977). Criteria, standards, norms – crucial terms in quality assurance. *Journal of Nursing Administration*, **7(7)**, 20–30.

Bloch, D. (1980). Interrelated issues in evaluation and evaluation research: a researcher's perspective. *Nursing Research*, **29(2)**, 69–73.

Butler, J. R. and Vaile, M. S. B. (1984). *Health and Health Services: an Introduction to Health Care in Britain*. Routledge & Kegan Paul, London.

Chapman, C. (1976). The use of sociological theories and models in nursing. *Journal of Advanced Nursing*, **1(2)**, 111–27.

Chapman, C. (1989). Research for action: the way forward. *Senior Nurse*, **9(6)**, 16–18.

Chapman, G. E. (1983). Ritual and rational action in hospitals. *Journal of Advanced Nursing*, **8(1)**, 13–20.

Committee on Nursing (1972). *Report*. HMSO, London. (Chairman: A. Briggs.)

Crow, R. A. (1981). Research and the standards of nursing care: what is the relationship? *Journal of Advanced Nursing*, **6(6)**, 491–6.

Davis, B. D. (1981). The training and assessment of social skills in nursing: the patient profile interview. *Nursing Times*, **77(15)**, 649–51.

Department of Health, Nursing Division. (1989). *A Strategy for Nursing: a Report of the Steering Committee*. DOH, London.

Dickoff, J. and James, P. (1968). A theory of theories: a position paper. *Nursing Research*, **17(3)**, 197–203.

Dolan, K. (1984). Building bridges between education and practice. In *From Novice to Expert*, P. Benner(Ed.), pp. 275–84. Addison-Wesley, Menlo Park.

Goldstone, L., Ball, J. A. and Collier, M. (1982). *Monitor – an Index of the Quality of Nursing Care for Acute Medical and Surgical Wards*. Newcastle Polytechnic Products, Newcastle-upon-Tyne.

Goodman, C. (1989). Nursing research: growth and development. In *Current Issues in Nursing*, M. Jolley and P. Allan (Eds), pp. 95–114. Chapman & Hall, London.

Hayward, J. (1975). *Information – a Prescription Against Pain*. Royal College of Nursing, London.

Heater, B. S., Becker, A. M. and Olson, R. K. (1988). Nursing interventions and patient outcomes: a meta-analysis of studies. *Nursing Research*, **37(5)**, 303–7.

Henderson, V. (1960). *Basic Principles of Nursing Care*. International Council of Nurses, London.

Henney, C. R. (1984). The use of computers for improvement and measurement of nursing care. In *Measuring the Quality of Care*, L. D. Willis and M. E. Linwood (Eds), pp. 174–91. Churchill Livingstone, Edinburgh. (Recent Advances in Nursing 10.)

Hilgard, E. R., Atkinson, R. C. and Atkinson, R. L. (1975). *Introduction to Psychology*, 6th edition. Harcourt, Brace, Jovanovich, New York.

Hockey, L. (1979). Collaborative research and its implementation in nursing. In *Collaborative Research and Its Implementation in Nursing: 1st Conference of the European Nurse Researchers*, European Nurse Researchers, pp. 83–94. National Hospital Institute, Utrecht.

Hockey, L. (1987). Issues in the communication of nursing research. In *Current Issues*, L. Hockey (Ed.), pp. 154–67. Churchill Livingstone, Edinburgh. (Recent Advances in Nursing 18.)

Jacox, A. (1974). Theory construction in nursing: an overview. *Nursing Research*, **23(1)**, 4–13.

King, I. M. (1981). *A Theory for Nursing*. Wiley, New York.

Kuhn, T. S. (1970). *The Structure of Scientific Revolutions*. University of Chicago Press, Chicago.

Lang, N. M. and Clinton, J. F. (1984). Quality assurance – the idea and its development in the United States. In *Measuring the Quality of Care*, L. Willis and M. E. Linwood (Eds), pp. 69–88. Churchill Livingstone, Edinburgh. (Recent advances in Nursing 10.)

Leddy, S. and Pepper, J. M. (1989). *Conceptual Bases of Professional Nursing*, 2nd edition. Lippincott, Philadelphia.

Longman (1984). *Longman Dictionary of the English Language*. Longman, London.

McFarlane, J. K. (1977). Developing a theory of nursing: the relation of theory to practice, education and research. *Journal of Advanced Nursing*, **2(3)**, 261–70.

Marram, G. (1976). The comparative costs of operating a team and primary nursing unit. *Journal of Nursing Administration*, **6(4)**, 21–4.

Menzies, I. E. P. (1960). A case study in the functioning of social systems as a defence against anxiety. *Human Relationships*, **13**, 95–121.

Miller, A. (1985a). Nurse/patient dependency – is it iatrogenic? *Journal of Nursing*, **10(1)**, 63–9.

Miller, A. (1985b). The relationship between nursing theory and nursing practice. *Journal of Advanced Nursing*, **10(5)**, 417–24.

Morrison, D. P. (1983). The Crichton Visual Analogue Scale for the assessment of behaviour in the elderly. *Acta Psychiatrica Scandinavica*, **68**, 408–13.

Nightingale, F. (1959). *Notes on Nursing*. Harrison, London.

Norton, D., McLaren, R. and Exton-Smith, A. N. (1962). *An Investigation of Geriatric Nursing Problems in Hospital*. National Corporation for the Care of Old People, London.

Orem, D. E. (1985). *Nursing: Concepts of Practice*, 3rd edition. McGraw-Hill, New York.

Patel, M. S., St. Ledger, A. S. and Schnieden, H. (1985). Process and outcome in the National Health Service. *British Medical Journal*, **291**, 1365–6.

Pearson, A. (Ed.) (1988). *Primary Nursing*. Croom Helm, London.

Peplau, H. E. (1952). *Interpersonal Relations in Nursing*. Putnam, New York.

Polanyi, M. (1958). *Personal Knowledge*. Routledge and Kegan Paul, London.

Rines, A. B. and Montag, M. L. (1976). *Nursing Concepts and Nursing Care*. Wiley, New York.

Rogers, M. E. (1980). Nursing: a science of unitary man. In *Conceptual Models for Practice*, 2nd edition. J. P. Riehl and C. Roy (Eds), pp. 329–37. Appleton-Century-Crofts, New York.

Rogers, M. E. (1983). *Nursing science – a science of unitary human beings*. Unpublished student handout.

Roper, N., Logan, W. W. and Tierney, A. J. (1980). *The Elements of Nursing*. Churchill Livingstone, Edinburgh.

Roy, C. (1984). *Introduction to Nursing: an Adaptation Model*, 2nd edition. Prentice Hall, Englewood Cliffs.

Sellick, K.J., Russell, S. and Beckmann, J. L. (1983). Primary nursing: an evaluation of its effects on patient perception of care and staff satisfaction. *International Journal of Nursing Studies*, **20(4)**, 265–73.

Sovie, M. D. (1989). Clinical nursing practices and patient outcomes: evaluation, evolution and revolution. *Nursing Economics*, **7(2)**, 79–85.

Statutory Instrument (1983). *The Nurses, Midwives and Health Visitors Rules Approval Order*. HMSO, London. (S.I. no. 873.)

Stevens, B. J. (1984). *Nursing Theory: Analysis, Application, Evaluation*, 2nd edition. Mosby, St. Louis.

Treece, E. W. and Treece, J. W. (1982). *Elements of Research in Nursing*, 3rd edition. Mosby, St. Louis.

United Kingdom Central Council for Nursing, Midwifery and Health Visiting. (1984). *Code of Professional Conduct for the Nurse, Midwife and Health Visitor*, 2nd edition. UKCC, London.

United Kingdom Central Council for Nursing, Midwifery and Health Visiting. (1986). *Project 2000: a New Preparation for Practice.* UKCC, London.

United Kingdom Central Council for Nursing, Midwifery and Health Visiting. (1987). *Confidentiality: a UKCC Advisory Paper.* UKCC, London.

United Kingdom Central Council for Nursing, Midwifery and Health Visiting. (1989). *Exercising Accountability: a Framework to Assist Nurses, Midwives and Health Visitors to Consider Ethical Aspects of Professional Practice: a UKCC Advisory Document.* UKCC, London.

Van Maanen, H. M. (1984). Evaluation of nursing care: quality of nursing evaluated within the context of health care and examined from a multinational perspective. In *Measuring the Quality of Care*, L. D. Willis and M. E. Linwood (Eds), pp. 3–42. Churchill Livingstone, Edinburgh. (Recent Advances in Nursing 10.)

Vaughan, B. and Pillmoor, M. (Eds) (1989). *Managing Nursing Work*. Scutari, London.

Wandelt, M. and Stewart, D. (1975). *Slater Nursing Competencies Rating Scale*. Appleton-Century-Crofts, New York.

Warnock, M. (1986). Why it is unthinkable to drop philosophy. (Letter.) *Daily Telegraph*, 15th July, 20.

Watkins, M. (1988). Lifting the burden. *Geriatric Nursing and Home Care*, **8(9)**, 18–20.

Wells, J. C. A. (1980). *Nursing: a Profession that Dislikes Innovation – an Investigation of the Reasons Why*. MA thesis, Dept. of Government, Brunel University.

White, T. H. (1939). *The Sword in the Stone*. Collins, London.

Wright, D. (1984). An introduction to the evaluation of nursing care: a review of the literature. *Journal of Advanced Nursing*, **9(5)**, 457–67.

Wright, S. G. (1990). *Building and Using a Model of Nursing*, second edition. Edward Arnold, Sevenoaks.

Zarit, S. H., Orr, N. K. and Zarit, S. M. (1985). *The Hidden Victims of Alzheimers Disease: Families Under Stress*. New York University Press, New York.

Index